TRADITIONAL CHINESE MEDICINE ATLAS

中药图册（上卷）

VOLUME 1

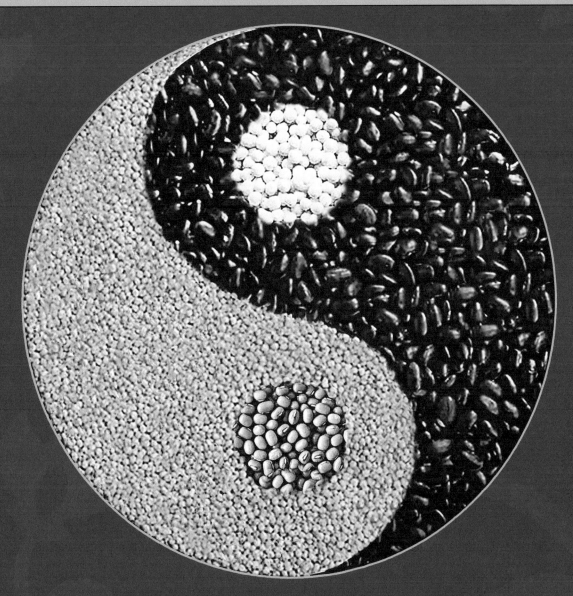

CHEN RUI

Traditional Chinese Medicine Atlas
Volume 1

iUniverse books may be ordered through booksellers or by contacting:

iUniverse
1663 Liberty Drive
Bloomington, IN 47403
www.iuniverse.com
1-800-Authors (1-800-288-4677)

ISBN: 978-1-5320-8142-2 (sc)
ISBN: 978-1-5320-8143-9 (e)

Library of Congress Control Number: 2019912741

Print information available on the last page.

iUniverse rev. date: 10/15/2019

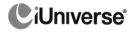

Traditional Chinese Medicine Atlas

中药图册（上卷）

(volume Ⅰ)

Menu

V

Attention

The Earth is the home of us and other creatures. Do not use the herb get from rare wildlife and rare wild plant. Use the herb abide by local laws.

Use with caution in people who are allergy to the component of the herb.

By
Chen Rui
(Qinghai Province Institute for Food Control, China)
Shu Tong
(Qinghai Province Institute for Food Control, China)
Zeng Yang
(Qinghai Normal University, China)
Yan Peiying
(Qinghai Normal University, China)
Yao Yilei
(OKAYAMA University, Japan)
Hongping Han
(Qinghai Normal University, China)
Luo Qiaoyu
(Qinghai Normal University, China)

General Introduction

Traditional Chinese Medicine (TCM) is the substance used to prevent, treat, diagnose diseases, and have the function of rehabilitation and health care under the guidance of the theory of Traditional Chinese Medicine. It is the wisdom fruit of the Chinese people's struggle against disease for thousands of years. Traditional Chinese Medicine mainly includes plant medicine (herb), mineral medicine, zoogenic medicine and their processed products. Sometime Traditional Chinese Medicine is referred as herb because most of the medicines is plants or processed products of plants.

Decocting method of Traditional Chinese Medicine

I. The selection of decocting apparatus

The quality of traditional Chinese medicine decoction is closely related to the choice of medicine decoction. It is good to use the earthenware casserole, because it doesn't react with the chemical composition of the drug and its thermal conductivity is slow and even. We can also use the enamel pan or the glass container. The iron and copper pot are not recommended, because the chemical properties of the iron or copper pot are unstable and easy to oxidize. In the decoction, it can react with the chemical composition of traditional Chinese medicine. Such as tannin, which can produce tannic acid and enhance the color of the liquid. The content of flavonoids can form a difficulty dissolved polymer, and Metal products also can react with organic acids to produce salts. These all can affect the quality of the decoction and affect the clinical efficacy of Chinese medicine decoction.

II. The amount of water of decocting

The amount of water decocting is very important too, quantity of water directly affects the quality of decoction. With less water, the drug cannot be boiled thoroughly and the effective ingredients are not fully leached. With more water, more liquid is cooked. It is not convenient for the patient to take the medicine. Chinese herbal medicine is a large difference in water absorption; the general amount of water is 5-10 times of herb. Loose textured medicinal herbs have much water absorption, tight textured medicinal herbs have less water absorption. Therefore, decocting the flowers, leaves, whole grass, add more water, decocting mineral, shell, add less water. Or you can put drugs into the pot. The first decoction, the amount of water added to the decoction is 3-5 centimeters above the surface of the medicine; the second decoction is 3 centimeters above the surface of the drug. This method of adding water is easy way to decocting.

III. Decocting attention

1. The immersion: drug must be soaked before decoction, it is because of traditional Chinese medicine always is dry herb, adding water soak can make medicinal materials become soft and it is easy to extract effective component during decoction. Generally, flowers, leaves, stem soaking time is 1-1.5 hours; root, seed, rhizome, and fruit soaking time is 2-3 hours.

2. Decoction times: it is better to cook more times than once cook for a long time. It has been proved that the twice decoction can get about 80% of the effective ingredients, so the number of decoctions should be two or three times.

3. Decoction temperature: decocting temperature in Chinese medicine is called "heat", generally which is commonly referred to as "Wenhuo" or "Wuhuo". "Wenhuo" is the weak fire, the temperature rises slowly and the water evaporation is slow. "Wuhuo" is the strong fire, the temperature rises fast and the water evaporates quickly. If the heat is too strong, water evaporates quickly, can reduce the leaching of effective composition, also easy to paste the pan. On the contrary, the heat is weak, the decoction of the medicine is poor. First boil with "Wuhuo" and then fry with "Wenhuo" for 20-60 minutes. That is the common way to decocting.

4. Decocting time: mainly according to the nature of the medicine and disease, as well as the situation of the drug. Generally, it takes 20-30 minutes for the first decocting after begin to boil, and second frying for 30-40 minutes. Herbs for antipyretic takes 10-15 minutes for the first time, and second time for 15-20 minutes. Tonic medicine, first fry is 30-40 minutes, second decocting is 40-50 minutes.

5. Dosage: generally, refers to the amount of liquid medicine after two decoctions combined. 400 to 600 milliliters are taken in two times a day for adults. 200 to 300 milliliters are taken in two or three times a day for children, or 30-40 milliliters per time, 5-6 times per day.

6. The medicine needs special decoction: It is the medicine which according to the patient's condition and the nature of the medicine, doctor prescribed with the footnote in the prescription.

(1) Medicine should be decocted first: Generally, it is some minerals, shells and corner drug, because of its hard texture is not easy to extract effective components, usually decoct for 30-40 minutes first, and then mixed with other drugs for decoction. They commonly are Gypsum, Abalone Shell, Hematite, Buffalo Horn and so on. Some toxic drugs first decocted for long time can reduce its poison and detoxify. For example, Kusnezoff Monkshood Root decocted first for a long time can make aconitine decomposite into hypaconitine, its toxicity is only 1/2000 of the original. Prepared Common Monkshood Daugher Root decocted first for a long time can not only reduce the toxicity, but also increase the effect of cardiotonic.

(2) Medicine added after other herbs: They are usually aromatic herbs with volatile oil, they are not suit for long time decocting. They usually are Rhubarb, Cablin Patchouli Herb, Gambir Plant and so on. Their effective components are volatile or easy to decompose.

(3) Medicine needs wrap-boiling: Generally, they are seeds, pollen and powder, packed it in gauze bags and then decocted together with other medicine. They usually are Plantain Seed, Inula Flower and so on. Plantain Seed is easy to paste and coker, so it needs wrap-boiling. The wrap-boiling can prevent the villus falling off from Inula Flower into the decoction and stimulate the throat.

(4) Melt Medicine: Some kinds of medicine can be dissolved by hot decoction. They are usually dissolvable salt and adhesive medicine, such as Sodium Sulfate, Donkey-Hide Glue and so on. For the adhesive medicine it should be dissolved by little hot water or wine and then added into decoction.

(5) Medicine needs Decocted separately: Some valuable medicine should be cooked separately and then added it into decoction, such as Ginseng, American Ginseng,

Pilose Antler.

(6) Some valuable medicine powder cannot be decocted with the group medicine, it should be mix with the already done decoction.

Altogether decocting of traditional Chinese medicine should pay attention to equipment selection, water quantity, decocting time, temperature and so on, especially the doctor's order.

Prescription of Traditional Chinese Medicine

Prescription of traditional Chinese medicine is a prescription which is prescribed by doctor based on the patient's condition and the rules of traditional Chinese Medicine. It often contains a variety of drugs or medicinal materials. Prescription of traditional Chinese medicine usually consists of Monarch Drug (Principal Herb), Ministerial Drug (Official Medicine), Adjuvant (Adjuvar) and Conductant Drug (Guide Herb).

Monarch Drug is a drug or a group of drugs which mainly treat the chief disease or syndrome. Its amount is usually larger than Ministerial Drug, Adjuvant and Conductant Drug. In a prescription, monarch drug is the most important and indispensable drug (medicine).

Ministerial Drug is a drug or a group of drugs which can auxiliary Monarch Drug to strengthen the treatment of the chief disease or syndrome, or can treat concurrent disease or syndromes. Its efficacy of the drug is less than Monarch Drug.

Adjuvant is a drug or a group of drugs which can auxiliary Monarch medicine and Ministerial Drug to strengthen the treatment disease or syndrome, or can eliminate or reduce the toxicity or intensity of the Monarch medicine or Ministerial Drug, or have the opposite nature and flavor (or Four states and Five Tastes) to play a complementary role in treatment. Its efficacy of the drug is less than Ministerial Drug.

Conductant Drug is a drug or a group of drugs which can guide other drugs to reach the focus, or coordinating the drug actions of a prescription. Its efficacy of the drug is less than Adjuvant and it is not essential drugs in the prescription.

Chinese Patent Medicine (Traditional Chinese Medicine Patent Prescription)

Chinese Patent Medicine is Chinese medicine products which is made by traditional Chinese Medicine. It includes various forms such as pill, powder, paste, pellet and so on. Compared with Traditional Chinese Medicine decoction, Chinese Patent Medicine does not need to be decocted and is convenient to carry. Since Chinese Patent Medicines are mostly processed and concentrated by special processing, the its dosage is far less than traditional Chinese medicine decoction, and it also reduces the bad stimulation of peculiar flavors. Therefore, it is easy to be accepted by the people. But the its defect is the composition and the proportion is constant, it cannot be flexible added or reduced with the disease like decoction.

Brief introduction of common terminology of Traditional Chinese Medicine

1. Four states (Properties) of human energy: *yang*(阳), *yin*(阴), *Qi*(气), blood (*xue*)

(血).

In terminology of Traditional Chinese Medicine *yang* is based on *yin-yang* theory. *yang* usually has one or more characterizations such as: male, dynamic, hot, upward, dry.

Symptom of *yang* deficiency/vacuity: aversion to cold, cold limbs, frequent (clear) urination, diarrhea, pale complexion, hypertrophy of tongue, and slow and weak pulse.

In terminology of Traditional Chinese Medicine *yin* is also based on *yin-yang* theory. *yin* usually have one or more characterizations such as: female, static, cold, downward, moist.

Symptom of *yin* deficiency/vacuity: heat sensations, easy to night sweating, insomnia, dry pharynx or mouth, dark urine, red tongue with less coating, and thready and rapid pulse.

Qi has five functions: actuation, warming, defense, containment and transformation. Usually, *Qi* is considered as the main driving force of human body.

Symptom of *Qi* deficiency/vacuity: lassitude of spirit, lack of strength, easy to catch cold, indigestion, shortness of breath.

Blood (*xue*) in terminology of Traditional Chinese Medicine usually refers to blood. Functions of Blood (*xue*) are nourishing all parts and tissues of the body, safeguarding an adequate degree of moisture, let people maintain invigoration and clear-mind, and ease of mind.

Symptom of blood (*xue*) deficiency/vacuity: pale or yellow complexion, dizziness, palpitations, insomnia, numbness of the limbs; pale tongue; thready pulse.

2. Six Excesses

Six Excesses are the six external factors which cause diseases (some doctors think they are allegorical terms used to describe disharmony patterns displaying certain typical symptoms.): wind(风), cold(寒), anemopyretic/heat/fire(热), dampness/moist(湿), dryness(燥), summerheat(暑).

Wind usually leads to disease such as: common cold (if it combined with cold we call it "chill (*Fenghan*) cold", if it combined with heat we call it "anemopyretic cold"), painful *bi* disorder (it is usually the muscle and bone pain, especially joint pain with stiffness in joints such as rheumatic arthritis), numbness of limbs, apoplexy, stroke, paralysis, coma, etc.

Cold usually leads to disease such as: abdominal pain, heart pain, stomachache, vomit, etc. It also can deteriorate the painful *bi* disorder, diarrhea, etc. Remarks: the "cold" in the indication of herb or medicine refers to common cold or influenza.

Anemopyretic (heat, fire) usually leads to disease such as: vexation, insomnia, red eyes, sore throat, oral ulcer, various kinds of hemorrhage, etc. It also can deteriorate convulsion, spasm, constipation, dry mouth and throat, etc.

Dampness (moist) usually leads to diseases such as: diarrhea, turbid urine, fullness and distention of the chest and abdomen, leucorrhea, edema, eczema, etc. It also can deteriorate the painful *bi* disorder, dermatophytosis, etc.

Dryness usually leads to diseases such as: dry mouth and throat, constipation, dry cough, dry and split of skin, etc.

Summerheat usually leads to diseases such as: heatstroke, dehydration, thirst, shortness of breath and tiredness (in summer), etc.

Main and collateral channels (Meridian tropism)

In traditional Chinese medicine, Main and collateral channels (Meridian tropism or

Jingluo) are channels that run *Qi* and blood. They connect each visceras, body surface and all parts of the body. They are the regulation system of human physical movement. Meridian is the basis of acupuncture and massage, and it is an important part of traditional Chinese medicine.

Part I Chinese Matera Medica and Prepared Slice of Traditional Chinese Drugs

Jie Biao Yao(解表药)-herbs for relieving exterior syndrome

Jie Biao Yao is a kind of herbs which's the major functions are to treat head and body pain, nasal obstruction, shed tears and sore throat; some of them can treat fever, relieve cough or induce perspiration.

Ephedra (Mahuang)

Chinese phonetic alphabet/pin yin: má huáng

Chinese characters simplified/traditional:麻黄/麻黄

Chinese nickname's alphabet (Nickname's Chinese characters): Longsha/ Guogu(龙沙/狗骨)

Latin: Ephedrae Herba (Common name: Ephedra)

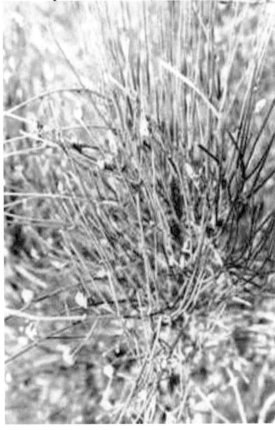 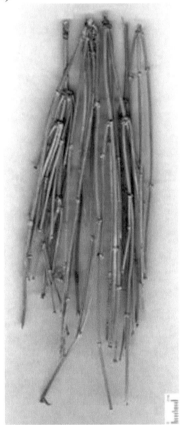

Plant: *Ephedra intermedia* Schrenk. et C. A. Mey. (or *Ephedra sinica* Stapf., *Ephedra equisetina* Bge.)

TCM prepared in ready-to-use forms (medicinal parts): it's dried herbaceous stem which harvested in autumn.

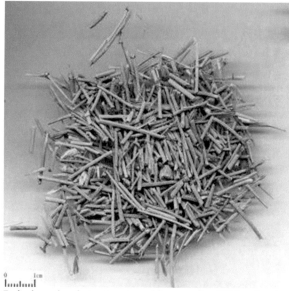

Property and flavor: warm; mild bitter, pungent.
Main and collateral channels: lung and bladder meridians.
Administration and dosage: 2-10 g.
Indication: chill (*Fenghan*) cold; relieve cough and asthma; induce diuresis to alleviate edema; promote sweating.

It is key herb to treat cold, cough, difficulty in micturition and induce perspiration.
Precaution and warnings: it is diaphoretic, used with caution in the people with auto-sweating or night sweating. Ephedra contains L-ephedrine and pseudoephedrine. They can be used to make methamphetamine (a kind of narcotics), don't prescribe it over 7 days dosage per prescription.
(The picture is only for learning and identification the herb; the specific use of the herb please consult the herbalist or health professionals)

Cassia Twig (Guizhi)
Chinese phonetic alphabet/pin yin: guì zhī
Chinese characters simplified/traditional:桂枝/桂枝
Chinese nickname's alphabet (Nickname's Chinese characters): Liugui/ Nenguizhi/ Guizhijian(柳桂/嫩桂枝/桂枝尖)
Latin: Cinnamomi Ramulus (Common name: Cassia Twig)

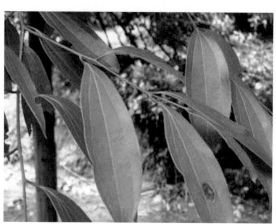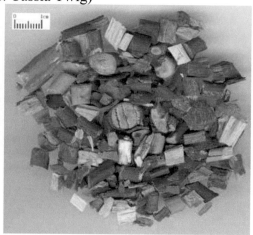

Plant: *Cinnamomum cassia* Presl.
TCM prepared in ready-to-use forms (medicinal parts): it is dried twig which harvested between November and December, remove leaves.
Property and flavor: warm; pungent, sweet.
Main and collateral channels: heart, lung and bladder meridians.
Administration and dosage: 3-10 g.
Indication: arthralgia, edema; relieve abdominal pain caused by chill (*Fenghan*) cold;

reduce phlegm; promote sweating.

Precaution and warning: use with caution during pregnancy.

Attention: to protect the rare wild plant, please don't use the herb from wild plant.

(The picture is only for learning and identification the herb; the specific use of the herb please consult the herbalist or health professionals)

Perilla Herb (Zisu)

Chinese phonetic alphabet/pin yin: zǐ sū

Chinese characters simplified/traditional:紫苏/紫蘇

Chinese nickname's alphabet (Nickname's Chinese characters): Guiren/ Baisu/ Chisu/ Suma(桂荏/白苏/赤苏/苏麻)

Latin: Perillae Herba (Common name: Perilla Herb or Purple Perilla Herb)

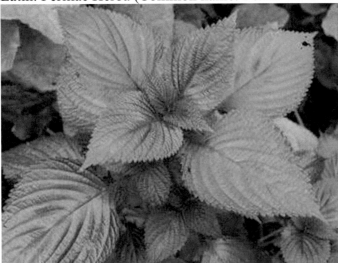

Plant: *Perilla frutescens* (L.) Britt.

Property and flavor: warm; pungent.
Main and collateral channels: lung and spleen meridians.
Administration and dosage: 5-10 g.
Indication: chill (*Fenghan*) cold, cough, nausea and vomiting; detoxify seafood poison.
It is commonly used in treating chill (*Fenghan*) cold.
It is taken as food in some part of China.
Attachment: Perilla Leaf Oil is volatile oil obtained by steam distillation from the plants of Perilla Herb.
(The picture is only for learning and identification the herb; the specific use of the herb please consult the herbalist or health professionals)

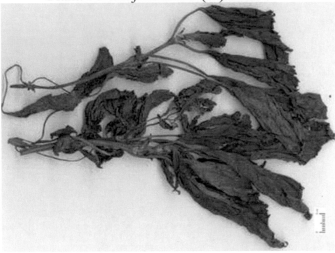

TCM prepared in ready-to-use forms (medicinal parts) :it's dried whole herb which harvested in summer.

Fresh Ginger (Shengjiang)

Chinese phonetic alphabet/pin yin: shēng jiāng

Chinese characters simplified/traditional:生姜/生薑

Chinese nickname's alphabet (Nickname's Chinese characters): Jianggen/ Bailayun/ Gouzhuangzhi/ Yindixin/ Yanliangxiaozi(姜根/百辣云/勾装指/因地辛/炎凉小子)

Latin: Zingiberis Rhizoma Recens (Common name: Fresh Ginger)

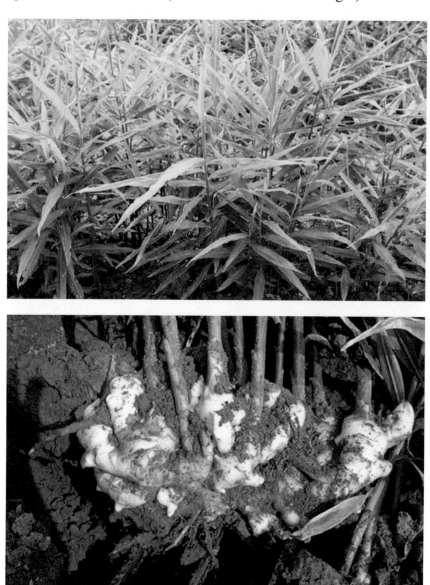

Plant: *Zingiber officinale* Roscoe.

1 cm

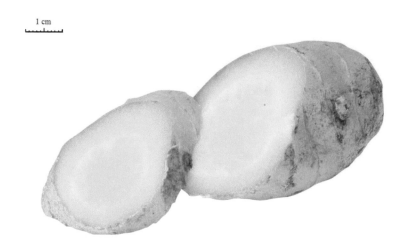

TCM prepared in ready-to-use forms (medicinalparts): it's fresh rhizome which harvested in autumn or winter.

Property and flavor: mild warm; pungent.

Main and collateral channels: lung, spleen and stomach meridians.

Administration and dosage: 3-10 g.

Indication: chill (*Fenghan*) cold, cough and vomiting; detoxify seafood poison.

It is key herb to treat vomiting.

It is taken as seasoning in some part of China.

Attention: to protect the rare wild plant, please don't use the herb from wild plant.
(The picture is only for learning and identification the herb; the specific use of the
herb please consult the herbalist or health professionals)

Fineleaf Schizonepeta Herb (Jingjie)

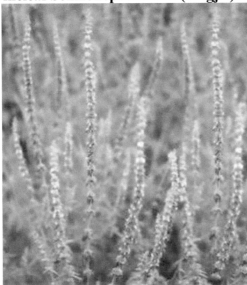

Chinese phonetic alphabet/
pin yin: jīng jiè
Chinese characters simplified/
traditional:荆芥/荊芥
Chinese nickname's alphabet
(Nickname's Chinese characters):
Xiangjingjie(香荆芥)
Latin: Schizonepetae Herba
(Common name: Fineleaf
Schizonepeta Herb)
Plant: *Schizomepeta tenuifolia*
Briq. (or *Nepeta cataria* L.)

TCM prepared in
ready-to-use forms
(medicinal parts): it's
dried above-ground part
of plant which harvested
when it is bloom.
Property and flavor:
mild warm; pungent.
Main and collateral
channels: lung and liver
meridians.
Administration and
dosage: 5-10 g.
Long-time decocted is
inadvisable.

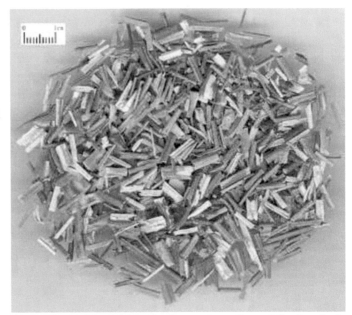

Indication: measles, mumps, rubella, cold and headache; external used for heal ulcer
and sore on the body surface.

It is commonly used in treating chill (*Fenghan*) cold.

Precaution and warnings: it is diaphoretic, used with caution in the people with
auto-sweating and night sweating.

(The picture is only for learning and identification the herb; the specific use of the herb please consult the herbalist or health professionals)

Divaricate Saposhnikovia Root (Fangfeng)

Chinese phonetic alphabet/
pin yin: fáng fēng
Chinese characters
simplified/traditional:
防风/防風
Chinese nickname's
alphabet(Nickname's
Chinese characters):
Pingfeng/ Guanfangfeng/
Dongfangfeng(屏风/
关防风/东防风)
Latin: Saposhnikoviae
Radix (Common name:
Divaricate Saposhnikovia
Root)
Plant: *Saposhnikovia
divaricata* (Trucz.) Schischk.

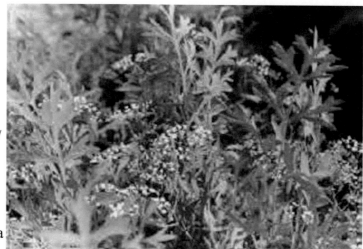

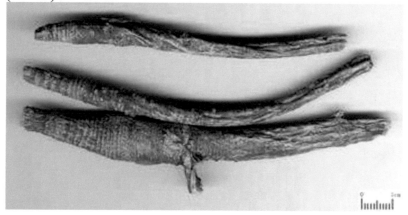

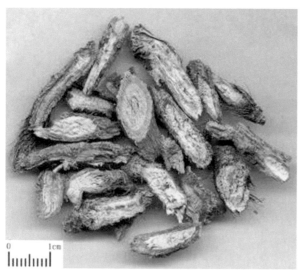

TCM prepared in ready-to-use forms (medicinal parts): it's dried root which harvested in spring or autumn.
Property and flavor: mild warm; pungent, sweet.
Main and collateral channels: bladder, liver and spleen meridians.
Administration and dosage: 5-10 g.
Indication: cold, painful *bi* disorder, rubella, tetanus and itching; relieve headache.

(The picture is only for learning and identification the herb; the specific use of the herb please consult the herbalist or health professionals)

Incised Notopterygium Rhizome or Root (Qianghuo)

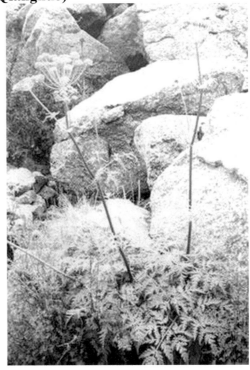

Chinese phonetic alphabet/
pin yin: qiāng huó
Chinese characters simplified/
traditional:羌活/羌活
Chinese nickname's alphabet
(Nickname's Chinese characters):
Chuanqiang/ Canqiang/ Zhujieqiang/
Datouqiang(川羌/蚕羌/竹节羌/
大头羌)
Latin: Notopterygii Rhizoma et
Radix
(Common name: Incised
Notopterygium Rhizome and Root)
Plant: *Notopterygium incisum* Ting.
ex H. T. Chang. (or *Notopterygium
franchetii* H. de Boiss.)

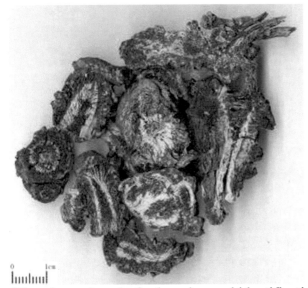

TCM prepared in ready-to-use
forms (medicinal parts): it's
dried root and rhizome which
harvested in spring or winter.
Property and flavor: warm;
bitter, pungent.
Main and collateral channels:
bladder and kidney meridians.
Administration and dosage:
3-10 g.
Indication: chill (*Fenghan*)
cold, stiff nape, arthralga and
rheumatism; relieve headache
and aching shoulder and back.

(The picture is only for learning and identification the herb; the specific use of the
herb please consult the herbalist or health professionals)

Manchurian Wildginger Root (Xixin)
Chinese phonetic alphabet/pin yin: xì xīn
Chinese characters simplified/traditional:细辛/細辛
Chinese nickname's alphabet (Nickname's Chinese characters): Xiaoxin/ Xicao/
Duyecao/ Jinpencao/ Shanrenshen(小辛/细草/独叶草/金盆草/山人参)
Latin: Asari Radix et Rhizoma (Common name: Manchurian Wildginger Root)

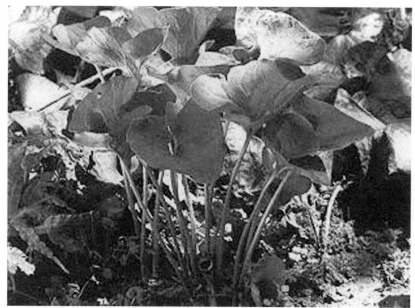

Plant: *Asarum sieboldii* Miq. (or *Asarum heterotropoides* Fr. Schmidt var. *mandshuricum* (Maxim.) Kitag., *Asarum sieboldii* Miq. var. *seoulense* Nakai.)

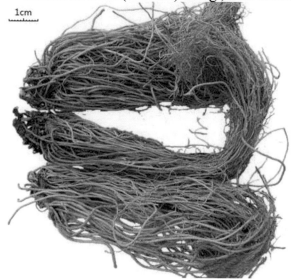

TCM prepared in ready-to-use forms (medicinal parts): it's dried root and rhizome which harvested in summer or autumn. Property and flavor: warm; pungent.
Main and collateral channels: heart, lung and kidney meridians.
Administration and dosage: 1-3 g; for powder administration: 0.5-1 g per time. Topical application in appropriate amount.

Indication: chill (*Fenghan*) cold, excessive phlegm, cough, rheumatic and arthralgia, painful *bi* disorder; relieve headache, toothache, nasal sinusitis and rhinitis.
It is key herb to treat pain, asthma and cough caused by chill (*Fenghan*) cold.
Precaution and warnings: slightly toxic. Incompatible with Black False Hellebore.
(The picture is only for learning and identification the herb; the specific use of the herb please consult the herbalist or health professionals)

Dahurian Angelica Root (Baizhi)
Chinese phonetic alphabet/pin yin: bái zhǐ
Chinese characters simplified/traditional:白芷/白芷
Chinese nickname's alphabet (Nickname's Chinese characters): Xiangbaizhi/ Chuanbaizhi/ Hangbaizhi/ Yubaizhi(香白芷/川白芷/杭白芷/禹白芷)
Latin: Angelicae Dahuricae Radix (English: Dahurian Angelica Root)

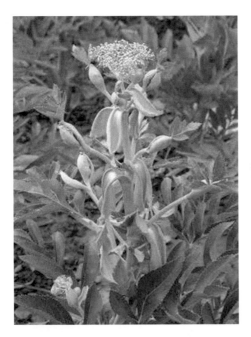

Plant: *Angelica dahurica* (Fisch. ex Hoffm.) Benth. et Hook. f. (or *Angelica dahurica* (Fisch. ex Hoffm.) Benth. et Hook. f. var. *formosana* (Boiss.) Shan. et Yuan.)

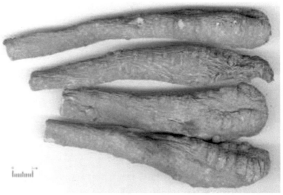

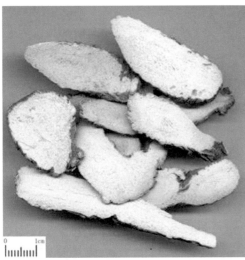

TCM prepared in ready-to-use forms (medicinal parts): it's dried root which harvested in summer or autumn.
Property and flavor: warm; pungent.
Main and collateral channels: stomach, large intestine and lung meridians.
Administration and dosage: 3-10 g.
Indication: cold, leucorrhea, allergic rhinitis; relieve headache, nasal congestion, sinusitis, eyebrow bone pain and toothache.
It is key herb to treat headache.
It is taken as food in some part of China.

(The picture is only for learning and identification the herb; the specific use of the herb please consult the herbalist or health professionals)

Chinese Mosla (Xiangru)

Chinese phonetic alphabet/pin yin: xiāng rú
Chinese characters simplified/traditional:香薷/香薷
Chinese nickname's alphabet (Nickname's Chinese characters): Xiangrong/Xiangrucao(香茸/香茹草)
Latin: Moslae Herba
(Common name: Chinese Mosla)

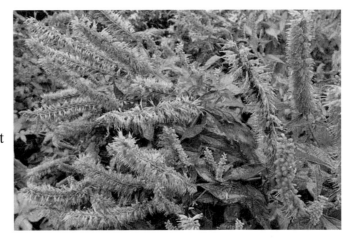

Plant: *Mosla chinensis* Maxim. (or *Elsholtzia ciliata* (Thunb.) Hyland., *Mosla chinensis* "Jiangxiangru").

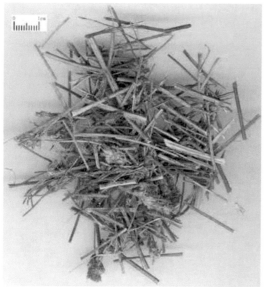

TCM prepared in ready-to-use forms (medicinal parts): it's dried all the grass which harvested in summer or autumn.

Property and flavor: mild warm; pungent.

Main and collateral channels: lung and stomach meridians.

Administration and dosage: 3-10 g.

Indication: cold, fever with no sweat, headache, abdominal pain, vomiting, diarrhea and edema; diuresis.

It has the similar function with Ephedra in summer.

It is taken as tea in some part of China.

Precaution and warnings: it is diaphoretic, used with caution in the people with auto-sweating or night sweating.

(The picture is only for learning and identification the herb; the specific use of the herb please consult the herbalist or health professionals)

Chinese Lovage (Gaoben)

Chinese phonetic alphabet/pin yin: gǎo běn

Chinese characters simplified/traditional:藁本/藁本

Chinese nickname's alphabet (Nickname's Chinese characters): Xixionggaoben/ Xianggaoben(西芎藁本/香藁本)

Latin: Ligustici Rhizoma et Radix (Common name: Chinese Lovage)

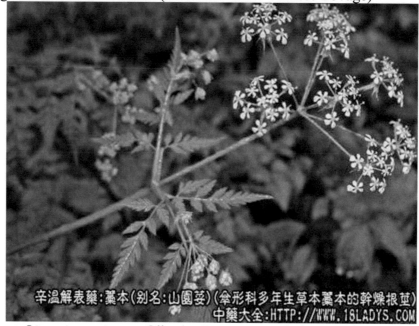

Plant: *Ligusticum sinense* Oliv. (or *Ligusticum jeholense* Nakai. et Kitag.)

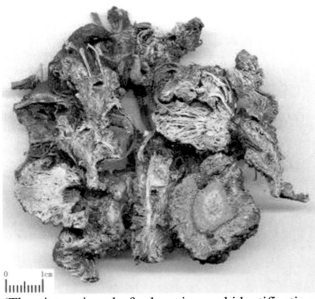

TCM prepared in ready-to-use forms (medicinal parts): it's dried root and rhizome which harvested in autumn.
Property and flavor: warm; pungent.
Main and collateral channels: bladder meridian.
Administration and dosage: 3-10 g.
Indication: chill (*Fenghan*) cold, rheumatism arthralgia; relieve parietal headache.

(The picture is only for learning and identification the herb; the specific use of the herb please consult the herbalist or health professionals)

Biond Magnolia Flower (Xinyi)

Chinese phonetic alphabet/pin yin: xīn yí
Chinese characters simplified/traditional:辛夷/ 辛夷
Chinese nickname's alphabet (Nickname's Chinese characters): Yingchun/ Mubihua/ Maoxinyi/ Jiangpuhua(迎 春/木笔花/毛辛夷/姜朴花)
Latin: Magnoliae Flos seu Magnolia Liliflora Flos (Common name: Biond Magnolia Flower or Lily Magnolia)

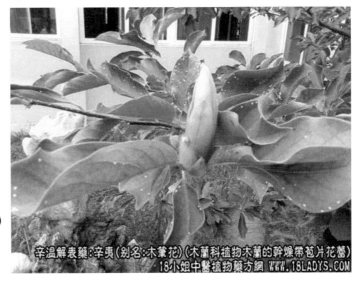

Plant: *Magnolia biondii* Pamp. (or *Magnolia denudata* Desr., *Magnolia sprengeri* Pamp.)

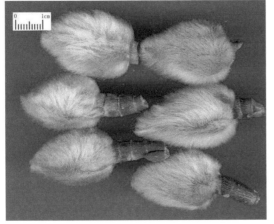

TCM prepared in ready-to-use forms (medicinal parts): it's dried (flower) bud.
Property and flavor: warm; pungent.
Main and collateral channels: lung and stomach meridians.
Administration and dosage: 3-10 g. wrap-boiling.
Indication: sinusitis, nasal pain and headache cause by chill (*Fenghan*) cold.

It is key herb to treat nasal obstruction, nasosinusitis and headache.
(The picture is only for learning and identification the herb; the specific use of the herb please consult the herbalist or health professionals)

Siberian Cocklebur Seed (Cang'erzi)
Chinese phonetic alphabet/pin yin: cāng ěr zǐ
Chinese characters simplified/traditional:苍耳子/蒼耳子
Chinese nickname's alphabet (Nickname's Chinese characters): Niushizi/ Hucangzi/ Canglangzhong/ Miantanglang(牛虱子/胡苍子/苍郎种/棉螳螂)
Latin: Xanthii Fructus (Common name: Siberian Cocklebur Seed)

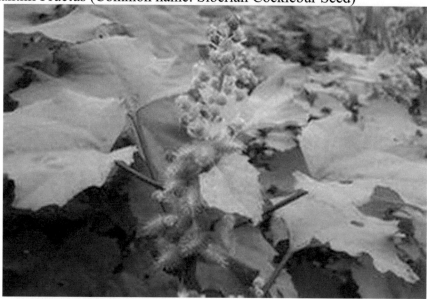

Plant: *Xanthium sibiricum* Patrin ex Widder.

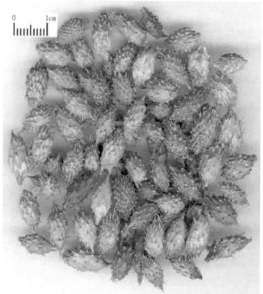

TCM prepared in ready-to-use forms (medicinal parts): it's dried mature seed.
Property and flavor: warm; bitter, pungent.
Main and collateral channels: lung meridian.
Administration and dosage: 3-10 g.
Indication: cold, headache, sinusitis, rhinorrhea, rubella itching and spasm.
Precaution and warnings: toxic, over dosage is inadvisable.

(The picture is only for learning and identification the herb; the specific use of the herb please consult the herbalist or health professionals)

Chinese Tamarisk Twig (Chengliu)
Chinese phonetic alphabet/pin yin: chēng liǔ
Chinese characters simplified/traditional:柽柳/檉柳

Chinese nickname's alphabet (Nickname's Chinese characters): Xiheliu/ Cheng/ Shanchuanliu(西河柳/柽/山川柳)

Latin: Tamaricis Cacumen (Common name: Chinese Tamarisk Twig)

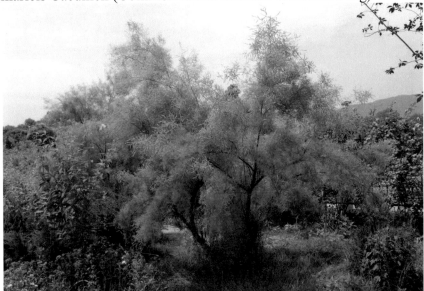

Plant: *Tamarix chinensis* Lour.

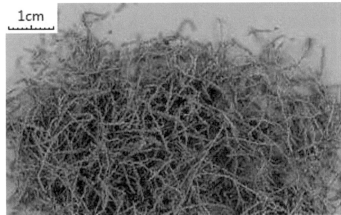

TCM prepared in ready-to-use forms (medicinal parts): it's dried twig and leaf which harvested in summer. Property and flavor: neutral; sweet, pungent. Main and collateral channels: heart, lung and stomach meridians.

Administration and dosage: 3-6 g. Its decoction can be used for rubbing-washing therapy.

Indication: measles, rheumatism, arthralgia and painful *bi* diorder.

(The picture is only for learning and the herb; the specific use of the herb please consult the herbalist or health professionals)

Peppermint (Bohe)

Chinese phonetic alphabet/ pin yin: bò he

Chinese characters simplified/traditional: 薄荷/薄荷

Chinese nickname's alphabet (Nickname's Chinese characters): Yindancao(银丹草)

Latin: Menthae Haplocalycis Herba (Common name:

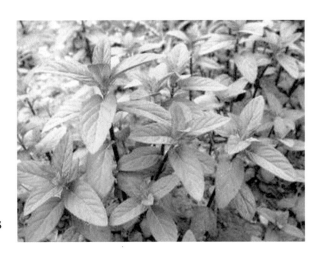

Peppermint or Mint)　　　　　Plant: *Mentha haplocalyx* Briq.

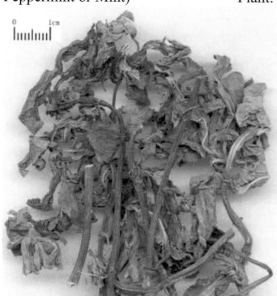

TCM prepared in ready-to-use forms (medicinal parts): it's dried stem and leaf which harvested in summer or autumn.

Property and flavor: cool; pungent.

Main and collateral channels: lung and liver meridians.

Administration and dosage: 3-6 g, added when the decoction is nearly done.

Indication: anemopyretic cold, febrile disease early, headache, red eyes, sore throat, mouth ulcers, rubella, measles, chest tightness and rise.

It is taken as seasoning in some part of China.

Precaution and warnings: it is diaphoretic, used with caution in the people with auto-sweating or night sweating.

Attachment: Peppermint Oil (Latin: Menthae Dementholatum Oleum)

Peppermint Oil is the volatile oil obtained by steam distillating, freezing, removing partly from menthol, which is got from fresh Peppermint.

(The picture is only for learning and identification the herb; the specific use of the herb please consult the herbalist or health professionals)

Great Burdock Achene (Niubangzi)

Chinese phonetic alphabet/pin yin: niú bàng zǐ

Chinese characters simplified/traditional:牛蒡子/牛蒡子

Chinese nickname's alphabet (Nickname's Chinese characters): Dalizi(大力子)

Latin: Arctii Fructus (Common name: Great Burdock Achene)

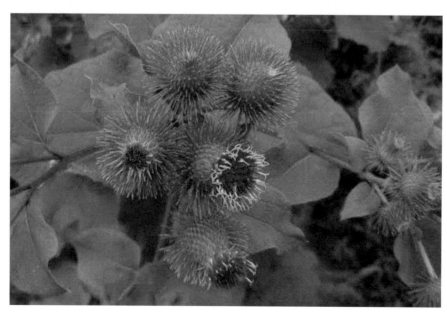

Plant: *Arctium lappa* L.

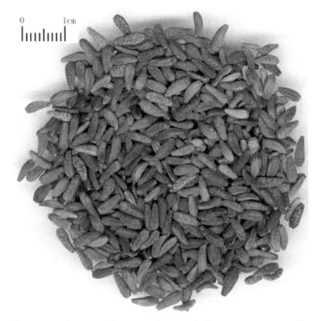

TCM prepared in ready-to-use forms (medicinal parts): it's ripe fruit.
Property and flavor: cold; pungent, bitter.
Main and collateral channels: lung and stomach meridians.
Administration and dosage: 6-12 g.
Indication: anemopyretic cold, cough, excessive phlegm, measles, rubella, mumps, erysipelas, sore throat and carbuncle sore.

Precaution and warnings: it has evacuant fuction, used with caution in the people with diarrhea or dysentery.
(The picture is only for learning and identification the herb; the specific use of the herb please consult the herbalist)

Cicada Slough (Chantui)

Chinese phonetic alphabet/pin yin: chán tuì
Chinese characters simplified/traditional: 蝉蜕/蟬蛻
Chinese nickname's alphabet (Nickname's Chinese characters): Chanke/ Kuchan/ Chanyi/ Zhiliaopi(蝉壳/枯蝉/蝉衣/知了皮)
Latin: Cicadae Periostracum (Common name: Cicada Slough)

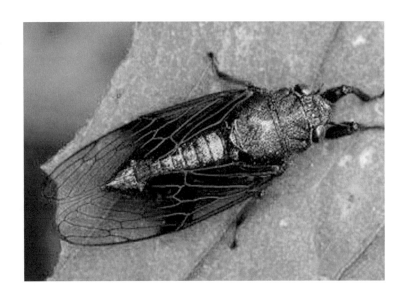

Animal: *Cryptotympana pustulata* Fabricius. (or *Cryptotympana atrata* Fabricus. , *Oncotumpana maculicollis*)

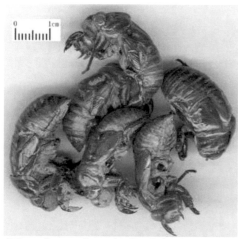

TCM prepared in ready-to-use forms (medicinal parts): it's the shell (slough) of cicada after the emergence.

Property and flavor: cold; sweet.

Main and collateral channels: lung and liver meridians.

Administration and dosage: 3-6 g.

Indication: anemopyretic cold, cough, sore throat, hoarseness, measles, rubella pruritus, red eye, cataract, convulsion and tetanus.

Precaution and warnings: use with cautiously during pregnancy.

(The picture is only for learning and identification the herb; the specific use of the herb please consult the herbalist or health professionals)

Mulberry Leaf (Sangye)

Chinese phonetic alphabet/pin yin: sāng yè

Chinese characters simplified/traditional: 桑叶/桑葉

Chinese nickname's alphabet (Nickname's Chinese characters): Dongsangye/ Shuangsangye/ Shuangye/ Tieshanzi(冬桑叶/霜桑叶/ 双叶/铁扇子)

Latin: Mori Folium (Common name: Mulberry Leaf)

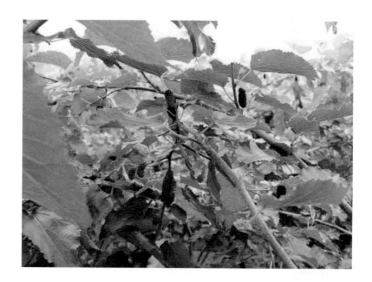

Plant: *Morus alba* L.

TCM prepared in ready-to-use forms (medicinal parts): it's dried leaf which harvested in autumn or winter.

Property and flavor: cold; sweet, bitter.

Main and collateral channels: lung and liver meridians.

Administration and dosage: 5-10 g.

Indication: anemopyretic cold, dry cough, dizziness, headache, red eyes and dazzle.

It is taken as food in some part of China.

(The picture is only for learning and identification the herb; the specific

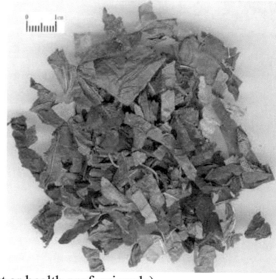

use of the herb please consult the herbalist or health professionals)

Chrysanthemum Flower (Juhua)
Chinese phonetic alphabet/pin yin: jú huā
Chinese characters simplified/traditional:菊花/菊花
Chinese nickname's alphabet (Nickname's Chinese characters): Baiju/ Ganju/ Hangju(白菊/甘菊/杭菊)
Latin: Chrysanthemi Flos (Common name: Chrysanthemum Flower or Chinese White Chrysanthemum)

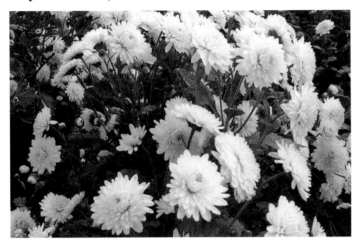

Plant: *Chrysanthemum morifolium* Ramat. (or *Dendranthema morifolium* (Ramat.) Tzvel.)

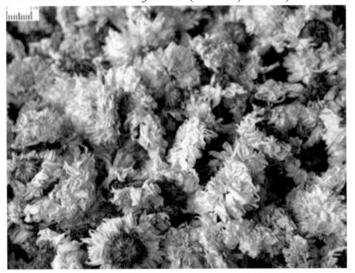

TCM prepared in ready-to-use forms (medicinal parts): it's dried capitulum. Property and flavor: mild cold; sweet, bitter. Main and collateral channels: lung and liver meridians. Administration and dosage: 5-10 g. Indication: anemopyretic cold, headache and dizziness, dim vision, sore, skin infection, swollen eyes, red eyes and dazzle. It is taken as tea in some part of China. (The picture is only for learning and identification the herb; the specific use of the herb please consult the herbalist or health professionals)

Kudzuvine Root (Gegen)
Chinese phonetic alphabet/pin yin: gě gēn
Chinese characters simplified/traditional:葛根/葛根
Chinese nickname's alphabet (Nickname's Chinese characters): Gange/ Gange/ Fenge/(干葛/甘葛/粉葛)
Latin: Puerariae Lobatae Radix (Common name: Kudzuvine Root)

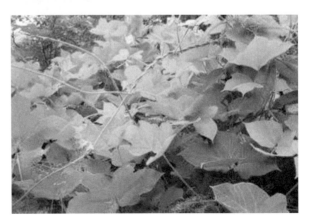

Plant: *Pueraria lobata* (Willd.) Ohwi. (or *Pueraria thomsonii* Benth.)

TCM prepared in ready-to-use forms (medicinal parts): it's dried root (cut into small pieces when it is fresh) which harvested in November or December.

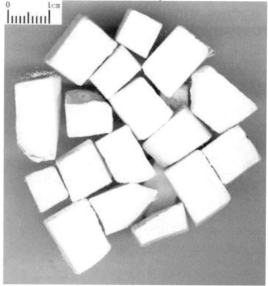

Property and flavor: cool; sweet, pungent.

Main and collateral channels: spleen, stomach and lung meridians.

Administration and dosage: 10-15 g.

Indication: fever, headache, stiff and pain of nape and back, thirst, diabetes, dysentery, measles without adequate eruption, strong neck pain, diarrhea, hemiplegia and hypertension.

It is key herb to treat pain and stiff nape and back.

It is taken as food in some part of China.

(The picture is only for learning and identification the herb; the specific use of the herb please consult the herbalist or health professionals)

Chinese Thorowax Root (Chaihu)

Chinese phonetic alphabet/pin yin: chái hú

Chinese characters simplified/traditional:柴胡/柴胡

Chinese nickname's alphabet (Nickname's Chinese characters): Chaicao/ Beichaihu/ Hongchaihu(柴草/北柴胡/红柴胡)

Latin: Bupleuri Radix (Common name: Chinese Thorowax Root)

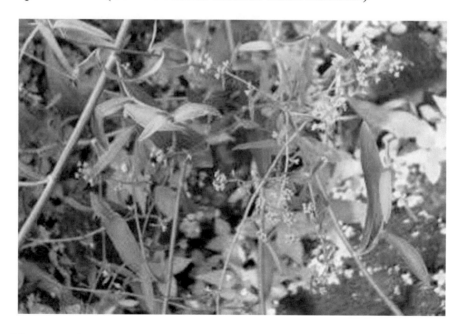

Plant: *Bupleurum chinense* DC. (or *Bupleurum scorzonerifolium* Willd.)

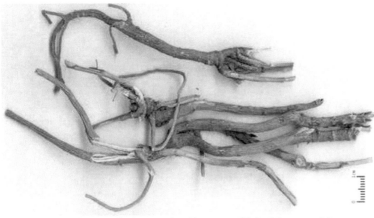

TCM prepared in ready-to-use forms (medicinal parts): it's dried root which harvested in spring or autumn. Property and flavor: mild cold; pungent, bitter.

Main and collateral channels: liver, gallbladder, and lung meridians.
Administration and dosage: 3-10 g.
Indication: fever caused by cold, cold feeling, chest pain, irregular menstruation, hepatitis, uterine prolapse and archoptosis.
It is key herb to treat fever, liver and gallbladder disease, bitter taste and dry throat.
Precaution and warnings: the dried rhizome of *Bupleurum longiradiatum* Turez., covered with numerous annular nodes externally, is poisonous and can not be used as Chinese Thorowax Root.
(The picture is only for learning and identification the herb; the specific use of the herb please consult the herbalist or health professionals)

Largetrifoliolious Bugbane Rhizome (Shengma)
Chinese phonetic alphabet/pin yin: shēng má
Chinese characters simplified/traditional:升麻/升麻
Chinese nickname's alphabet (Nickname's Chinese characters): Longyangen/ Zhouma/ Kulongyagen(龙眼根/周麻/窟窿牙根)
Latin: Cimicifugae Rhizoma (Common name: Largetrifoliolious Bugbane Rhizome)

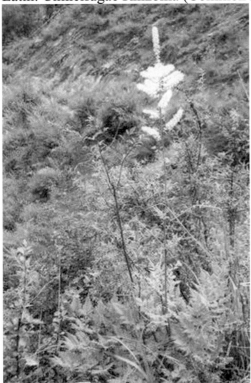

Plant: *Cimicifuga heracleifolia* Kom. (or *Cimicifuga foetida* L., *Cimicifuga dahurica* (Turcz.) Maxim.)

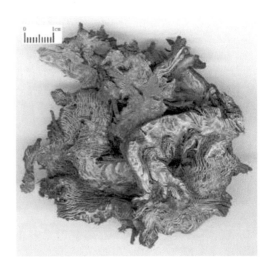

TCM prepared in ready-to-use forms (medicinal parts): it's dried rhizome and root which harvested in autumn.

Property and flavor: mild cold; pungent, mild sweet.

Main and collateral channels: lung, spleen, stomach and large intestine meridians.

Administration and dosage: 3-10 g.

Indication: fever, headache, toothache, sore throat, mouth ulcers, measles without adequate eruption, swelling and spots of the skin, archoptosis and prolapse of uterus. It is key herb to treat gastroptosis, prolapse of the anus and uterus.

(The picture is only for learning and identification the herb; the specific use of the herb please consult the herbalist or health professionals)

Shrub Chastetree Fruit (Manjingzi)

Chinese phonetic alphabet/
pin yin: màn jīng zǐ
Chinese characters simplified/
traditional:蔓荆子/蔓荊子
Chinese nickname's alphabet
(Nickname's Chinese characters):
Manjingshi/ Manqingzi/
Wanjingzi(蔓荆实/蔓青子/
万荆子)
Latin: Viticis Fructus
(Common name: Shrub
Chastetree Fruit)
Plant: *Vitex trifolia* L. (or *Vitex trifolia* L. var. *simplicifolia* Cham.)

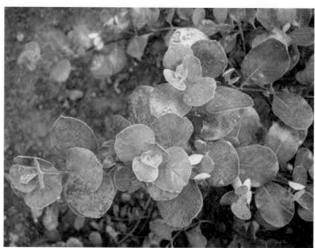

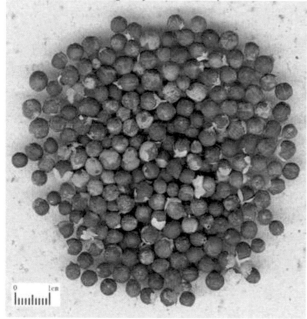

TCM prepared in ready-to-use forms (medicinal parts): it's dried ripe fruit.

Property and flavor: mild cold; bitter, pungent.

Main and collateral channels: bladder, liver and stomach meridians.

Administration and dosage: 5-10 g.

Indication: headache caused by anemopyretic cold, anemopyretic cold, swelling and aching of gum, eyes red and with more tears, dim vision and dizzy.

(The picture is only for learning and identification the herb; the specific use of the herb please consult the herbalist or health professionals)

Fermented Soybean (Dandouchi)

Chinese phonetic alphabet/pin yin: dàn dòu chǐ
Chinese characters simplified/traditional:淡豆豉/淡豆豉

Chinese nickname's alphabet (Nickname's Chinese characters): Douchi/ Xiangchi(豆豉/香豉)

Latin: Sojae Semen Praeparatum (Common name: Fermented Soybean)

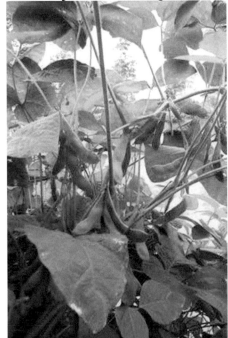

Plant: *Glycine max* (Linn.) Merr.

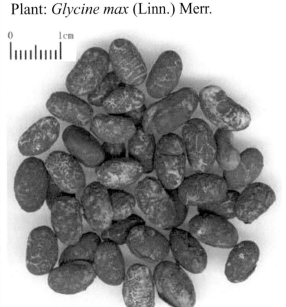

TCM prepared in ready-to-use forms (medicinal parts): it's ferment seed after washed and cooked.

Property and flavor: cool; bitter, pungent.

Main and collateral channels: lung and stomach meridians.

Administration and dosage: 6-12 g.

Indication: cold, headache caused by cold, fever, chest tightness and insomnia. It is taken as food in some part of China.

(The picture is only for learning and identification the herb; the specific use of the herb please consult the herbalist or health professionals)

Common Ducksmeat Herb (Fuping)

Chinese phonetic alphabet/ pin yin: fú píng

Chinese characters simplified/ traditional:浮萍/浮萍

Chinese nickname's alphabet (Nickname's Chinese characters): Shuiping/ Tianping(水萍/田萍)

Latin: Spirodelae Herba (Common name: Common Ducksmeat Herb)

Plant: *Spirodela polyrrhiza* (L.) Schleid. (or *Lemna minor* L.)

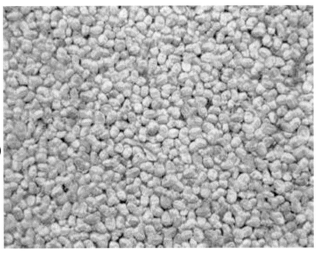

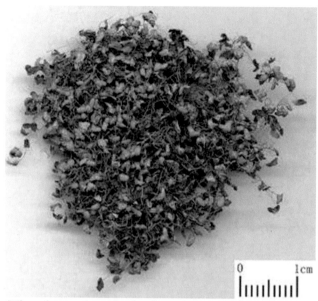

TCM prepared in ready-to-use forms (medicinal parts): it's dried whole grass which harvested between July and September.
Property and flavor: cold; pungent.
Main and collateral channels: lung meridian.
Administration and dosage: 3-9 g. It can be decocted for bathing.
Indication: measles, rubella pruritus, itching caused by rubella, edema and oliguria.

(The picture is only for learning and identification the herb; the specific use of the herb please consult the herbalist or health professionals)

Common Scouring Rush Herb (Muzei)

Chinese phonetic alphabet/pin yin: mù zéi
Chinese characters simplified/traditional: 木贼/木賊
Chinese nickname's alphabet (Nickname's Chinese characters): Qianfengcao/ Cuocao/ Bitoucao(千峰草/锉草/笔头草)
Latin: Equiseti Hiemalis Herba (Common name: Common Scouring Rush Herb)

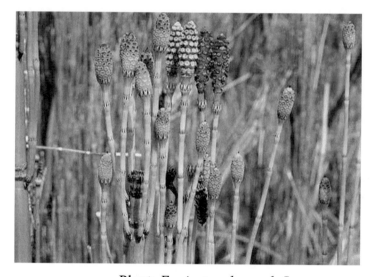

Plant: *Equisetum hyemale* L.

TCM prepared in ready-to-use forms (medicinal parts): it's dried whole grass which harvest in summer or autumn.
Property and flavor: neutral; bitter, sweet.
Main and collateral channels: lung and liver meridians.
Administration and dosage: 3-9 g.
Indication: red eyes cause by anemopyretic, epiphora induced by wind and cataract.

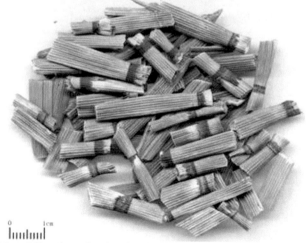

(The picture is only for learning and identification the herb; the specific use of the

herb please consult the herbalist or health professionals)

Coriader Seed (Yansuizi)
Chinese phonetic alphabet/pin
yin: yán suì zǐ
Chinese characters simplified/
traditional:芫荽子/芫荽子
Chinese nickname's alphabet
(Nickname's Chinese characters):
Husuizi/ Xiangcaizi(胡荽子/香菜子)
Latin: Coriandri Semen
(Common name: Coriader
Seed, Cilantro Seed or
Caraway Seed.

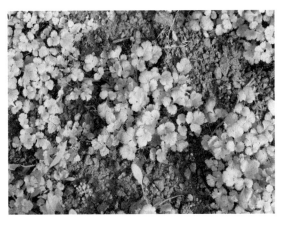

Plant: *Coriandrum sativum* L.

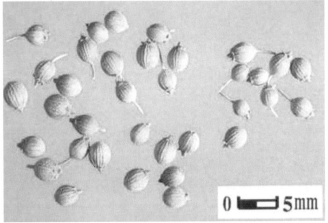

TCM prepared in
ready-to-use forms
(medicinal parts): it's dried
mature fruit.
Property and flavor:
neutral; pungent.
Main and collateral
channels: lung and stomach
meridians.
Administration and dosage:
5-10 g.

Indication: cold and fever; promoting eruption; appetizer.
Precaution and warning: contraindicated in measles with out rash on surface.
(The picture is only for learning and identification the herb; the specific use of the
herb please consult the herbalist or health professionals)

Shallot Herb (Congbai)
Chinese phonetic alphabet/pin yin: cōng bái
Chinese characters simplified/traditional:葱白/蔥白
Chinese nickname's alphabet (Nickname's Chinese characters): Dacongbai/
Xiangcongbai (大葱白/香葱白)

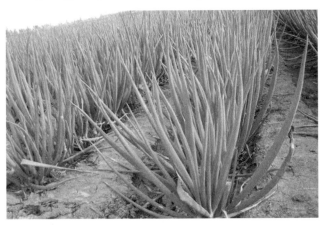

Latin: Fistulosi Herba
(Common name: Shallot
Herb or Chinese Green
Onion Herb)
Plant: *Allium fistulosum* L.

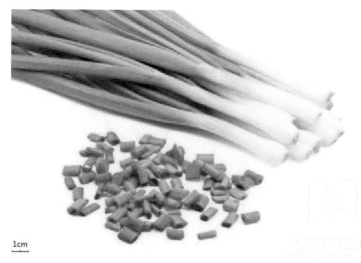

TCM prepared in ready-to-use forms (medicinal parts): it's fresh stalk which harvested all year round.
Property and flavor: warm; sweet, pungent.
Main and collateral channels: lung and stomach meridians.

1cm

Administration and dosage: 3-15 g. Topical application in appropriate amount, mashed and mixed with honey, applied to *pars affecta*. (not taken with honey by oral administration)
Indication: common cold; detoxing; external used for boil, carbuncle and ulcer.
It is taken as food in some part of China.
(The picture is only for learning and identification the herb; the specific use of the herb please consult the herbalist or health professionals)

Small Centipeda Herb (Ebushicao)
Chinese phonetic alphabet/pin yin: é bù shí cǎo
Chinese characters simplified/traditional:鹅不食草/鵝不食草
Chinese nickname's alphabet(Nickname's Chinese characters): Shihusui(石胡荽)
Latin: Centipedae Herba (Common name: Small Centipeda Herb)

Plant: *Centipeda minima* (L.) Br et Aschers

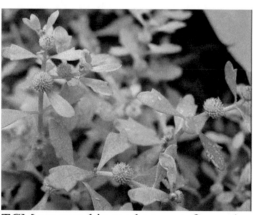

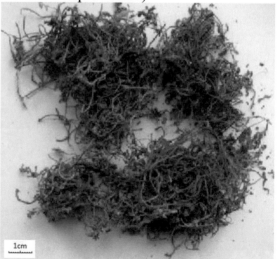

1cm

TCM prepared in ready-to-use forms (medicinal parts): it's dried whole herb which harvested in summer or autumn.
Property and flavor: warm; pungent.
Main and collateral channels: lung meridian.
Administration and dosage: 6-9 g. Appropriate amount for topical application.
Indication: headache caused by chill (*Fenghan*) cold, cough, excessive phlegm and stuffy nose.
(The picture is only for learning and identification the herb; the specific use of the herb please consult the herbalist or health professionals)

Wingedtooth Laggera Leaf (Choulingdancao)

Chinese phonetic alphabet/pin yin: chòu líng dān cǎo

Chinese characters simplified/traditional:臭灵丹草/臭靈丹草

Chinese nickname's alphabet (Nickname's Chinese characters): Shizicao/ Chouyezi/ Liulengju(狮子草/臭叶子/六棱菊)

Latin: Laggerae Herba (Common name: Wingedtooth Laggera Leaf)

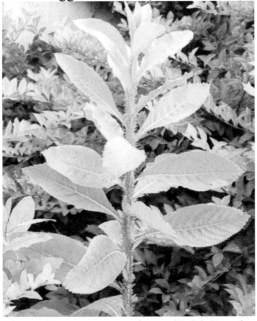

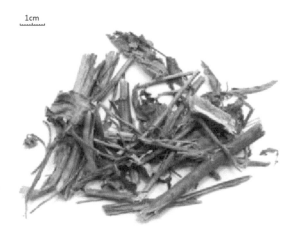

TCM prepared in ready-to-use forms (medicinal parts): it's dried up-ground-part which harvested in autumn.

Plant: *Laggera pterodonta* (DC.) Benth.

Property and flavor: cold; bitter, pungent.

Main and collateral channels: lung meridian.

Administration and dosage: 9-15 g.

Indication: anemopyretic cold, sore throat and cough.

Precaution and warning: toxic.

(The picture is only for learning and identification the herb; the specific use of the herb please consult the herbalist or health professionals)

Common Goldenrod Herb (Yizhihuanghua)

Chinese phonetic alphabet/ pin yin: yī zhī huáng huā

Chinese characters simplified/ traditional:一枝黄花/ 一枝黃花

Chinese nickname's alphabet (Nickname's Chinese characters): Yehuangju/ Manshanhuang (野黄菊/满山黄)

Latin: Solidaginis Herba (Common name: Common Goldenrod Herb)

Plant: *Solidago decurrens* Lour.

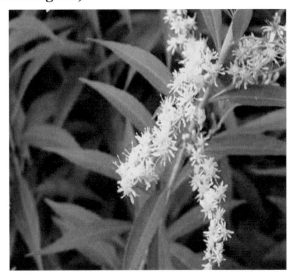

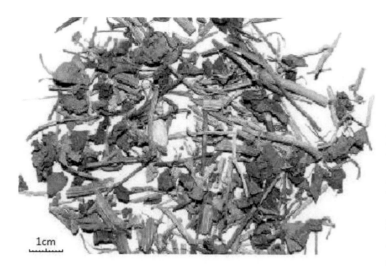

TCM prepared in ready-to-use forms (medicinal parts): it's dried whole herb which harvested in autumn. Property and flavor: cool; bitter, pungent. Main and collateral channels: lung and liver meridians. Administration and dosage: 9-15 g.

Indication: tonsillitis, sore and swollen throat, anemopyretic cold, sore and boil. (The picture is only for learning and identification the herb; the specific use of the herb please consult the herbalist or health professionals)

Qing Re Yao(清热药)-herbs for antipyretic

Qing Re Yao is a kind of herbs which's the major functions are to treat fever, some of them can treat dysentery, carbuncle, abscess.

Gypsum (Shigao)

Chinese phonetic alphabet/pin yin: shí gāo

Chinese characters simplified/traditional:石膏/石膏

Chinese nickname's alphabet (Nickname's Chinese characters): Xilishi/ Baihu(细理石/白虎)

Latin: Gypsum Fibrosum (Common name: Gypsum)

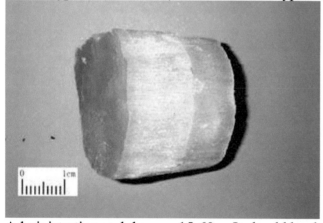

Mineral: main component $CaSO_4 \cdot 2H_2O$
TCM prepared in ready-to-use forms (medicinal parts): it's cleaned mineral.
Property and flavor: highly cold; sweet, pungent.
Main and collateral channels: lung and stomach meridians.

Administration and dosage: 15-60 g. It should be decocted first. Topical application in appropriate amount (usually the calcined gypsum).

Indication: fever caused by cold, cough caused by lung hyperactivity, stomach hyperactivity, headache and toothache.

It is key herb to treat fever, thirst, profuse sweating, dry and hard stool.

(The picture is only for learning and identification the herb; the specific use of the herb please consult the herbalist or health professionals)

Common Anemarrhena Rhizome (Zhimu)

Chinese phonetic alphabet/pin yin: zhī mǔ

Chinese characters simplified/ traditional:知母/知母

Chinese nickname's alphabet (Nickname's Chinese characters): Chimu/ Lianmu/ Yeliao/ Dishen(蚔母/连母/野蓼/地参)

Latin: Anemarrhenae Rhizoma (Common name: Common Anemarrhena Rhizome)

Plant: *Anemarrhena asphodeloides* Bunge.

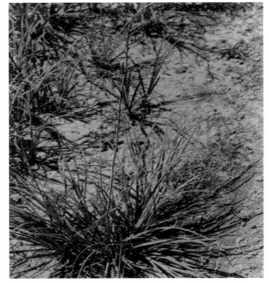

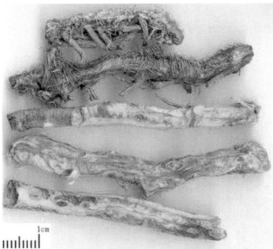

TCM prepared in ready-to-use forms (medicinal parts): it's dried rhizome which harvested in spring or autumn.

Property and flavor: cold; bitter and sweet.

Main and collateral channels: lung, stomach and kidney meridians.

Administration and dosage: 6-12 g.

Indication: fever caused by cold, dry cough, diabetes and constipation.

It is key herb to treat fever.

(The picture is only for learning and identification the herb; the specific use of the herb please consult the herbalist or health professionals)

Snakegourd Root (Tianhuafen)

Chinese phonetic alphabet/pin yin: tiān huā fěn

Chinese characters simplified/traditional:天花粉/ 天花粉

Chinese nickname's alphabet (Nickname's Chinese characters): Gualougen(栝楼根)

Latin: Trichosanthis Radix (Common name: Snakegourd Root)

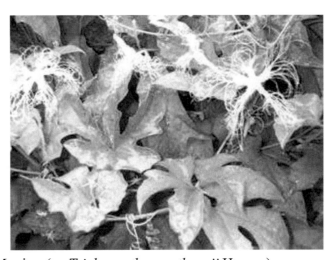

Plant: *Trichosanthes kirilowii* Maxim. (or *Trichosanthes rosthornii* Harms.)

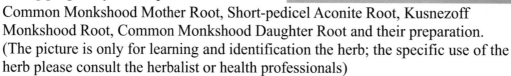

TCM prepared in ready-to-use forms (medicinal parts): it's dried root which harvested in autumn or winter.

Property and flavor: mild cold; sweet, mild bitter.

Main and collateral channels: lung and stomach meridians.

Administration and dosage: 10-15 g.

Indication: fever caused by cold, dry cough, vexation, diabetes, carbuncle, sore and ulcer.

Precaution and warning: use with caution during pregnancy. Incompatible with Common Monkshood Mother Root, Short-pedicel Aconite Root, Kusnezoff Monkshood Root, Common Monkshood Daughter Root and their preparation.

(The picture is only for learning and identification the herb; the specific use of the herb please consult the herbalist or health professionals)

Cape Jasmine Fruit (Zhizi)

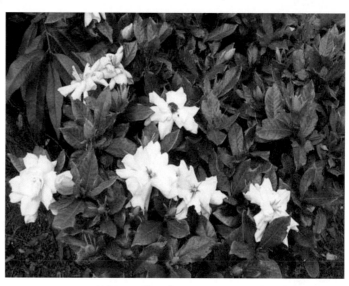

Chinese phonetic alphabet/pin yin: zhī zǐ

Chinese characters simplified/traditional: 栀子/栀子

Chinese nickname's alphabet (Nickname's Chinese characters): Shanzhizi/ Zhizi/ Mudan(山栀子/枝子/木丹)

Latin: Gardeniae Fructus (Common name: Cape Jasmine Fruit)

Plant: *Gardenia jasminoides* Ellis.

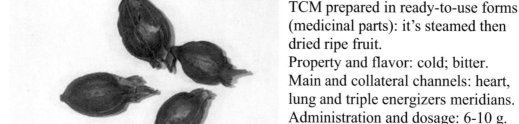

TCM prepared in ready-to-use forms (medicinal parts): it's steamed then dried ripe fruit.

Property and flavor: cold; bitter.

Main and collateral channels: heart, lung and triple energizers meridians.

Administration and dosage: 6-10 g. Ground into powder for topical application.

Indication: fever, fret, jaundice, urine red, swollen and sore; external use for sprain and contusions.

It is key herb to treat vexation and heat.

(The picture is only for learning and identification the herb; the specific use of the

herb please consult the herbalist or health professionals)

Common Selfheal Fruit-Spike (Xiakucao)
Chinese phonetic alphabet/pin yin: xià kū cǎo
Chinese characters simplified/traditional:夏枯草/夏枯草
Chinese nickname's alphabet (Nickname's Chinese characters): Tiexianxiaku/
Datouhua(铁线夏枯/大头花)
Latin: Prunellae Spica (Common name: Common Selfheal Fruit-Spike)

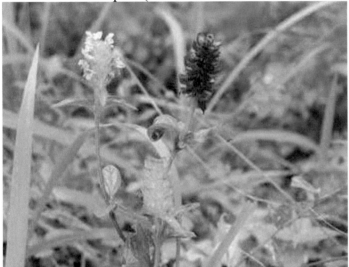

Plant: *Prunella vulgaris* L.

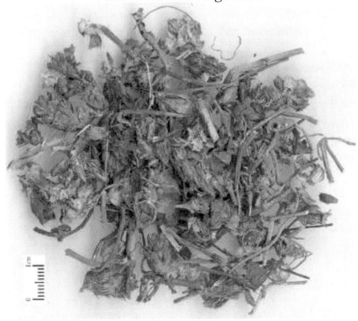

TCM prepared in ready-to-use forms (medicinal parts): it's dried up-ground-part with ear which harvested in summer.

Property and flavor: cold; bitter, pungent. Main and collateral channels: liver and gallbladder meridians.

Administration and dosage: 9-15 g. Indication: red eye, headache, dizziness, scrofula, gall, goiter and tuberculosis, lymph node hyperplasia, hypertension.

It is key herb to treat vertigo, scrofula and eyeball pain at night. It is taken as tea in some part of China.

(The picture is only for learning and identification the herb; the specific use of theherb please consult the herbalist or health professionals)

Reed Rhizome (Lugen)
Chinese phonetic alphabet/pin yin: lú gēn
Chinese characters simplified/traditional:芦根/蘆根
Chinese nickname's alphabet (Nickname's Chinese characters): Weigen/ Lutou(苇根/芦头)
Latin: Phragmitis Rhizoma (Common name: Reed Rhizome)

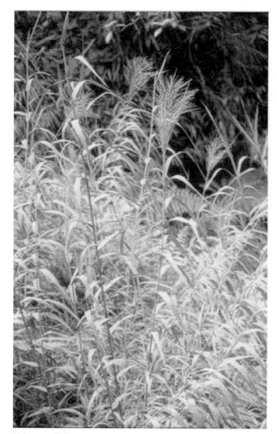

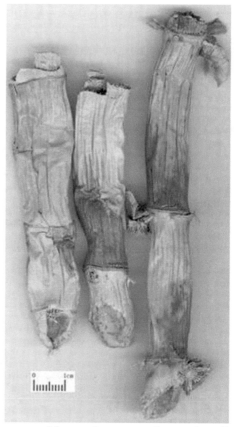

Plant: *Phragmites communis* Trin. (or *Phragmites australias* Trin.)

TCM prepared in ready-to-use forms (medicinal parts): it's fresh or dried rhizome which harvested in November or December.

Property and flavor: cold; sweet.

Main and collateral channels: lung and stomach meridians.

Administration and dosage: 15-30 g, double the dosage for the fresh one.

Indication: fever, vomiting, pyemesis and difficulty in micturition with pain.

The fresh one is taken as food in some part of China.

(The picture is only for learning and identification the herb; the specific use of the herb please consult the herbalist or health professionals)

Bamboo Leaf (Zhuye)

Chinese phonetic alphabet/ pin yin: zhú yè

Chinese characters simplified/traditional:竹叶/ 竹葉

Chinese nickname's alphabet (Nickname's Chinese characters): Danzhuye(淡竹叶)

Latin: Bambusae Folium seu Henonis Folium (Common name: Bamboo Leaf)

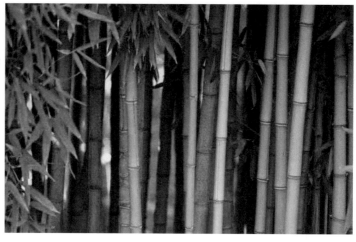

Plant: *Phyllostachys nigra* (Lodd. ex Lindl.) Munro. var. *henonis* (Mitf.) Stapf. et Rendle.(or other species of *Phyllostachys*)

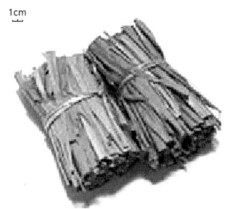

1cm

TCM prepared in ready-to-use forms (medicinal parts): it's dried fresh leaf (with twig) which harvested all year round.
Property and flavor: cold; sweet, bland.
Main and collateral channels: heart, lung and stomach meridians.
Administration and dosage: 6-12 g.
Indication: fever, thirst, coma and delirium; promote urination.

(The picture is only for learning and identification the herb; the specific use of the herb please consult the herbalist or health professionals)

Lophatherum Herb (Danzhuye)

Chinese phonetic alphabet/ pin yin: dàn zhú yè
Chinese characters simplified/ traditional:淡竹叶/淡竹葉
Chinese nickname's alphabet (Nickname's Chinese characters): Zhuyemaidong/ Jinzhuye/ Danzhumi(竹叶麦冬/金竹叶/淡竹米)
Latin: Lophatheri Herba (Common name: Lophatherum Herb)

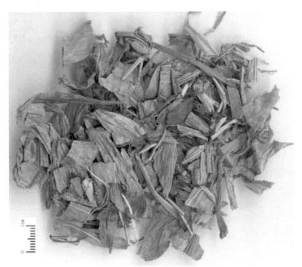

Plant: *Lophatherum gracile* Brongn.

TCM prepared in ready-to-use forms (medicinal parts): it's dried stem and leaf which harvested in summer before it ears.
Property and flavor: cold; sweet and bland.
Main and collateral channels: heart, stomach and small intestine meridians.
Administration and dosage: 6-10 g.
Indication: fever, thirst, vexation, urinating with pain and mouth sores.

It is taken as food in some part of China.
(The picture is only for learning and identification the herb; the specific use of the herb please consult the herbalist or health professionals)

Cassia Seed (Juemingzi)

Chinese phonetic alphabet/pin yin: jué míng zǐ

Chinese characters simplified/traditional: 决明子/决明子

Chinese nickname's alphabet (Nickname's Chinese characters): Caojueming/ Jialvdou (草决明/ 假绿豆)

Latin: Cassiae Semen (Common name: Cassia Seed)

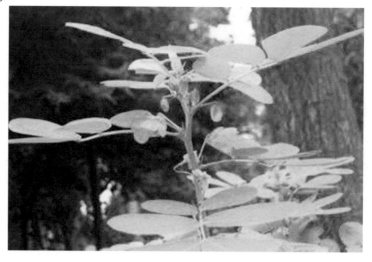

Plant: *Cassia tora* Linn. (or *Cassia obtusifolia* L.)

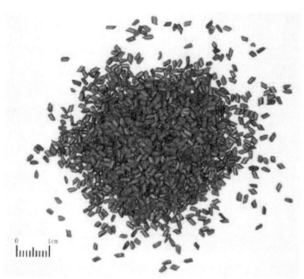

TCM prepared in ready-to-use forms (medicinal parts): it's dried mature seed.

Property and flavor: mild cold; sweet, bitter and salty.

Main and collateral channels: liver and large intestine meridians.

Administration and dosage: 9-15 g.

Indication: red eye with pain, hyperdacryosis, headache, dizziness, dim vision and constipation.

It is taken as tea in some part of China.

(The picture is only for learning and identification the herb; the specific use of the herb please consult the herbalist or health professionals)

Pale Butterflybush Flower (Mimenghua)

Chinese phonetic alphabet/pin yin: mì méng huā

Chinese characters simplified/traditional:密蒙花/密蒙花

Chinese nickname's alphabet (Nickname's Chinese characters): Ranfanhua/ Jiulixiang/ Xiaojinhua(染饭花/九里香/小锦花)

Latin: Buddlejae Flos (Common name: Pale Butterflybush Flower)

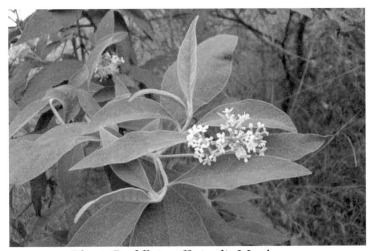

Plant: *Buddleja officinalis* Maxim.

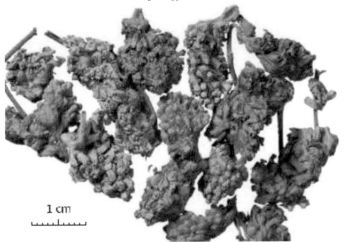

1 cm

TCM prepared in ready-to-use forms (medicinal parts): it's dried bud and inflorescence.
Property and flavor: mild cold; sweet.
Main and collateral channels: liver meridian.
Administration and dosage: 3-9 g.
Indication: swollen red eyes, hyperdacryosis, cataract and dim vision.
(The picture is only for learning and identification the herb; the specific use of the herb please consult the herbalist or health professionals)

Pipewort Flower (Gujingcao)

Chinese phonetic alphabet/
pin yin: gǔ jīng cǎo
Chinese characters simplified/traditional:
谷精草/谷精草
Chinese nickname's alphabet (Nickname's Chinese characters):
Yuyancao/ Zhenzhucao
(鱼眼草/珍珠草)
Latin: Eriocauli Flos
(Common name: Pipewort Flower)
Plant: *Eriocaulon buergerianum* Koern.

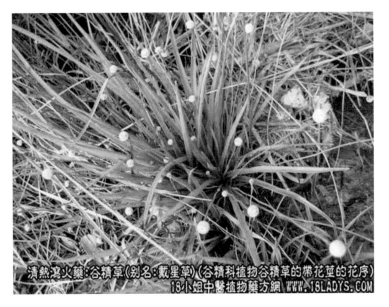

清熱瀉火藥:谷精草(別名:戴星草)(谷精科植物谷精草的帶花莖的花序)
18小姐中醫植物藥方網 WWW.18LADYS.COM

38

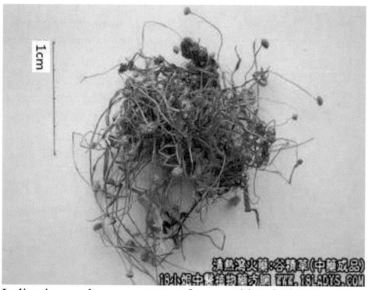

TCM prepared in ready-to-use forms (medicinal parts): it's dried capitulum with scape/peduncle.
Property and flavor: neutral; bitter, pungent.
Main and collateral channels: lung and liver meridians.
Administration and dosage: 5-10 g.

Indication: red eyes, cataract, fever and headache.
(The picture is only for learning and identification the herb; the specific use of the herb please consult the herbalist or health professionals)

Feather Cockscomb Seed (Qingxiangzi)
Chinese phonetic alphabet/pin yin: qīng xiāng zǐ
Chinese characters simplified/traditional:青葙子/青葙子
Chinese nickname's alphabet (Nickname's Chinese characters): Gouweicao/ Jiguanxian (狗尾草/鸡冠苋)
Latin: Celosiae Semen (Common name: Feather Cockscomb Seed)

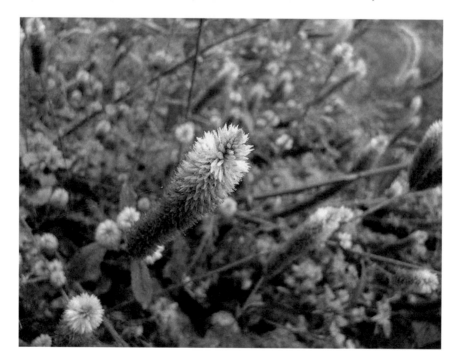

Plant: *Celosia argentea* L.

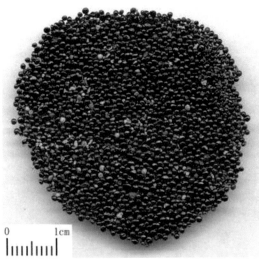

TCM prepared in ready-to-use forms (medicinal parts): it's dried fruit which harvested in autumn.
Property and flavor: mild cold; bitter.
Main and collateral channels: liver meridian.
Administration and dosage: 9-15 g.
Indication: red eyes, eye congest, dim vision, dizziness and turbid urine; mydriasis.
Precaution and warning: contraindicated for patient with glaucoma.

(The picture is only for learning and identification the herb; the specific use of the herb please consult the herbalist or health professionals)

Baical Skullcap Root (Huangqin)

Chinese phonetic alphabet/pin yin: huáng qín
Chinese characters simplified/traditional:黄芩/黃芩
Chinese nickname's alphabet (Nickname's Chinese characters): Shanchagen/ Tujinchagen(山茶根/土金茶根)
Latin: Scutellariae Radix (Common name: Baical Skullcap Root)

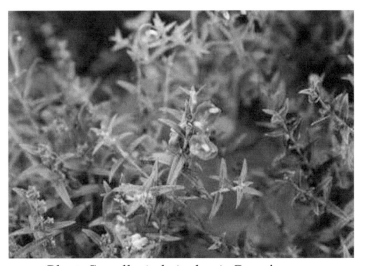

Plant: *Scutellaria baicalensis* Georgi.

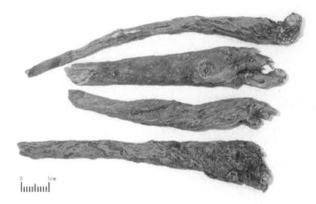

TCM prepared in ready-to-use forms (medicinal parts): it's sun dried root removed fibrous and mud, peel rough skin which harvested in November or December.
Property and flavor: cold; bitter.

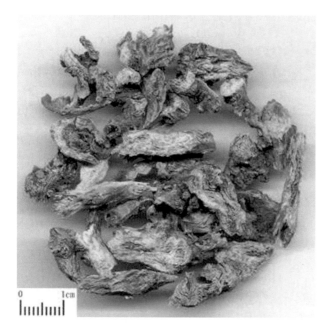

Main and collateral channels: lung, gallbladder, spleen, large intestine and small intestine meridians.

Administration and dosage: 3-10 g.

Indication: stuffy chest and vomiting, distention and fullness, jaundice, diarrhea, cough, fever, vomit blood, carbuncle sore and fetal irritability.

(The picture is only for learning and identification the herb; the specific use of the herb please consult the herbalist or health professionals)

Golden Thread (Huanglian)

Chinese phonetic alphabet/ pin yin: huáng lián

Chinese characters simplified /traditional:黄连/黃連

Chinese nickname's alphabet (Nickname's Chinese characters): Weilian/ Chuanlian/ Jizhualia(味连/ 川连/鸡爪连)

Latin: Coptidis Rhizoma (Common name: Golden Thread)

Plant: *Coptis chinensis* Franch. (or *Coptis deltoidea* C. Y. Cheng et Hsiao., *Coptis teeta* Wall.)

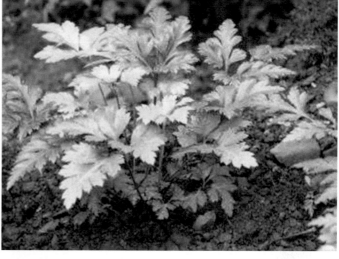

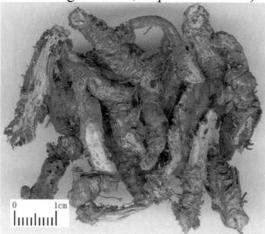

TCM prepared in ready-to-use forms (medicinal parts): it's root or rhizome removed fibrous and mud, sun dried peel rough skin which harvested in autumn.

Property and flavor: cold; bitter.

Main and collateral channels: heart, spleen, stomach, liver, gallbladder and large intestine meridians.

Administration and dosage: 2-5 g. Topical application in appropriate amount.

Indication: distention and fullness, acid regurgitation and vomiting, dysentery and diarrhea, jaundice, fever, coma caused by fever, insomnia, palpitation, vomit, red eyes, toothache and thirst; external use for eczema, ear pus.

It is key herb to treat abdominal distention and pain, bitter taste and dry throat, nausea, diarrhea and dysentery.

(The picture is only for learning and identification the herb; the specific use of the herb please consult the herbalist or health professionals)

Chinese Cork-tree (Huangbai)

Chinese phonetic alphabet/pin yin: huáng bǎi

Chinese characters simplified/traditional:黄柏/黃柏

Chinese nickname's alphabet (Nickname's Chinese characters): Huangnie/ Chuanhuangbo(黄蘗/川黄柏)

Latin: Phellodendri Chinensis Cortex (Common name: Chinese Cork-tree or Cypress Bark)

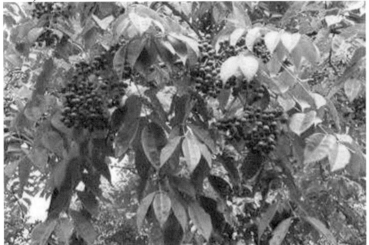

Plant: *Phellodendron chinensis* Schneid.

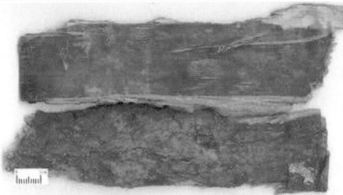

TCM prepared in ready-to-use forms (medicinal parts): it's dried bark which removed the rough skin.
Property and flavor: cold; bitter.
Main and collateral channels: kidney and bladder meridians.
Administration and dosage: 3-12 g. External used in appropriate amount.
Indication: fever, dysentery, jaundice, leucorrhea, beriberi, deficiency to heat, night sweating, sores, eczema and itching.
Attention:
to protect the rare wild plant, please don't use the herb from wild plant.

(The picture is only for learning and identification the herb; the specific use of the herb please consult the herbalist or health professionals)

Chinese Gentian (Longdan)

Chinese phonetic alphabet/pin yin: lóng dǎn

Chinese characters simplified/traditional:龙胆/龍膽

Chinese nickname's alphabet (Nickname's Chinese characters): Longdancao/ Didantou/ Modidan(龙胆草/地胆头/磨地胆)

Latin: Gentianae Radix et Rhizoma (Common name: Chinese Gentian)

Plant: *Gentiana scabra* Bunge. (or *Gentiana manshurica* Kitag.,*Gentiana triflora* Pall., *Gentiana rigescens* Franch.)

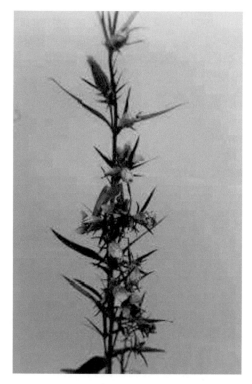
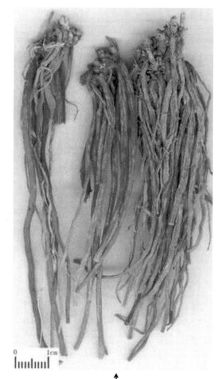

↑
root

TCM prepared in ready-to-use forms (medicinal parts): it's root and rhizome (with leaf) which harvested in spring or autumn.

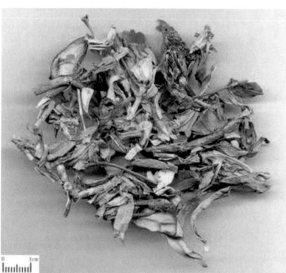

←— branch with leaf

Property and flavor: cold; bitter.
Main and collateral channels: liver and gallbladder meridians.
Administration and dosage: 3-6 g.
Indication: jaundice, swelling of the vulva, pruritus vulvae, leucorrhea, eczema, red eyes, deafness, hypochondriac pain, mouth pain and convulsion.
It is key herb to treat jaundice, fever, sticky and stinky leucorrhea.
(The picture is only for learning and identification the herb; the specific use of the herb please consult the herbalist or health professionals)

Lightyellow Sophora Root (Kushen)

Chinese phonetic alphabet/
pin yin: kǔ shēn
Chinese characters
simplified/
traditional:苦参/苦參
Chinese nickname's alphabet
(Nickname's Chinese
characters): Dihuai/
Haohanzhi/ Shanhuaizi
(地槐/好汉枝/山槐子)
Latin: Sophorae Flavescentis
Radix (Common name:
Lightyellow Sophora Root or
Kuh-Seng)

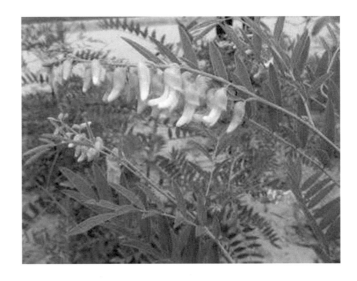

Plant: *Sophora flavescens* Ait.

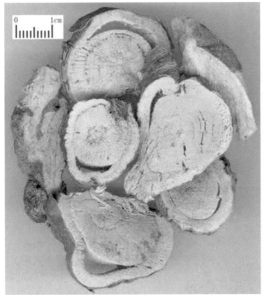

TCM prepared in ready-to-use forms
(medicinal parts): it's dried root which
harvested in spring or autumn.
Property and flavor: cold; bitter.
Main and collateral channels: heart,
stomach, large intestine and bladder
meridians.
Administration and dosage: 4.5-9 g.
Topical application in appropriate
amount, decocted for rinsing.
Indication: dysentery, jaundice,
hematochezia, anuria, leucorrhea,
swelling vulva, pruritus vulvae, eczema,
skin itching, scabies, and leprosy;
external use for curing trichomonas
vaginitis.

It is commonly used in treating morbid leucorrhea.
Precaution and warning: incompatible with Black False Hellebore.
(The picture is only for learning and identification the herb; the specific use of the
herb please consult the herbalist or health professionals)

Rehmannia Root (Shengdihuang)
Chinese phonetic alphabet/pin yin: shēng dì huáng
Chinese characters simplified/traditional:生地黄/生地黄
Chinese nickname's alphabet (Nickname's Chinese characters): Shendi/ Dihuang(生
地/地黄)
Latin: Rehmanniae Radix (Common name: Rehmannia Root)

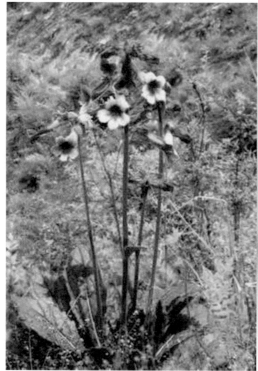

Plant: *Rehmannia glutinosa*
(Gaetn.) Libosch. ex Fisch. et Mey.

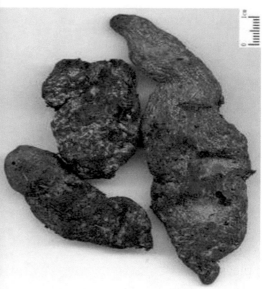

TCM prepared in ready-to-use forms (medicinal parts): it's dried root tuber which harvested in autumn.
Property and flavor: cold; sweet, bitter.
Main and collateral channels: heart, liver and kidney meridians.
Administration and dosage: 10-15 g.
Indication: fever, hematemesis, thirst, vexation, dryness, bleeding from five sense organs or subcutaneous tissue, sore throat and dermexanthesis.
It is key herb to treat xerosis cutis, thirst, hair withered and yellow.
(The picture is only for learning and identification the herb; the specific use of the herb please consult the herbalist or health professionals)

Figwort Root (Xuanshen)

Chinese phonetic alphabet/pin yin: xuán shēn
Chinese characters simplified/ traditional:玄参/玄參
Chinese nickname's alphabet (Nickname's Chinese characters): Yuanshen/ Heishen/ Zhongtai/ Guizang(元参/黑参/重台/鬼藏)
Latin: Scrophulariae Radix (Common name: Figwort Root)
Plant: *Scrophularia ningpoensis* Hemsl.

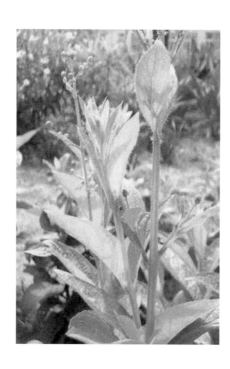

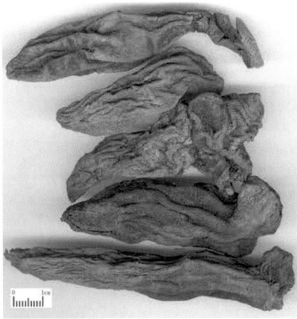

TCM prepared in ready-to-use forms (medicinal parts): it's dried root which harvested in winter.

Property and flavor: mild cold; sweet, bitter and salty.

Main and collateral channels: lung, stomach and kidney meridians.

Administration and dosage: 9-15 g.

Indication: fever, red eyes, sore throat, scrofula, diphtheria, carbuncle sore and constipation.

Precaution and warning: incompatible with Black False Hellebore.

(The picture is only for learning and identification the herb; the specific use of the herb please consult the herbalist or health professionals)

Tree Peony Bark (Mudanpi)

Chinese phonetic alphabet/
pin yin: mǔ dān pí
Chinese characters simplified/
traditional:牡丹皮/牡丹皮
Chinese nickname's alphabet
(Nickname's Chinese characters):
Danpi/ Dangen(丹皮/丹根)
Latin: Moutan Cortex (Common name: Tree Peony Bark)
Plant: *Paeonia suffruticosa* Andr.

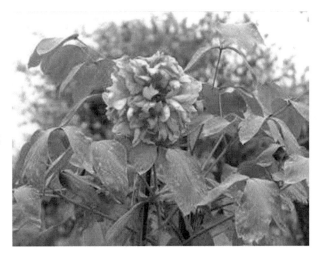

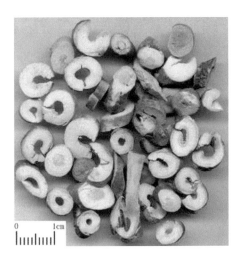

TCM prepared in ready-to-use forms (medicinal parts): it's dried root bark which harvested in autumn.

Property and flavor: mild cold; bitter, pungent.

Main and collateral channels: heart, liver and kidney meridians.

Administration and dosage: 6-12 g.

46

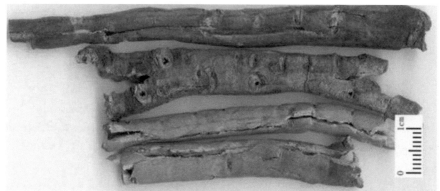

Indication: macula and papule, bleeding from five sense organs or subcutaneous tissue, no sweat fever, amenorrhea, dysmenorrhea, carbuncle sore and traumatic injury.
It is key herb to treat fever without sweating.
Precaution and warning: use with caution during pregnancy.
(The picture is only for learning and identification the herb; the specific use of the herb please consult the herbalist or health professionals)

Red Peony Root (Chishao)
Chinese phonetic alphabet/pin yin: chì sháo
Chinese characters simplified/traditional:赤芍/赤芍
Chinese nickname's alphabet (Nickname's Chinese characters): Mushaoyao/
Caoshaoyao(木芍药/草芍药)
Latin: Paeoniae Radix Rubra (Common name: Red Peony Root)
Plant: *Paeonia veitchii* Lynch. (or *Paeonia lactiflora* Pall.)

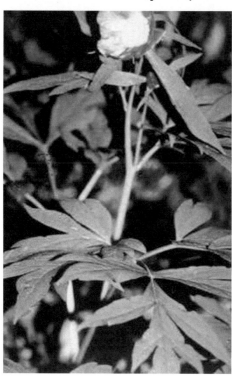
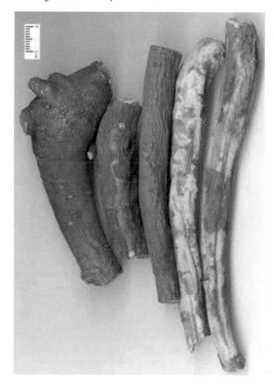

TCM prepared in ready-to-use forms (medicinal parts): it's dried root which harvested in spring or autumn.

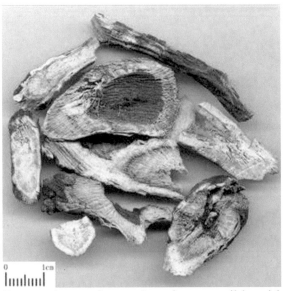

Property and flavor: mild cold; bitter.
Main and collateral channels: liver meridian.
Administration and dosage: 6-12 g.
Indication: macula and papule caused by warm toxin, bleeding from five sense organs or subcutaneous tissue, swollen, liver or chest or abdominal pain, dysmenorrhea, amenorrhea, traumatic injury and sore carbuncle.

Precaution and warning: incompatible with Black False Hellebore.
(The picture is only for learning and identification the herb; the specific use of the herb please consult the herbalist or health professionals)

Arnebia Root (Zicao)

Chinese phonetic alphabet/pin yin: zǐ cǎo
Chinese characters simplified/traditional:紫草/紫草
Chinese nickname's alphabet (Nickname's Chinese characters): Zicao/Zidan/ Dixue(茈草/紫丹/地血)
Latin: Arnebiae Radix seu Lithospermi Radix (Common name: Arnebia Root or Puccoon Root)

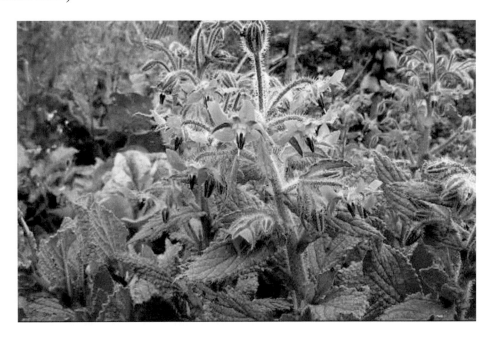

Plant: *Arnebia euchroma* (Royle.) Johnst. (or *Arnebia guttata* Bunge., *Lithospermum erythrorhizon* Sieb. et Zucc.)

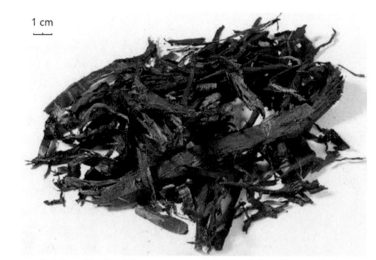

1 cm

TCM prepared in ready-to-use forms (medicinal parts): it's dried root which harvested in spring or autumn.

Property and flavor: cold; sweet, salty.

Main and collateral channels: heart and liver meridians.

Administration and dosage: 5-10 g. Boiled into paste or soaked in plant oil for external used.

Indication: maculae caused by virulent heat pathogen, jaundice, purpura, ulcers, eczema, beginning of measles, burns and scalds.

(The picture is only for learning and identification the herb; the specific use of the herb please consult the herbalist or health professionals)

Buffalo Horn (Shuiniujiao)

Chinese phonetic alphabet/pin yin: shuǐ niǔ jiǎo

Chinese characters simplified/traditional:水牛角/水牛角

Chinese nickname's alphabet(Nickname's Chinese characters): Niujiaojian/ Shaniujiao(牛角尖/沙牛角)

Latin: Bubali Cornu (Common name: Buffalo Horn)

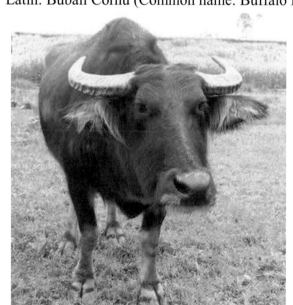

Animal: *Bubalus bubalis* L. (or *Bubalus arnee* L., *Bubalus depressicornis* H. Smith., *Bubalus quarlesi* (Ouwens.))

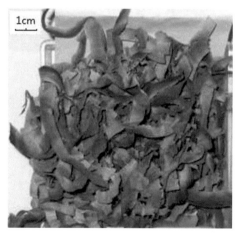

1cm

TCM prepared in ready-to-use forms (medicinal parts): it's Chinese buffalo's horn cut into slice.

Property and flavor: cold; bitter.

Main and collateral channels: heart and liver meridians.

Administration and dosage: 15-30 g. It should be decocted first for more than 3 hours. Indication: fever, coma, delirium, hematemesis, bleeding from five sense organs or subcutaneous tissue, epilepsy and mania.

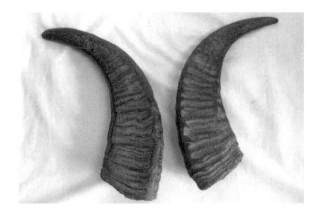

Attention: to protect the rare wild animals, please don't use it from wild animal.
Attachment: Powdered Buffalo Horn Extract (Latinal: Pulvis Cornus Bubali Concentratus)
Procedure: take the clean Buffalo Horn, saw off and discard the horn plug, and cleave in pieces. Take the solid core part of horn tip (commonly known as "Jiaojian"), soak in 75% alcohol or sterilize with steam, and pulverize to fine powder. Take the remained part (commonly known as "Jiaozhuang"), pulverize to coarse granules or chip into slices, decoct with 10 quantities of water twice, 7 to 10 hours for each time, and replenishing the water loss in decoction process momentarily. Combine the decoctions, filter, and concentrate to 80-160 mL (per 810 g "Jiaozhuang"). mix well with the fine powder of "Jiaojian" (20% "Jiaojian" to 80% concentration of "Jiaozhuang"), dry not more than 80°C, pulverize to fine powder and sift.
(The picture is only for learning and identification the herb; the specific use of the herb please consult the herbalist or health professionals)

Japanese Honeysuckle Flower (Jinyinhua)

Chinese phonetic alphabet/ pin yin: jīn yín huā
Chinese characters simplified/ traditional:金银花/金銀花
Chinese nickname's alphabet (Nickname's Chinese characters):
Jinyinteng/ Zifengteng/ Erhua (金银藤/子风藤/二花)
Latin: Lonicerae Japonicae Flos
(Common name: Japanese Honeysuckle Flower)
Plant: *Lonicera japonica* Thunb.

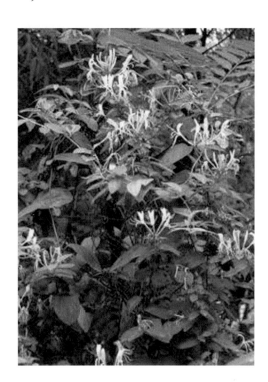

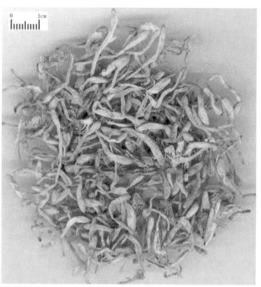

TCM prepared in ready-to-use forms (medicinal parts): it's dried flower or bud.
Property and flavor: cold; sweet.
Main and collateral channels: lung, heart and stomach meridians.
Administration and dosage: 6-15 g.
Indication: abscess, sore carbuncle, sore throat, erysipelas, dysentery, fever caused by anemopyretic cold.
It is key herb to treat carbuncle and sore swelling.
It is taken as tea in some part of China.

(The picture is only for learning and identification the herb; the specific use of the herb please consult the herbalist or health professionals)

Honeysuckle Flower (Shanyinhua)
Chinese phonetic alphabet/pin yin: shā yín huā
Chinese characters simplified/traditional:山银花/山銀花
Chinese nickname's alphabet (Nickname's Chinese characters): Shanhua/Nanyinhua(山花/南银花)
Latin: Lonicerae Flos (Common name: Honeysuckle Flower)

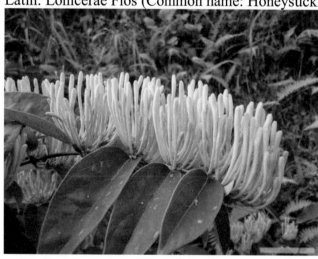

Plant: *Lonicera marcranthoides* Hand. -Mazz. (or *Lonicera hypoglauca* Miq., *Lonicera confusa* DC., *Lonicera fulvotomentosa* Hsu et S. C. Cheng)

TCM prepared in ready-to-use forms (medicinal parts): it's dried flower bud or flower which harvested in summer.
Property and flavor: cold; sweet.
Main and collateral channels: lung, heart and stomach meridians.
Administration and dosage: 6-15 g.
Indication: abscess, swelling, sore, erysipelas, blood dysentery and anemopyretic cold.

It is taken as food in some part of China.

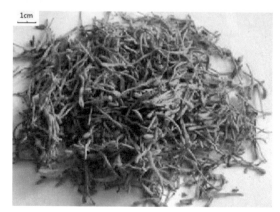

(The picture is only for learning and identification the herb; the specific use of the herb please consult the herbalist or health professionals)

Weeping Forsythia Capsule (Lianqiao)

Chinese phonetic alphabet/pin yin: lián qiào
Chinese characters simplified/traditional: 连翘/連翹
Chinese nickname's alphabet (Nickname's Chinese characters): Huanghuagan/ Huangshoudan(黄花杆/黄寿丹)
Latin: Forsythiae Fructus (Common name: Weeping Forsythia Capsule)

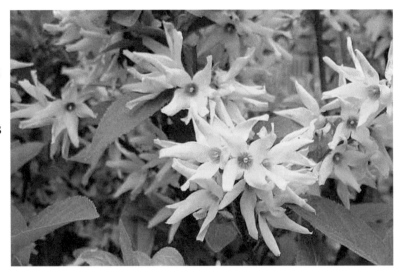

Plant: *Forsythia suspensa* (Thunb.) Vahl.

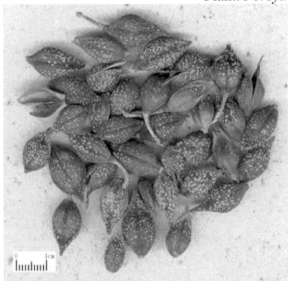

TCM prepared in ready-to-use forms (medicinal parts): it's dried nearly ripe and still greenish fruit.
Property and flavor: mild cold; bitter.
Main and collateral channels: lung, heart and small intestine meridians.
Administration and dosage: 6-15 g.
Indication: carbuncle, mastitis, scrofula, erysipelas, anemopyretic cold, beginning of fever, dizziness and pyretic strangury.
It is key herb to treat sore.

(The picture is only for learning and identification the herb; the specific use of the herb please consult the herbalis or health professionals)

Dandelion (Pugongying)
Chinese phonetic alphabet/pin yin: pú gōng yīng
Chinese characters simplified/traditional:蒲公英/蒲公英
Chinese nickname's alphabet (Nickname's Chinese characters): Huahualang/ Pugongcao/ Popoding(华花郎/蒲公草/婆婆丁)
Latin: Taraxaci Herba (Common name: Dandelion)

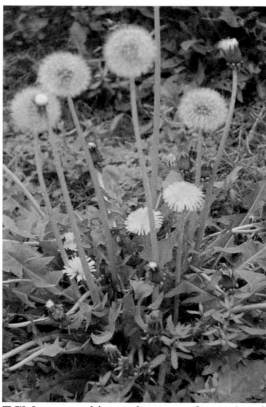

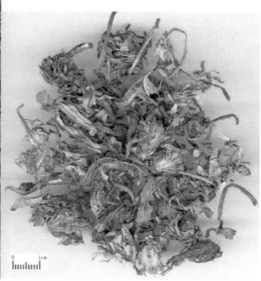

Plant: *Taraxacum mongolicum* Hand.-Mazz. (or *Taraxacum sinicum* Kitag.)

TCM prepared in ready-to-use forms (medicinal parts): it's dried whole herb which harvested from spring to autumn.
Property and flavor: cold; bitter, sweet.
Main and collateral channels: liver and stomach meridians.
Administration and dosage: 10-15 g.
Indication: carbuncle sore, mastitis, scrofula, red-eyes, sore throat, jaundice and pyretic strangury.
It is key herb to treat mastitis.
It is taken as food in some part of China.
(The picture is only for learning and identification the herb; the specific use of the herb please consult the herbalist or health professionals)

Dyers Woad Leaf (Daqingye)
Chinese phonetic alphabet/pin yin: dà qīng yè
Chinese characters simplified/traditional:大青叶/大青葉
Chinese nickname's alphabet (Nickname's Chinese characters): Lanye/ Lancai(蓝叶/蓝菜)
Latin: Isatidis Folium (Common name: Dyers Woad Leaf or Indigowoad Leaf)
Plant: *Isatis indigotica* Fortune.

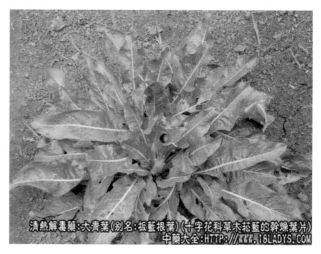

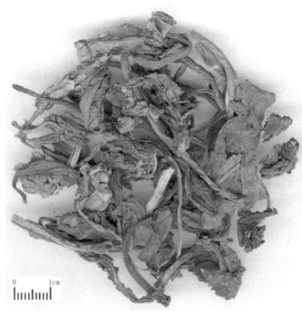

TCM prepared in ready-to-use forms (medicinal parts): it's dried leaf which harvested in summer or autumn.
Property and flavor: cold; bitter.
Main and collateral channels: heart and stomach meridians.
Administration and dosage: 9-15 g.
Indication: fever, coma, macule, jaundice, dysentery, mumps, sore throat and erysipelas.

It is key herb to treat thirsty, vexation, aphtha, distention and pain in the head. (The picture is only for learning and identification the herb; the specific use of the herb please consult the herbalist or health professionals)

Isatis Root (Banlangen)
Chinese phonetic alphabet/pin yin: bǎn lán gēn
Chinese characters simplified/traditional:板蓝根/板藍根
Chinese nickname's alphabet (Nickname's Chinese characters): Shanlan/Dianqinggen/Daqingge(山蓝/靛青根/大青根)
Latin: Isatidis Radix (Common name: Isatis Root)

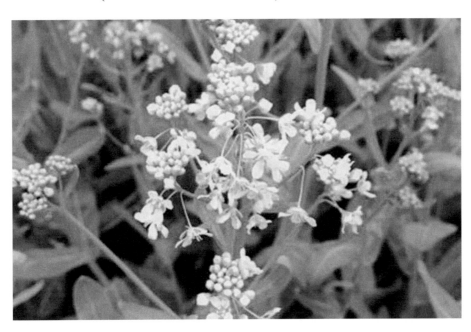

Plant: *Isatis indigotica* Fort. (or *Isatis tinctoria* L.,*Cleredendrum cwtophyllum* Turcz.)

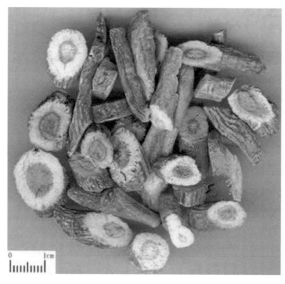

TCM prepared in ready-to-use forms (medicinal parts): it's dried root which harvested in autumn.
Property and flavor: cold; bitter.
Main and collateral channels: heart and stomach meridians.
Administration and dosage: 9-15 g.
Indication: sore throat, fever, macula, papule, erysipelas, mumps and cold (caused by viruses infection); clear away heat and toxic material.
(The picture is only for learning and identification the herb; the specific use of the herb please consult the herbalist or health professionals)

Cow-bezoar (Niuhuang)

Chinese phonetic alphabet/pin yin: niú huáng
Chinese characters simplified/traditional:牛黄/牛黃
Chinese nickname's alphabet (Nickname's Chinese characters): Xihuang/ Choubao(犀黄/丑宝)
Latin: Bovis Calculus (Common name: Cow-bezoar or Bezoar of Cattle)

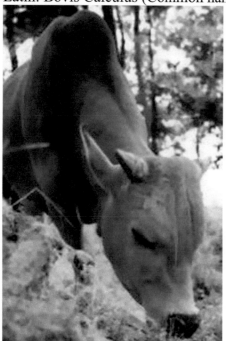

Animal: *Bos taurus domesticus* Gmelin.(or *Bubalus bubalis* L.)
Property and flavor: cool; sweet.

TCM prepared in ready-to-use forms (medicinal parts): it's gallstone of the animal (cattle).

Main and collateral channels: heart and liver meridians.
Administration and dosage: 0.15-0.35 g, usually used in pill or powder. Topical application in appropriate amount, after grounding into power.
Indication: fever, coma caused by fever, convulsion, apoplexy, sore throat, carbuncle sore and manic psychosis.
It is commonly used in treating coma, convulsions and twitch caused by heat.
Precaution and warning: used with caution in pregnant woman.

Attention: to protect the rare wild animals, please don't use it from wild animal. (The picture is only for learning and identification the herb; the specific use of the herb please consult the herbalist or health professionals)

Artificial Cow-bezoan (Rengong Niuhuang)
Chinese phonetic alphabet/pin yin: rén gōng niú huáng
Chinese characters simplified/traditional:人工牛黄/人工牛黃
Latin: Bovis Calculus Artifactus (Common name: Artificial Cow-bezoan)

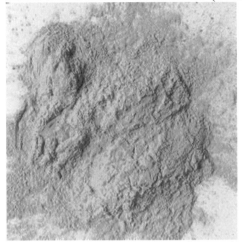

TCM prepared in ready-to-use forms (medicinal parts): it's mixed powder of cow bile, cholic acid, hyodeoxycholic acid, taurine, bilirubin, cholesterol and trace elements, etc.
Property and flavor: cool; sweet.
Main and collateral channels: heart and liver meridians.
Administration and dosage: 0.15-0.35 g per time, usually used for combination of medicinals. Topical application in appropriate amount.

Indication: delirium and manic psychosis, loss of consciousness and speech, acute convulsion, sore throat and abscess.
Precaution and warning: use with caution during pregnancy.
(The picture is only for learning and identification the herb; the specific use of the herb please consult the herbalist or health professionals)

Heartleaf Houttuvnia Herb (Yuxingcao)

Chinese phonetic alphabet/
pin yin: yú xīng cǎo
Chinese characters simplified/traditional:鱼腥草/魚腥草
Chinese nickname's alphabet (Nickname's Chinese characters): Gouxincao/ Zhe'ergen/ Goudian'er(狗心草/折耳根/狗点耳)
Latin: Houttuyniae Herba (Common name: Heartleaf Houttuynia Herb)

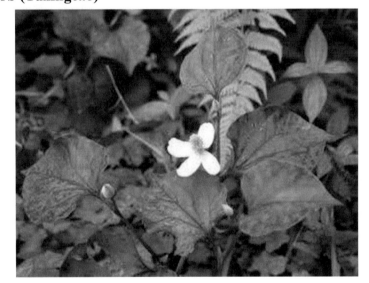

Plant: *Houttuynia cordata* Thunb.

TCM prepared in ready-to-use forms (medicinal parts): it's dried whole herb which harvested in summer.
Property and flavor: mild cold; pungent.
Main and collateral channels: lung meridian.
Administration and dosage: 15-25 g. It should not be decocted for a long time. Topical application in appropriate amount.

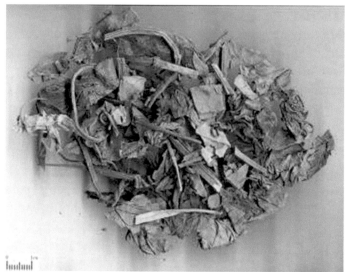

Indication: phlegm and retained fluid, cough with asthma, dysentery, pyretic strangury, carbuncle, sore and skin infection.
It is key herb to treat lung abscess.
It is taken as food in some part of China.
(The picture is only for learning and identification the herb; the specific use of the herb please consult the herbalist or health professionals)

Blackberrylily Rhizome (Shegan)

Chinese phonetic alphabet/pin yin: shè gān
Chinese characters simplified/traditional:射干/射幹
Chinese nickname's alphabet (Nickname's Chinese characters): Wushan/Huangyuan/Caojiang(乌扇/黄远/草姜)
Latin: Belamcandae Rhizoma (Common name: Blackberrylily Rhizome or Leopard Flower Rhizome)

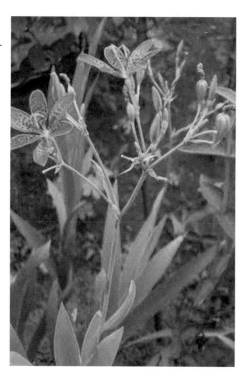

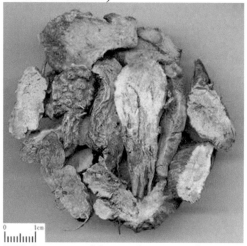

Plant: *Belamcanda chinensis* (L.) DC.

TCM prepared in ready-to-use forms (medicinal parts): it's dried rhizome which harvested in spring or autumn.
Property and flavor: cold; bitter.
Main and collateral channels: lung meridian.
Administration and dosage: 3-10 g.

Indication: fever, excessive phlegm, cough and wheezing; clear and detoxify; relieve sore throat.

It is commonly used in treating sore throat.

Precaution and warning: use with caution during pregnancy.

(The picture is only for learning and identification the herb; the specific use of the herb please consult the herbalist or health professionals)

Roof Iris Rhizome (Chuanshegan)

Chinese phonetic alphabet/pin yin: chuān shè gān
Chinese characters simplified/traditional:川射干/川射干
Chinese nickname's alphabet (Nickname's Chinese characters): Lanhudie/ Tiebiandan/ Shanbacao(蓝蝴蝶/铁扁担/扇把草)
Latin: Iridis Tectori Rhizoma (Common name: Roof Iris Rhizome)

Plant: *Iris tectorum* Maxim.

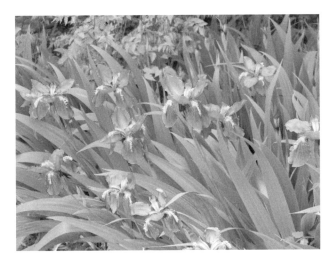

TCM prepared in ready-to-use forms (medicinal parts): it's dried rhizome which harvested all year around.
Property and flavor: cold; bitter.
Main and collateral channels: lung meridian.
Administration and dosage: 6-10 g.
Indication: excessive phlegm and slobber, swelling and sore throat, cough and wheezing.

(The picture is only for learning and identification the herb; the specific use of the herb please consult the herbalist or health professionals)

Chinese Pulsatilla Root (Baitouweng)

Chinese phonetic alphabet/pin yin: bái tóu wēng
Chinese characters simplified/traditional:白头翁/白頭翁
Chinese nickname's alphabet (Nickname's Chinese characters): Baitoupo/ Naihecao (白头婆/奈何草)
Latin: Pulsatillae Radix (Common name: Chinese Pulsatilla Root)

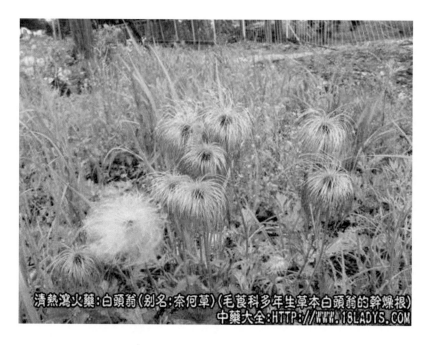

Plant: *Pulsatilla chinensis* (Bunge.) Regel.

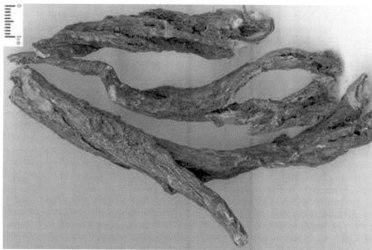

TCM prepared in ready-to-use forms (medicinal parts): it's dried root which harvested in spring or autumn.
Property and flavor: cold; bitter.
Main and collateral channels: stomach and large intestine meridians.

Administration and dosage: 9-15 g.
Indication: dysentery, diarrhea, leucorrhea, colpitis and pudendal itching.
(The picture is only for learning and identification the herb; the specific use of the herb please consult the herbalist or health professionals)

Boor's Mustard (Baijiangcao)
Chinese phonetic alphabet/pin yin: bài jiàng cǎo
Chinese characters simplified/traditional:败酱草/敗醬草
Chinese nickname's alphabet (Nickname's Chinese characters): Subaijiang/ Elancao/ Ximing(苏败酱/遏蓝菜/菥蓂)
Latin: Thlaspi Herba seu Patriniae Herba (Common name: Boor's Mustard Herb or Patrinia Herb)

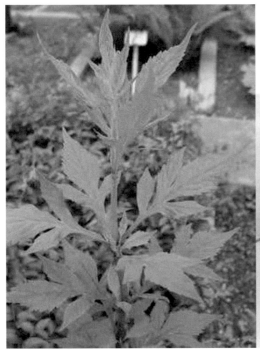

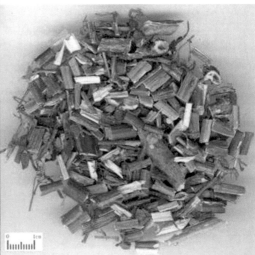

Plant: *Thlaspi arvense* Linn.

TCM prepared in ready-to-use forms (medicinal parts): it's dried whole herb which harvested in summer.
Property and flavor: mild cold; pungent.
Main and collateral channels: liver, stomach and large intestine meridians.
Administration and dosage: 9-15 g.
Indication: abdominal pain, carbuncle sore, edema and abnormal vaginal discharge. It is key herb to treat acute appendicitis and enteritis.
(The picture is only for learning and identification the herb; the specific use of the herb please consult the herbalist or health professionals)

Natural Indigo (Qingdai)
Chinese phonetic alphabet/pin yin: qīng dài
Chinese characters simplified/traditional:青黛/青黛
Chinese nickname's alphabet (Nickname's Chinese characters): Dianhua/ Qinggefen/ Lanlu(靛花/青蛤粉/蓝露)
Latin: Indigo Naturalis (Common name: Natural Indigo)

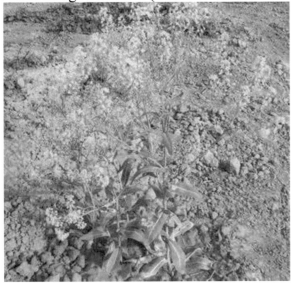

Plant: *Baphicacanthus cusia* (Nees.) Bremek. (or *Isatis indigotica* Fort., *Polygonum tinctorium* Ait., *Isatis tinctoria* L., *Cleredendrum cwtophyllum* Turcz.)

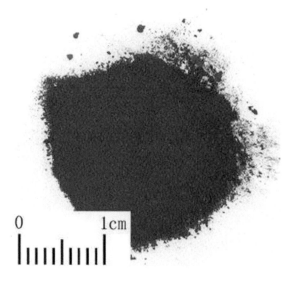

0   1cm

TCM prepared in ready-to-use forms (medicinal parts): a dry powder or lump made by processed leaves or stems.

Processing: put the stem and leaf into the earthen vessel, add the water, soaking in 2 ~ 3 days, until leaf fall off from the branch, removed the branch, add lime (stone) (1 kg lime per 10 kg herb), stirred thoroughly until the immersion become deep purple red, fished out of the liquid blue foam, sun-dry.

Property and flavor: cold; salty.

Main and collateral channels: liver meridian.

Administration and dosage: 1-3 g, used in pills or powder. Topical application in appropriate amount.

Indication: macula caused by virulent heat pathogen, hematemesis, bleeding from five sense organs or subcutaneous tissue, chest pain, aphtha, mumps, sore throat, epilepsy. (The picture is only for learning and identification the herb; the specific use of the herb please consult the herbalist or health professionals)

Paris Rhizome (Chonglou)

Chinese phonetic alphabet/pin yin: chóng lóu

Chinese characters simplified/traditional:重楼/重樓

Chinese nickname's alphabet (Nickname's Chinese characters): Qiyelian/ Tiedengtai/ Zaoxiu(七叶莲/铁灯台/蚤休)

Latin: Paridis Rhizoma (Common name: Paris Rhizome)

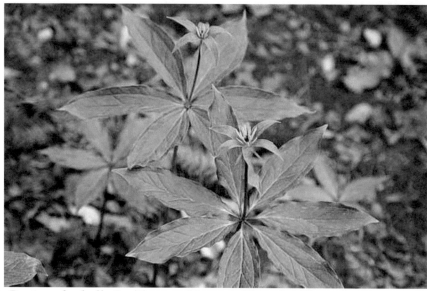

Plant: *Paris polyphylla* Smith var. *chinensis* (Franch.) Hara. (or *Paris polyphylla* Smith var. *yunnanensis* (Franch.) Hand. -Mazz.)

TCM prepared in ready-to-use forms (medicinal parts): it's dried rhizome which harvested in autumn.
Property and flavor: mild cold; bitter.
Main and collateral channels: liver meridian.
Administration and dosage: 3-9 g. Topical application in appropriate amount, ground into powder for application.
Indication: carbuncle sore, sore throat, snake bites, traumatic injury, convulsion and twitch.

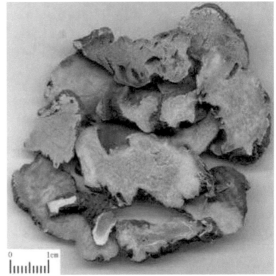

It is key herb to treat abscess and furunculosis.
Precaution and warning: slightly toxic. Use with caution during pregnancy.
(The picture is only for learning and identification the herb; the specific use of the herb please consult the herbalist or health professionals)

Common Andrographis Herb (Chuanxinlian)
Chinese phonetic alphabet/pin yin: chuān xīn lián
Chinese characters simplified/traditional:穿心莲/穿心蓮
Chinese nickname's alphabet (Nickname's Chinese characters): Yijianxi/ Lanhelian/ Kudancao/ Jinxiangcao(一见喜/榄核莲/苦胆草/金香草)
Latin: Andrographis Herba (Common name: Common Andrographis Herb)

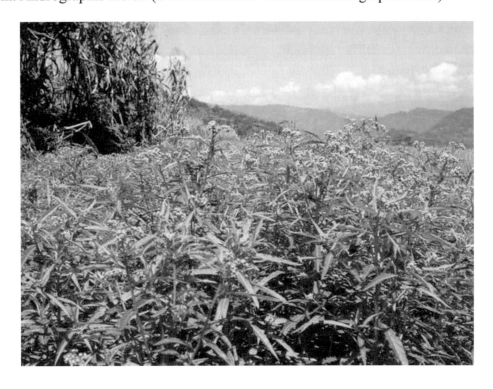

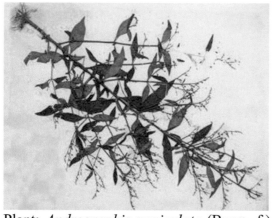
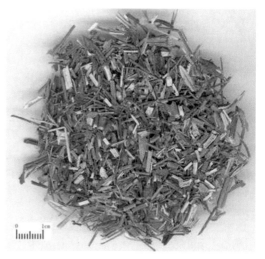
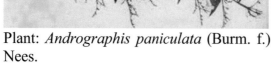

Plant: *Andrographis paniculata* (Burm. f.) Nees.

TCM prepared in ready-to-use forms (medicinal parts): it's dried whole herb which harvested in autumn.

Property and flavor: cold; bitter.

Main and collateral channels: heart, lung, large intestine and bladder meridians.

Administration and dosage: 6-9 g. Topical application in appropriate amount.

Indication: cold, fever, sore throat, aphtha, cough with asthma, diarrhea, dysentery, pyretic strangury, carbuncle sore and snake or insect bites.

(The picture is only for learning and identification the herb; the specific use of the herb please consult the herbalist or health professionals)

Densefruit Pittany Root-bark (Baixianpi)

Chinese phonetic alphabet/pin yin: bái xiǎn pí

Chinese characters simplified/traditional:白鲜皮/白鮮皮

Chinese nickname's alphabet (Nickname's Chinese characters): Baguniu/ Shanmudan/ Yangxiancao(八股牛/山牡丹/羊鲜草)

Latin: Dictamni Cortex (Common name: Densefruit Pittany Root-bark)

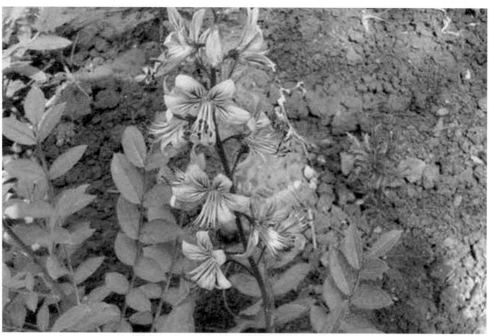

Plant: *Dictamnus dasycarpus* Turcz.

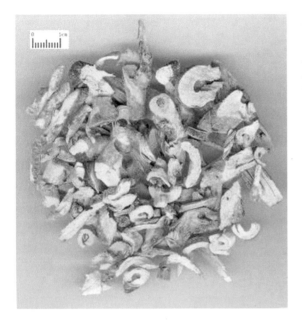

TCM prepared in ready-to-use forms (medicinal parts): it's dried root bark which harvested in spring or autumn.
Property and flavor: cold; bitter.
Main and collateral channels: spleen, stomach and bladder meridians.
Administration and dosage: 5-10 g. Topical application in appropriate amount, decocted for bathing.
Indication: carbuncle, rubella, eczema, scabies, rheumatic, arthralgia, jaundice and skin infection.
(The picture is only for learning and identification the herb; the specific use of the herb please consult the herbalist or health professionals)

Chinese Lobelia Herb (Banbianlian)

Chinese phonetic alphabet/pin yin: bàn biān lián
Chinese characters simplified/ traditional:半边莲/半邊蓮
Chinese nickname's alphabet (Nickname's Chinese characters): Guarencao/ Jijiesuo/ Ximicao(瓜仁草/急解索/细米草)
Latin: Lobeliae Chinensis Herba (Common name: Chinese Lobelia Herb)

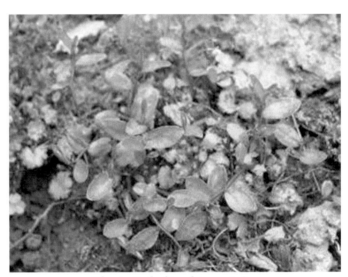

Plant: *Lobelia chinensis* Lour.

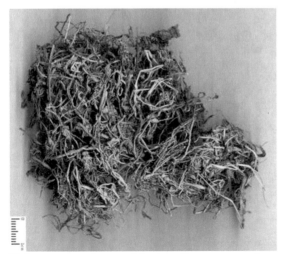

TCM prepared in ready-to-use forms (medicinal parts): it's dried whole herb which harvested in summer.
Property and flavor: neutral; pungent.
Main and collateral channels: heart, small intestine and lung meridians.
Administration and dosage: 9-15 g.
Indication: carbuncle, edema, jaundice, eczema and snake or insect bites; diuresis.

It is commonly used in treating sore carbuncle and swollen.
(The picture is only for learning and identification the herb; the specific use of the herb please consult the herbalist or health professionals)

Glabrous Greenbrier Rhizome (Tufuling)

Chinese phonetic alphabet/pin yin: tǔ fú líng
Chinese characters simplified/traditional: 土茯苓/土茯苓
Chinese nickname's alphabet (Nickname's Chinese characters): Lengfantuan/ Yingfantou/ Hongtuling (冷饭团/硬饭头/红土苓)

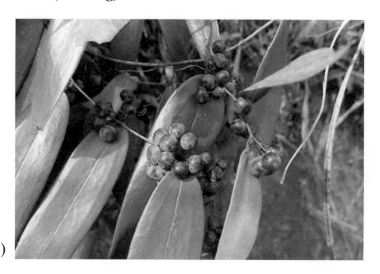

Plant: *Smilax glabra* Roxb.

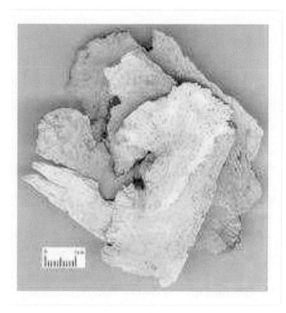

Latin: Smilacis Glabrae Rhizoma (Common name: Glabrous Greenbrier Rhizome)
TCM prepared in ready-to-use forms (medicinal parts): it's dried rhizome which harvested in summer or autumn.
Property and flavor: neutral; sweet, bland.
Main and collateral channels: liver and stomach meridians.
Administration and dosage: 15-16 g.

Indication: syphilis, limb spasm, mercury poisoning, turbid urine, aching pain, leucorrhea, carbuncle, scrofula, scabies and tinea.
It is key herb to treat syphilis.
(The picture is only for learning and identification the herb; the specific use of the herb please consult the herbalist or health professionals)

Vietnamese Sophora Root (Shandougen)
Chinese phonetic alphabet/pin yin: shān dòu gēn
Chinese characters simplified/traditional:山豆根/山豆根
Chinese nickname's alphabet (Nickname's Chinese characters): Guangdougen/ Kudougen(广豆根/苦豆根)
Latin: Sophorae Tonkinensis Radix et Rhizoma (Common name: Vietnamese Sophora Root)

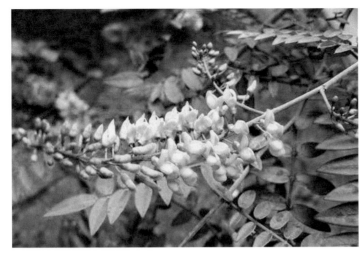

Plant: *Sophora tonkinensis* Gagnep. (or *Euchresta japonica* Hook. f. et Regel.)

TCM prepared in ready-to-use forms (medicinal parts): it's dried root and rhizome which harvested in autumn.
Property and flavor: cold; bitter.
Main and collateral channels: lung and stomach meridians.
Administration and dosage: 3-6 g.
Indication: sore throat, swelling and aching of gum.
It is key herb to treat sore throat.
Precaution and warning: toxic.
(The picture is only for learning and identification the herb; the specific use of the herb please consult the herbalist or health professionals)

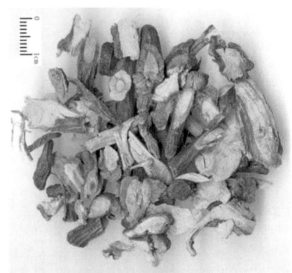

Purslane Herb (Machixie)
Chinese phonetic alphabet/ pin yin: mǎ chǐ xiè
Chinese characters simplified/traditional: 马齿苋/馬齒莧
Chinese nickname's alphabet (Nickname's Chinese characters): Wuxingcao/ Changmingcai/ Machicai(五行草/长命菜/马齿菜)
Latin: Portulacae Herba (Common name: Purslane Herb)

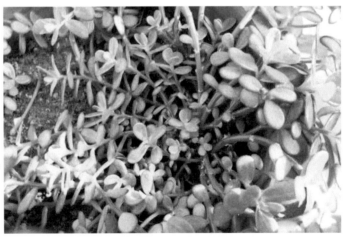

Plant: *Portulaca oleracea* L.

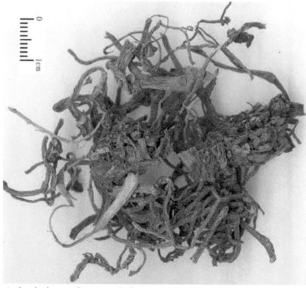

TCM prepared in ready-to-use forms (medicinal parts): it's (dried) twig.
Property and flavor: cold; acidity.
Main and collateral channels: liver and large intestine meridians.

Administration and dosage: 9-15 g. Topical application in appropriate amount, ground into paste for application.

Indication: dysentery with blood, hemafecia, eczema, erysipelas, hemorrhoid bleeding, menstrual flooding and spotting and snake or insect bites; anti-inflammatory; diuresis. It is commonly used in treating dysentery.

It is taken as food in some part of China.

(The picture is only for learning and identification the herb; the specific use of the herb please consult the herbalist or health professionals)

Sargentgloryvine Stem (Daxueteng)

Chinese phonetic alphabet/pin yin: dà xuě téng

Chinese characters simplified/traditional:大血藤/大血藤

Chinese nickname's alphabet (Nickname's Chinese characters): Hongpiteng/ Dahuoxue/ Hongteng(红皮藤/大活血/红藤)

Latin: Sargentodoxae Caulis (Common name: Sargentgloryvine Stem)

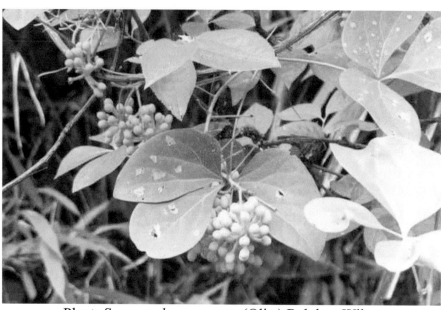

Plant: *Sargentodoxa cuneata* (Oliv.) Rehd. et Wils.

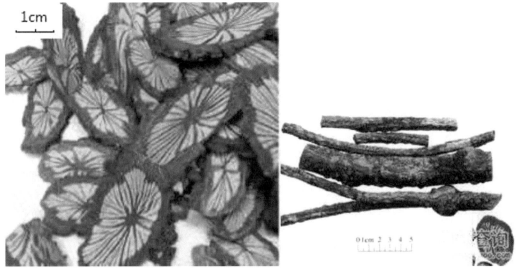

TCM prepared in ready-to-use forms (medicinal parts): it's dried lianoid stem which harvested in autumn or winter.

Property and flavor: neutral; bitter.

Main and collateral channels: large intestine and liver meridians.

Administration and dosage: 9-15 g.

Indication: rheumatic, arthralgia, dysentery, hematuria, irregular menstruation, malnutrition, traumatic injury, painful *bi* disorder, sore and ulcer.

Precaution and warning: use with caution during pregnancy.

(The picture is only for learning and identification the herb; the specific use of the herb please consult the herbalist or health professionals)

Spreading Hedvotis Herb (Baihuasheshecao)

Chinese phonetic alphabet/pin yin: bái huā shé shé cǎo
Chinese characters simplified/traditional: 白花蛇舌草/白花蛇舌草
Chinese nickname's alphabet (Nickname's Chinese characters): Sheshecao/ Yangxucao/ Shezongguan(蛇舌草/羊须草/蛇总管)
Latin: Hedyotis Diffusae Herba (Common name: Spreading Hedvotis Herb)

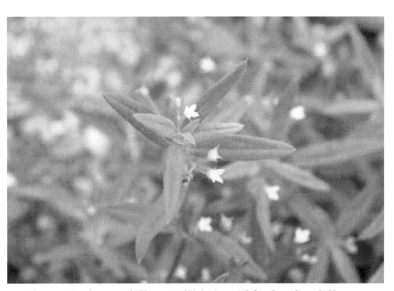

Plant: *Hedyotis diffusa* Willd. (or *Oldenlandia diffusa* (Willd.) Roxb.)

TCM prepared in ready-to-use forms (medicinal parts): it's dried whole herb which harvested in autumn or summer.
Property and flavor: cold; mild bitter.
Main and collateral channels: stomach, large intestine and small intestine meridians.
Administration and dosage: 15-30 g. Appropriate amount for topical application .

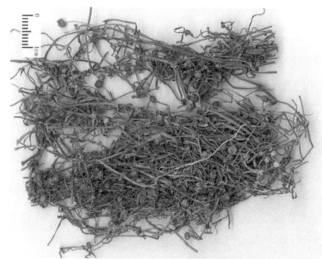

Indication: carbuncle sore, sore throat, snake or insect bites, edema and pain.
Precaution and warning: use with caution during pregnancy.
(The picture is only for learning and identification the herb; the specific use of the herb please consult the herbalist or health professionals)

Wild Chrysanthemum Flower (Yejuhua)

Chinese phonetic alphabet/pin yin: yě jú huā
Chinese characters simplified/traditional:野菊花/野菊花
Chinese nickname's alphabet(Nickname's Chinese characters): Kuyi(苦薏)
Latin: Chrysanthemi Indici Flos (Common name: Wild Chrysanthemum Flower or Mother Chrysanthemum)

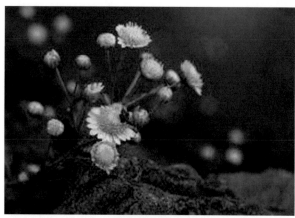

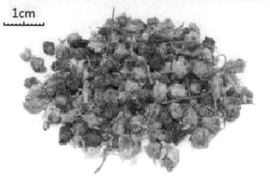

1cm

Plant: *Chrysanthemum indicum* L. (or *Dendranthema indicum* (L.) Des Moul.)
TCM prepared in ready-to-use forms (medicinal parts): it's dried flower or capitulum.
Property and flavor: mild cold; bitter, pungent.
Main and collateral channels: liver and heart meridians.
Administration and dosage: 9-15 g. Topical application in appropriate amount. Decocted for bathing or made into paste for topical application.
Indication: carbuncle, sore throat, red eyes, headache and dizziness.
(The picture is only for learning and identification the herb; the specific use of the herb please consult the herbalist or health professionals)

Bear Gall (Xiongdan)

Chinese phonetic alphabet/
pin yin: xióng dǎn
Chinese characters simplified/
traditional:熊胆/熊膽
Latin: Fel Ursi (Common
name: Bear Gall)
Animal: *Ursus thibetanus* G.
 (or *Ursus arctos*)

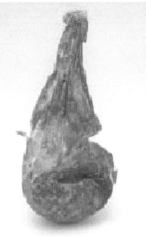

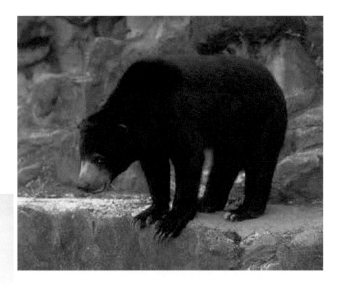

TCM prepared in ready-to-use forms
(medicinal parts): it's bear's gallbladder.
Property and flavor: cold; bitter.
Main and collateral channels: heart, liver
and gallbladder meridians.
Administration and dosage: 0.3-1.5 g
(artificial synthesis products).

Indication: cough with asthma, excessive phlegm, convulsion, blur vision; sedative;
cholagogic.
Attention: to protect the rare wild animals, don't use it from wild animal, please use
artificial synthesis products to substitute.
(The picture is only for learning and identification the herb; the specific use of the
herb please consult the herbalist or health professionals)

Tokoy Violet Herb (Zihuadiding)

Chinese phonetic alphabet/
pin yin: zǐ huā dì dīng
Chinese characters
simplified/traditional:紫花地
丁/紫花地丁
Chinese nickname's alphabet
(Nickname's Chinese
characters): Yejincai/
Guangbanjincai(野菫菜/
光瓣菫菜)
Latin: Violae Herba
(Common name: Tokoy
Violet Herb or Chinese
Violet)
Plant: *Viola yedoensis* Makino.

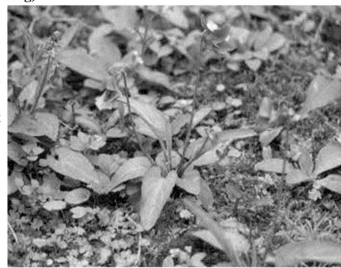

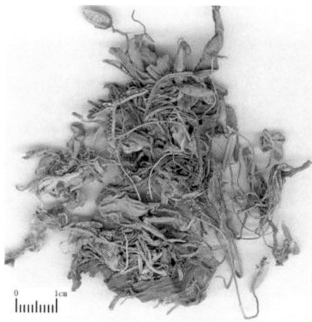

TCM prepared in ready-to-use forms (medicinal parts): it's dried whole herb which harvested in spring or autumn.
Property and flavor: cold; bitter, pungent.
Main and collateral channels: heart and liver meridians.
Administration and dosage: 15-30 g.

Indication: sore swollen poison, furunculosis, erysipelas and snake bite.
It is good at treating furunculosis.
(The picture is only for learning and identification the herb; the specific use of the herb please consult the herbalist or health professionals)

Golden Buckwheat Rhizome (Jinqiaomai)

Chinese phonetic alphabet/pin yin: jīn qiáo mài
Chinese characters simplified/traditional:金荞麦/金蕎麥
Chinese nickname's alphabet (Nickname's Chinese characters): Kuqiaomai/ Tianqiaomai(苦荞麦/天荞麦)
Latin: Fagopyri Dibotryis Rhizoma (Common name: Golden Buckwheat Rhizome)

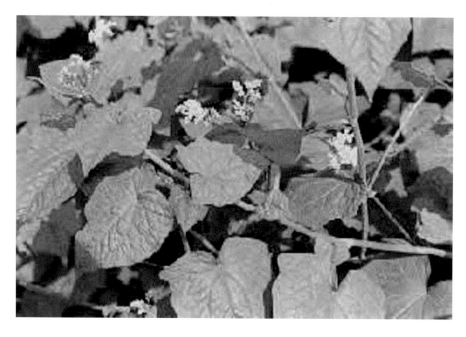

Plant: *Fagopyrum dibotrys* (D. Don) Hara.

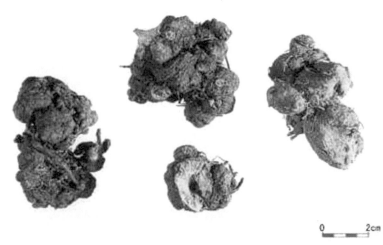

TCM prepared in ready-to-use forms (medicinal parts): it's dried rhizome which harvested in winter.
Property and flavor: cool; mild pungent, astringent.
Main and collateral channels: lung meridian.

0 _____ 2cm

Administration and dosage: 15-45 g, mixed with water or yellow rice wine, and simmered in an airtight container for oral administration.

Indication: measles, pneumonia, amygdalitis, cough and wheezing.

Attention: to protect the rare wild plant, please don't use the herb from wild plant. (The picture is only for learning and identification the herb; the specific use of the herb please consult the herbalist or health professionals)

Java Brucea Fruit (Yadanzi)

Chinese phonetic alphabet/pin yin: yā dǎn zi

Chinese characters simplified/traditional:鸦胆子/鴉膽子

Chinese nickname's alphabet (Nickname's Chinese characters): Laoyadan/ Kuzhenzi/ Xiaokulian(老鸦胆/苦榛子/小苦楝)

Latin: Bruceae Fructus (Common name: Java Brucea Fruit or Khosam)

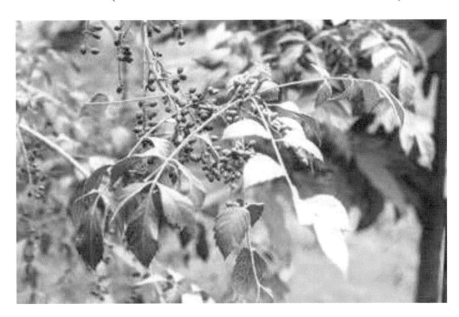

Plant: *Brucea javanica* (L.) Merr.

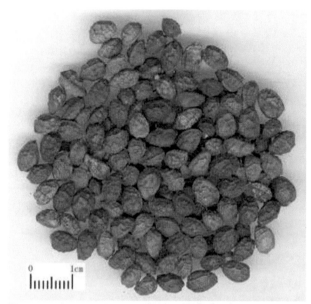

TCM prepared in ready-to-use forms (medicinal parts): it's dried mature seed.
Property and flavor: cold; bitter.
Main and collateral channels: large intestine and liver meridians.
Administration and dosage: 0.5-2 g, wrapped by Longan Aril or capsuled for oral administration. Topical application in appropriate amount.
Indication: dysentery, malaria; external use for warts, heloma.

Precaution and warning: slightly toxic. Use with caution during pregnancy.
(The picture is only for learning and identification the herb; the specific use of the herb please consult the herbalist or health professionals)

Stringy Stonecrop Herb (Chuipencao)

Chinese phonetic alphabet/pin yin: chúi pén cǎo
Chinese characters simplified/traditional: 垂盆草/垂盆草
Chinese nickname's alphabet (Nickname's Chinese characters): Gouyacao/ Guazicao/ Shizhijia(狗牙草/瓜子草/石指甲)
Latin: Sedi Herba (Common name: Stringy Stonecrop Herb)

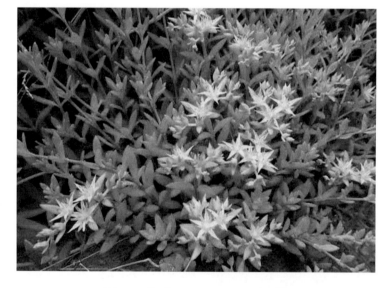

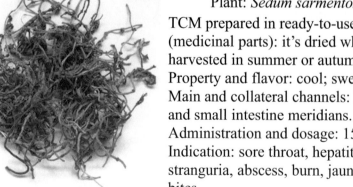

Plant: *Sedum sarmentosum* Bunge.
TCM prepared in ready-to-use forms (medicinal parts): it's dried whole grass which harvested in summer or autumn.
Property and flavor: cool; sweet, bland.
Main and collateral channels: liver, gallbladder and small intestine meridians.
Administration and dosage: 15-30 g.
Indication: sore throat, hepatitis, pyretic stranguria, abscess, burn, jaundice and snake bites.
(The picture is only for learning and identification the herb; the specific use of the herb please consult the herbalist or health professionals)

Ash Bark (Qinpi)

Chinese phonetic alphabet/pin yin: qín pí

Chinese char acters simplified/traditional: 秦皮/秦皮

Chinese nickname's alphabet (Nickname's Chinese characters): Qinpi/ Lashupi(岑皮/蜡树皮)

Latin: Fraxini Cortex (Common name: Ash Bark)

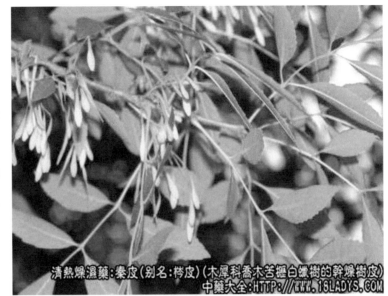

清熱燥濕藥:秦皮(別名:梣皮)(木犀科喬木苦櫪白蠟樹的幹燥樹皮)
中藥大全:HTTP://WWW.18LADYS.COM

Plant: *Fraxinus chinensis* Roxb. (or *Fraxinus rhynchophylla* Hance., *Fraxinus szaboana* Lingelsh., *Fraxinus stylosa* Lingelsh.)

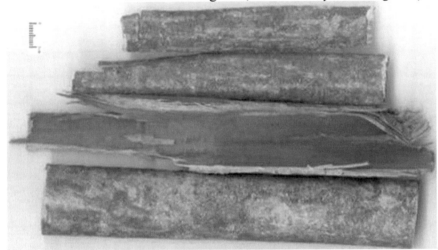

TCM prepared in ready-to-use forms (medicinal parts): it's dried bark which harvested in spring or autumn. Property and flavor: cold; bitter, astringent.

Main and collateral channels: liver, gallbladder and large intestine meridians.
Administration and dosage: 6-12 g. Topical application in appropriate amount, decocted for rinsing.
Indication: diarrhea and dysentery, leucorrhea, red eyes, cataract.
(The picture is only for learning and identification the herb; the specific use of the herb please consult the herbalist or health professionals)

Puff-ball (Mabo)

Chinese phonetic alphabet/pin yin: mǎ bó

Chinese characters simplified/traditional:马勃/馬勃

Chinese nickname's alphabet (Nickname's Chinese characters): Mafenbao/ Mapipao(马粪包/马屁泡)

Latin: Lasiosphaera seu Calvatia (Common name: Puff-ball)

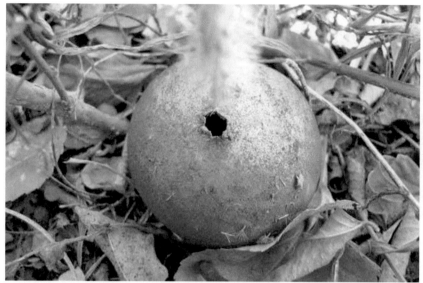

Fungus: *Lasiosphaera fenzlii* Reich. (or *Calvatia gigantea* (Batsch ex Pers.) Lloyd., *Calvatia lilacina* (Mont. et Berk.) Lloyd., *Lycoperdon spp.*)

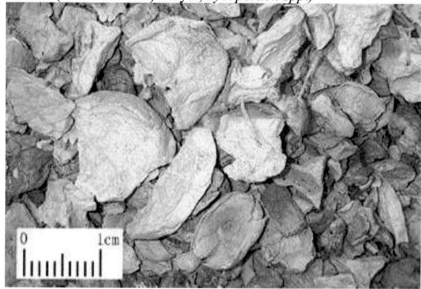

TCM prepared in ready-to-use forms (medicinal parts): it's dried sporocarp (of fungus).

Property and flavor: neutral; pungent.

Main and collateral channels: lung meridian.

Administration and dosage: 2-6 g. Topical application in appropriate amount.

Indication: pneumonia, sore throat, cough with asthma, hoarseness and bleeding from five sense organs or subcutaneous tissue; external use for epistaxis and bleeding.

It is good at treating sore throat with bleeding and fester.

(The picture is only for learning and identification the herb; the specific use of the herb please consult the herbalist or health professionals)

Indian Trumpetflower Seed (Muhudie)

Chinese phonetic alphabet/pin yin: mù hú dié

Chinese characters simplified/traditional:木蝴蝶/木蝴蝶

Chinese nickname's alphabet (Nickname's Chinese characters): Qianzhangzhi/ Maoyachuan(千张纸/毛鸦船)

Latin: Oroxyli Semen (Common name: Indian Trumpetflower Seed)

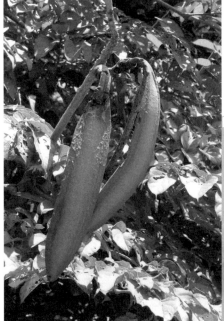
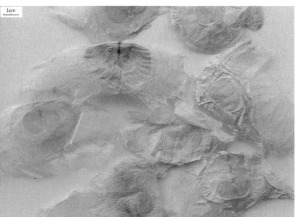

Plant: *Oroxylum indicum* (Linn.) Vent.

TCM prepared in ready-to-use forms (medicinal parts): it's dried mature seed.
Property and flavor: cool; bitter, sweet.
Main and collateral channels: lung, liver and stomach meridians.
Administration and dosage: 1-3 g.
Indication: cough with asthma, hoarseness and sore throat.
(The picture is only for learning and identification the herb; the specific use of the herb please consult the herbalist or health professionals)

Barbated Skullcup Herb (Banzhilian)
Chinese phonetic alphabet/pin yin: bàn zhī lián
Chinese characters simplified/traditional:半枝莲/半枝蓮
Chinese nickname's alphabet (Nickname's Chinese characters): Bingtoucao/
Hanxincao/ Ganshanbian(并头草/韩信草/赶山鞭)
Latin: Scutellariae Barbatae Herb (Common name: Barbated Skullcup Herb)

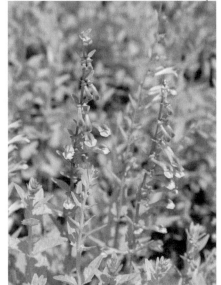
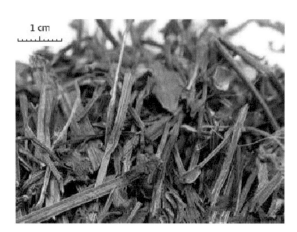

Plant: *Scutellaria barbata* D. Don.
TCM prepared in ready-to-use forms (medicinal parts): it's dried whole herb which

harvested in summer or winter.
Property and flavor: cold; bitter, pungent.
Main and collateral channels: lung, liver and kidney meridians.
Administration and dosage: 15-30 g.
Indication: detumescence, sore throat, traumatic injuries, edema and jaundice; diuresis; disperse blood stasis; relieve pain.
Precaution and warning: use with caution during pregnancy.
(The picture is only for learning and identification the herb; the specific use of the herb please consult the herbalist or health professionals)

Sweet Wormwood Herb (Qinghao)

Chinese phonetic alphabet/pin yin: qīng hāo
Chinese characters simplified/traditional: 青蒿/青蒿
Chinese nickname's alphabet (Nickname's Chinese characters): Caohao/ Linhao(草蒿/廩蒿)
Latin: Artemisiae Annuae Herba (Common name:Sweet Wormwood Herb)

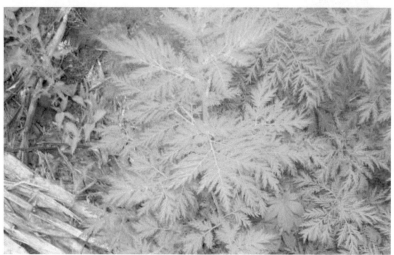

Plant: *Artemisia annua* L. (*or Artemisia carvifolia* Buch.-Ham. ex Roxb.)

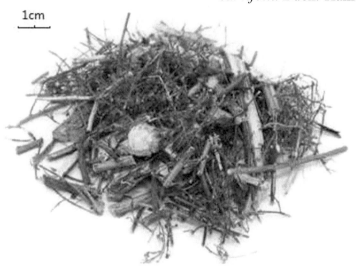

TCM prepared in ready-to-use forms (medicinal parts): it's dried the aerial part removed old stem which harvested in autumn.
Property and flavor: cold; bitter, pungent.
Main and collateral channels: liver and gallbladder meridians.
Administration and dosage: 6-12 g, added when the decoction is nearly done.

Indication: malaria, fever, jaundice.
It is good at treating malaria.
(The picture is only for learning and identification the herb; the specific use of the herb please consult the herbalist or health professionals)

Chinese Wolfberry Root-bark (Digupi)

Chinese phonetic alphabet/pin yin: dì gǔ pí

Chinese characters simplified/traditional:地骨皮/地骨皮
Chinese nickname's alphabet (Nickname's Chinese characters): Gouqipi(枸杞皮)
Latin: Lycii Cortex (Common name: Chinese Wolfberry Root-bark)

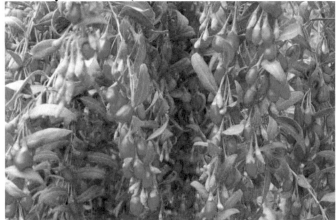

Plant: *Lycium barbarum* L. (or *Lycium chinense* Mill.) TCM prepared in ready-to-use forms (medicinal parts): it's dried root-bark which harvested in spring or autumn.

Property and flavor: cold; sweet.
Main and collateral channels: lung, liver and kidney meridians.
Administration and dosage: 9-15 g.
Indication: fever, cough with asthma, hematemesis, hemoptysis, epistaxis, hematuria, diabetes, hypertension and carbuncle.
It is good at treating fever.

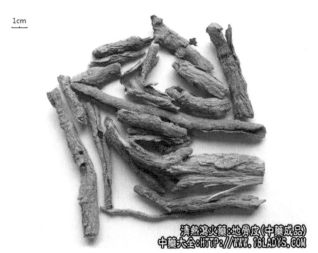

(The picture is only for learning and identification the herb; the specific use of the herb please consult the herbalist or health professionals)

Blackend Swallowwort Root (Baiwei)
Chinese phonetic alphabet/ pin yin: bái wēi
Chinese characters simplified/ traditional:白薇/白薇
Chinese nickname's alphabet (Nickname's Chinese characters): Baiwei/ Bailongxu(白尾/白龙须)
Latin: Cynanchi Atrati Radix et Rhizoma (Common name: Blackend Swallowwort Root)
Plant: *Cynanchum atratum* Bunge. (or *Cynanchum versicolour* Bunge.)

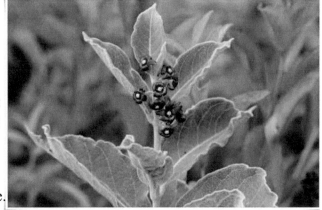

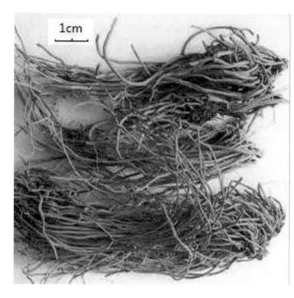

1cm

TCM prepared in ready-to-use forms (medicinal parts): it's dried root and rhizome which harvested in spring or autumn.

Property and flavor: cold; bitter, salty.

Main and collateral channels: stomach, liver and kidney meridians.

Administration and dosage: 5-10 g.

Indication: fever, pyretic strangury, hematuria, abscess and skin infection.

(The picture is only for learning and identification the herb; the specific use of the herb please consult the herbalist or health professionals)

Figwortflower Picrorhiza Rhizome (Huhuanglian)

Chinese phonetic alphabet/ pin yin: hú huáng lián

Chinese characters simplified/ traditional:胡黄连/胡黄連

Chinese nickname's alphabet (Nickname's Chinese characters): Hulian/ Geguluze (胡连/割孤露泽)

Latin: Picrorhizae Rhizoma (Common name: Figwortflower Picrorhiza Rhizome)

Plant: *Picrorhiza scrophulariiflora* Pennell.

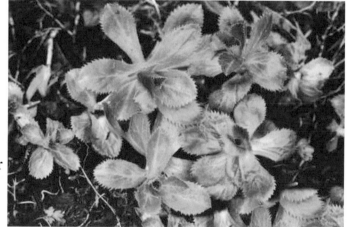

TCM prepared in ready-to-use forms (medicinal parts): it's dried rhizome which harvested in autumn.

Property and flavor: cold; bitter.

Main and collateral channels: liver, stomach and large intestine meridians.

Administration and dosage: 3-10 g.

Indication: dysentery and diarrhea, jaundice, hemorrhoid, infantile malnutrition and fever in children.

Attention: to protect the rare wild plant, please don't use the herb from wild plant.

(The picture is only for learning and identification the herb; the specific use of the herb please consult the herbalist or health professionals)

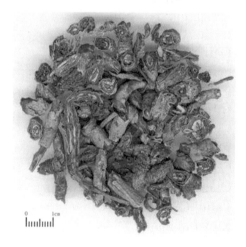

0   1cm

Starwort Root (Yinchaihu)

Chinese phonetic alphabet/ pin yin: yín chái hú

Chinese characters simplified/traditional:银柴胡/ 銀柴胡

Chinese nickname's alphabet (Nickname's Chinese characters): Xiyinchaihu/ Yinhu/ Shancaigen/ Niudugen(西银柴胡/银胡/山 菜根/牛肚根)

Latin: Stellariae Radix (Common name: Starwort Root)

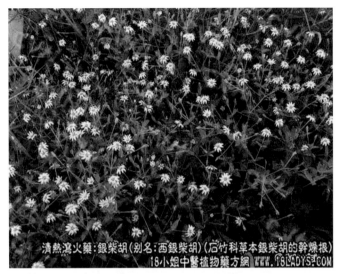

Plant: *Stellaria dichotoma* L. var. *lanceolata* Bunge.

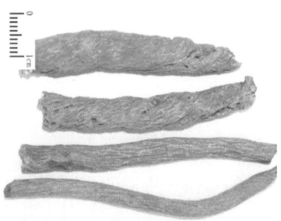
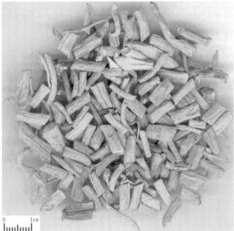

TCM prepared in ready-to-use forms (medicinal parts): it's dried root which harvested in spring or summer.

Property and flavor: mild cold; sweet.

Main and collateral channels: liver and stomach meridians.

Administration and dosage: 3-10 g.

Indication: fever, infantile malnutrition and fever in children.

It is commonly used in treating fever.

(The picture is only for learning and identification the herb; the specific use of the herb please consult the herbalist or health professionals)

Calcitum (Hanshuishi)

Chinese phonetic alphabet/pin yin: hán shǔi shí

Chinese characters simplified/traditional:寒水石/寒水石

Chinese nickname's alphabet (Nickname's Chinese characters): Ningshuishi/ Shuishi/ Queshi(凝水石/水石/鹊石)

Latin: Gypsum Rubrum (Common name: Calcitum)

Mineral: main component $CaCO_3$ with some $CaSO_4$

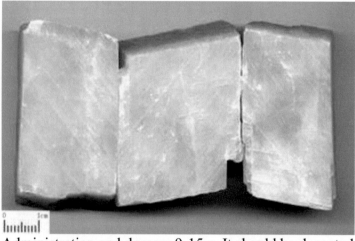

TCM prepared in ready-to-use forms (medicinal parts): it's cleaned mineral (powder).
Property and flavor: mild cold; pungent, salty.
Main and collateral channels: heart, kidney and stomach meridians.

Administration and dosage: 9-15 g. It should be decocted first. Appropriate amount for topical application.

Indication: fever caused by cold, erysipelas, burn, scald.

(The picture is only for learning and identification the herb; the specific use of the herb please consult the herbalist or health professionals)

Appendiculate Cremastra Pseudobulb (Shancigu)

Chinese phonetic alphabet/pin yin: shān cí gū

Chinese characters simplified/traditional:山慈菇/山慈菇

Chinese nickname's alphabet (Nickname's Chinese characters):Jindenghua/Luticao/Bingqiuzi(金灯花/鹿蹄草/冰球子)

Latin: Cremastrae Pseudobulbus seu Pleiones Pseudobulbus (Common name: Appendiculate Cremastra Pseudobulb or Common Pleione Pseudobulb)

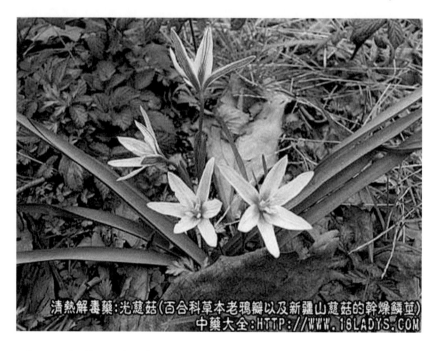

Plant: *Pleione bulbocodioides* (Franch.) Rolfe. (or *Pleione yunnanensis* Rolfe., *Cremastra appendiculata* (D. Don) Makino., *Iphigenia indica* Kunth.)

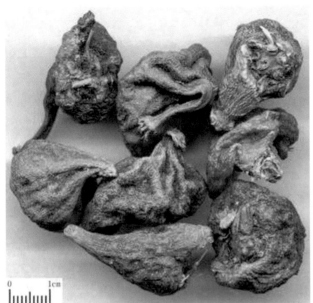

TCM prepared in ready-to-use forms (medicinal parts): it's dried pseudobulb which harvested in summer or autumn.

Property and flavor: cool; sweet, mild pungent.

Main and collateral channels: spleen and liver meridians.

Administration and dosage: 3-9 g. Topical application in appropriate amount.

Indication: scrofula, lymphadenitis, glomus, abscess, insect and snake bites.

Precaution and warning: slightly toxic.

Attention: to protect the rare wild plant, please don't use the herb from wild plant. (The picture is only for learning and identification the herb; the specific use of the herb please consult the herbalist or health professionals)

Bistort Rhizome (Quanshen)

Chinese phonetic alphabet/pin yin: quán shēn

Chinese characters simplified/traditional:拳参/拳參

Chinese nickname's alphabet (Nickname's Chinese characters): Zishen/ Shican(紫参/石蚕)

Latin: Bistortae Rhizoma (Common name: Bistort Rhizome)

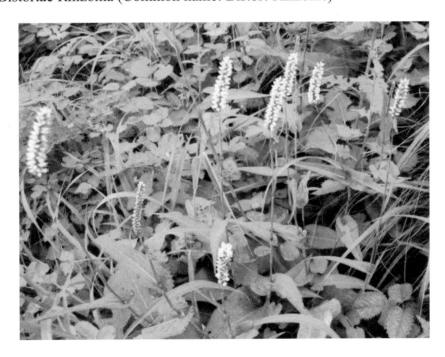

Plant: *Polygonum bistorta* L.

TCM prepared in ready-to-use forms (medicinal parts): it's dried rhizome which harvested in spring or autumn.

Property and flavor: mild cold; bitter, astringent.

Main and collateral channels: lung, liver and lager intestine meridians.

Administration and dosage: 5-10 g. Topical application in appropriate amount.

Indication: diarrhea, dysentery with blood, cough, carbuncle, scrofula, mouth and tongue sore, insect and snake bites.

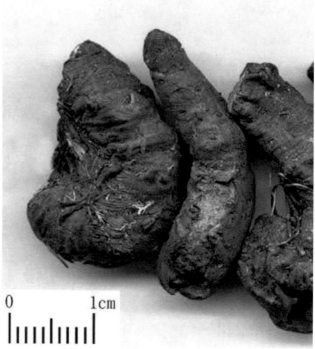

(The picture is only for learning and identification the herb; the specific use of the herb please consult the herbalist or health professionals)

Grosvenor Momordica Fruit (Luohanguo)

Chinese phonetic alphabet/pin yin: luó hàn guǒ

Chinese characters simplified/traditional:罗汉果/羅漢果

Chinese nickname's alphabet (Nickname's Chinese characters): Shenxianguo(神仙果)

Latin: Siraitiae Fructus seu Momordicae Fructus (Common name: Grosvenor Momordica Fruit)

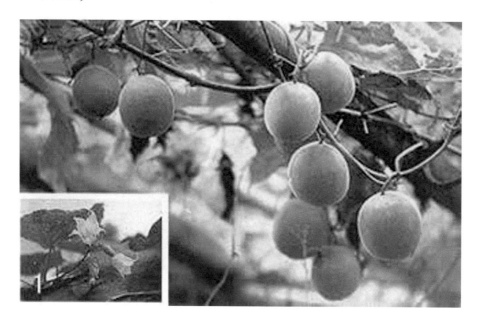

Plant: *Siraitia grosvenorii* (Swingle.) C. Jeffrey ex A. M. Lu et Z. Y. Zhang.

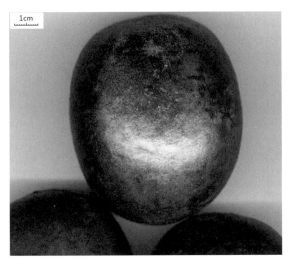

TCM prepared in ready-to-use forms (medicinal parts): it's dried fruit.
Property and flavor: cool; sweet.
Main and collateral channels: lung and large intestine meridians.
Administration and dosage: 9-15 g.
Indication: dry cough, sore throat, hoarseness, constipation.
It is taken as food in some part of China.
(The picture is only for learning and identification the herb; the specific use of the herb please consult the herbalist or health professionals)

Canton Love-pea Vine (Jigucao)

Chinese phonetic alphabet/pin yin: jī gǔ cǎo
Chinese characters simplified/traditional:鸡骨草/雞骨草
Chinese nickname's alphabet (Nickname's Chinese characters): Huangtoucao/ Dahuangcao (黄头草/大黄草)
Latin: Abri Herba (Common name: Canton Love-pea Vine or Abrus Mollis Hance)

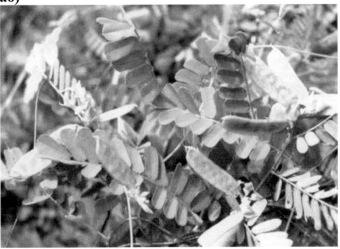

Plant: *Abrus cantoniensis* Hance.

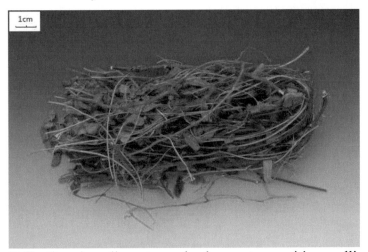

TCM prepared in ready-to-use forms (medicinal parts): it's dried whole herb which harvested all year round.
Property and flavor: cool; sweet and mild bitter.
Main and collateral channels: liver and stomach meridians.
Administration and dosage: 15-30 g.

Indication: jaundice, stomachache, acute mastitis, swelling and pain; remove toxin.
(The picture is only for learning and identification the herb; the specific use of the herb please consult the herbalist or health professionals)

Japanese Ampelopsis Root (Bailian)

Chinese phonetic alphabet/pin yin: bái liàn

Chinese characters simplified/traditional:白蔹/白蘞
Chinese nickname's alphabet (Nickname's Chinese characters): Shandigua/
Shanputaoyang/ Baigen/ Wuzhuateng(山地瓜/山葡萄秧/白根/五爪藤)
Latin: Ampelopsis Radix (Common name: Japanese Ampelopsis Root)

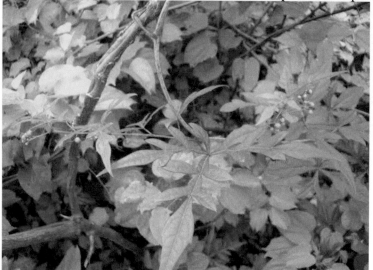

Plant: *Ampelosis japonica* (Thunb.) Makino.

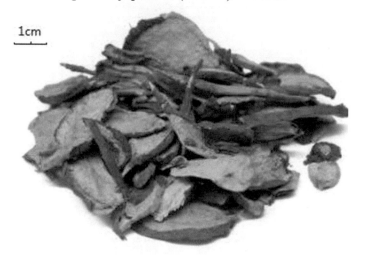

TCM prepared in ready-to-use forms (medicinal parts): it's dried root tuber which harvested in spring or autumn. Property and flavor: mild cold; bitter. Main and collateral channels: heart and stomach meridians. Administration and dosage: 5-10 g. Appropriate amount for topical application, decocted for bathing or ground into extreme fine powder to apply on the *pars affecta*. Indication: abscess, cellulitis, carbuncle of the back, scrofula, burn and scald. It is commonly used in treating burn and scald.

Precaution and warning: incompatible with Common Monkshood Mother Root, Kusnezoff Monkshood Root, Common Monkshood Daughter Root, Short-pedicel Aconite Root and their prepared one.
(The picture is only for learning and identification the herb; the specific use of the herb please consult the herbalist or health professionals)

Baphicacanthus Root (Nan Banlangen)
Chinese phonetic alphabet/pin yin: nán bǎn lán gēn
Chinese characters simplified/traditional:南板蓝根/南板藍根
Chinese nickname's alphabet (Nickname's Chinese characters): Tubanlangen/
Landiangen/ Dalangen/ Daqinggen(土板蓝根/蓝靛根/大蓝根/大青根)
Latin: Baphicacanthis Cusiae Rhizoma et Radix (Common name: Baphicacanthus Root)

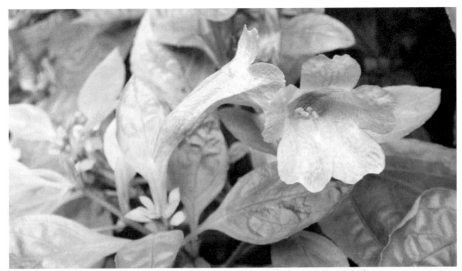

Plant: *Baphicacanthus cusia* (Nees.) Bremek.

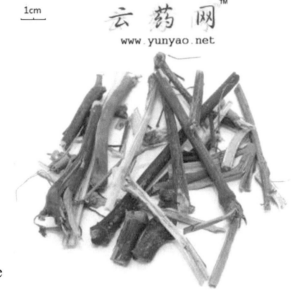

TCM prepared in ready-to-use forms (medicinal parts): it's dried rhizome and root which harvested in summer or autumn.
Property and flavor: cold; bitter.
Main and collateral channels: heart and stomach meridians.
Administration and dosage: 9-15 g.
Indication: epidemic disease, fever with sore throat, erysipelas, macula and papule.

(The picture is only for learning and identification the herb; the specific use of the herb please consult the herbalist or health professionals)

Chinese White Olive (Qingguo)

Chinese phonetic alphabet/pin yin: qīng guǒ
Chinese characters simplified/traditional:青果/青果
Chinese nickname's alphabet (Nickname's Chinese characters): Ganlan(橄榄)
Latin: Canarii Fructus (Common name: Chinese White Olive)

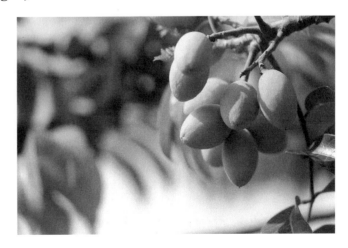

Plant: *Canarium album* Raeusch.

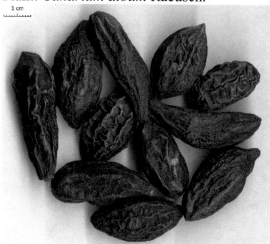

TCM prepared in ready-to-use forms (medicinal parts): it's dried ripe fruit.
Property and flavor: neutral; sweet, acidity.
Main and collateral channels: lung and stomach meridians.
Administration and dosage: 5-10 g.
Indication: sore throat, cough, excessive phlegm, sticky sputum, thirst and sea food poisoning.
It is taken as food in some part of China.

(The picture is only for learning and identification the herb; the specific use of the herb please consult the herbalist or health professionals)

Chicory Herb (Juju)

Chinese phonetic alphabet/pin yin: jú jù
Chinese characters simplified/traditional: 菊苣/菊苣
Chinese nickname's alphabet (Nickname's Chinese characters): Kuju/ Mingmucai/ Kafeicao(苦苣/明目菜/咖啡草)
Latin: Cichorii Herba seu Cichorii Radix (Common name: Chicory Herb or Chicory Root)

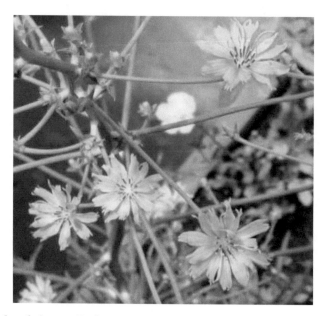

Plant: *Cichorium glandulosum* Boiss. et Hoet. (or *Cichorium intybus* L.)

TCM prepared in ready-to-use forms (medicinal parts): it's dried aerial part or root which harvested in autumn.
Property and flavor: cool; mild bitter, salty.
Main and collateral channels: liver, gallbladder and stomach meridians.
Administration and dosage: 9-18 g.

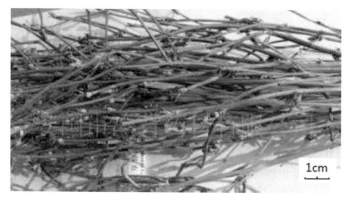

Indication: jaundice, stomachache and edema; diuresis.
It is taken as food in some part of China.

(The picture is only for learning and identification the herb; the specific use of the herb please consult the herbalist or health professionals)

Common Davflower Herb (Yazhicao)

Chinese phonetic alphabet/pin yin: yā zhī cǎo
Chinese characters simplified/traditional: 鸭跖草/鴨跖草
Chinese nickname's alphabet (Nickname's Chinese characters): Bizhuzi/ Cuihudie/ Lanhuacao/ Zhuyecao(碧竹子/翠蝴蝶/兰花草/竹叶草)
Latin: Commelinae Herba (Common name: Common Dayflower Herb)

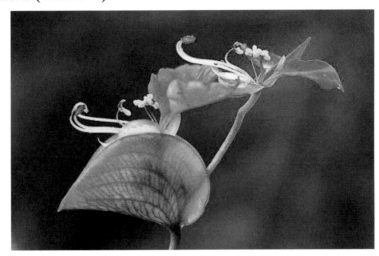

Plant: *Commelina communis* L.

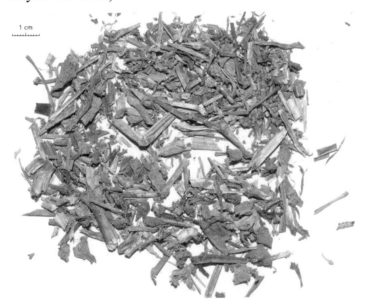

TCM prepared in ready-to-use forms (medicinal parts): it's dried aerial part which harvested in summer or autumn. Property and flavor: cold; sweet, bland. Main and collateral channels: stomach, lung and small intestine meridians. Administration and dosage: 15-30 g. Topical application in appropriate amount.

Indication: cold with fever, vexation and thirst, swollen sore throat, edema, pyretic stranguria with difficult and pain, swelling abscess.
(The picture is only for learning and identification the herb; the specific use of the herb please consult the herbalist or health professionals)

Conyza Herb (Jinlongdancao)

Chinese phonetic alphabet/pin yin: jīn lóng dǎn cǎo
Chinese characters simplified/traditional:金龙胆草/金龍膽草
Chinese nickname's alphabet (Nickname's Chinese characters): Aijiaokuhao/ Xiongdancao(矮脚苦蒿/熊胆草)
Latin: Conyzae Herba (Common name: Conyza Herb)

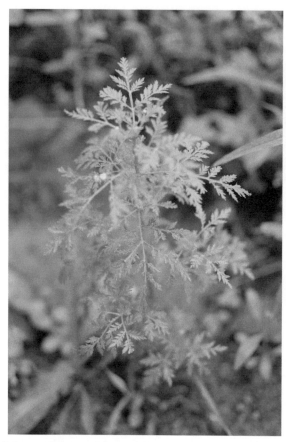

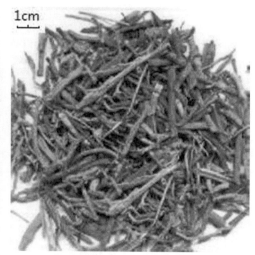

TCM prepared in ready-to-use forms (medicinal parts): it's dried aerial part which harvested in summer or autumn.
Property and flavor: cold; bitter.
Main and collateral channels: lung and liver meridians.
Administration and dosage: 6-9 g.

Plant: *Conyza blinii* Lévl.
Indication: cough, excessive phlegm and wheezing, mouth and throat sore, jaundice, epistaxis, bloody stool, menstrual flooding and spotting, external bleeding and rheumatoid arthritis.
(The picture is only for learning and identification the herb; the specific use of the herb please consult the herbalist or health professionals)

Red Gentian Herb (Honghualongdan)

Chinese phonetic alphabet/pin yin:
hóng huā lóng dǎn
Chinese characters
simplified/traditional:红花龙胆/
紅花龍膽
Chinese nickname's alphabet
(Nickname's Chinese characters):
Honglongdan/ Xiaoqingyudan/
Xingxiuhua(红龙胆/小青鱼胆/星
秀花)
Latin: Gentianae Rhodanthae Herb
(Common name: Red Gentian
Herb)
Plant: *Gentiana rhodantha* Franch.

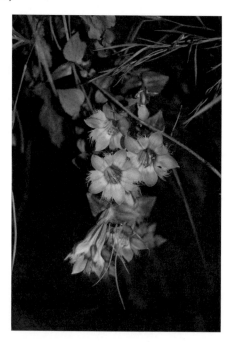

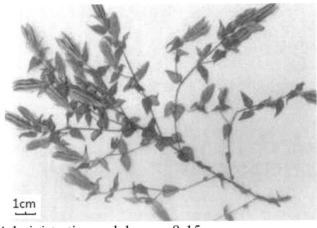

TCM prepared in ready-to-use forms (medicinal parts): it's dried herb which harvested in autumn or winter.
Property and flavor: cold; bitter.
Main and collateral channels: liver and gallbladder meridians.

Administration and dosage: 9-15 g.
Indication: jaundice, anuria and cough.
(The picture is only for learning and identification the herb; the specific use of the herb please consult the herbalist or health professionals)

Bunge Corydalis Herb (Kudiding)

Chinese phonetic alphabet/pin yin: kǔ dì dīng
Chinese characters simplified/traditional:苦地丁/苦地丁
Chinese nickname's alphabet (Nickname's Chinese characters): Didingzijin(地丁紫堇)
Latin: Corydalis Bungeanae Herba (Common name: Bunge CorydalisHerb)

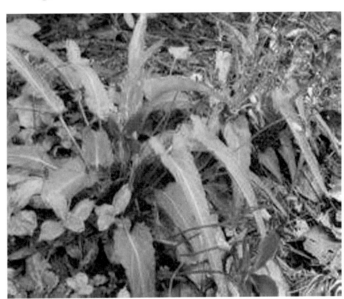

Plant: *Corydalis bungeana* Turcz.

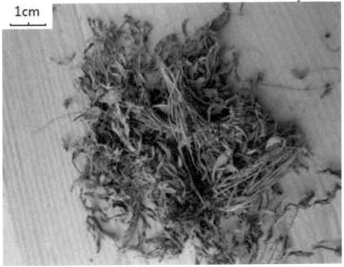

TCM prepared in ready-to-use forms (medicinal parts): it's dried whole grass which harvested in summer or autumn.
Property and flavor: cold; bitter.
Main and collateral channels: heart, liver, large intestine meridians.

Administration and dosage: 9-15 g. Topical application in appropriate amount, decocted for bathing.

Indication: influenza, sore throat, boil and sore, swelling and pain, abscesses and cellulites, carbuncle, mumps and erysipelas.

(The picture is only for learning and identification the herb; the specific use of the herb please consult the herbalist or health professionals)

Globethistle Root (Yuzhou Loulu)

Chinese phonetic alphabet/pin yin: yǔ zhōu lòu lú

Chinese characters simplified/traditional: 禹州漏芦/禹州漏蘆

Chinese nickname's alphabet (Nickname's Chinese characters): Huazhouloulu/Lancitou(华州漏芦/蓝刺头)

Latin: Echinopsis Radix (Common name: Globethistle Root)

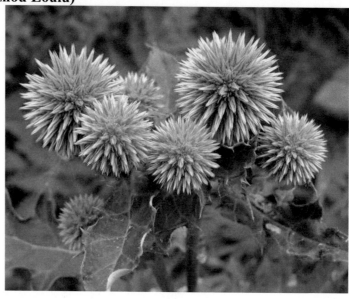

Plant: *Echinops latifolius* Tausch. (or *Echinops grijisii* Hance.)

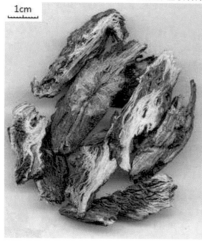

TCM prepared in ready-to-use forms (medicinal parts): it's dried root which harvested in spring or autumn.

Property and flavor: cold; bitter.

Main and collateral channels: stomach meridian.

Administration and dosage: 5-10 g.

Indication: acute mastitis, abscesses and cellulites, scrofula, sore and toxin; lactagogue.

Precaution and warning: use with caution during pregnancy.

(The picture is only for learning and identification the herb; the specific use of the herb please consult the herbalist or health professionals)

Garden Euphorbia Herb (Feiyangcao)

Chinese phonetic alphabet/pin yin: fēi yáng cǎo

Chinese characters simplified/traditional:飞扬草/飛揚草

Chinese nickname's alphabet (Nickname's Chinese characters): Dafeiyang/Jiejiehua(大飞羊/节节花)

Latin: Euphorbiae Hirtae Herba (Common name: Garden Euphorbia Herb)

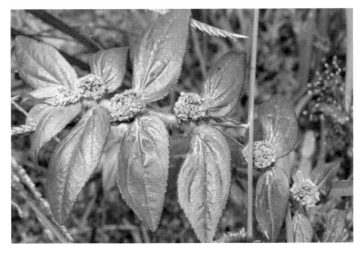

Plant: *Euphorbia hirta* L.
TCM prepared in ready-to-use forms (medicinal parts): it's dried whole plant which harvested in summer or autumn.

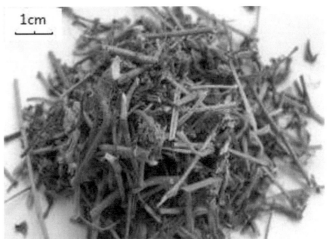

Property and flavor: cool; acidity, pungent.
Main and collateral channels: lung, bladder and large intestine meridians.
Administration and dosage: 6-9 g. Appropriate amount for topical application, decocted for rinsing.

Indication: lung abscess, mastitis, boil and sore, ulcerative gingivitis, dysentery, diarrhea, pyretic stranguria, eczema, beriberi, itch of skin and postpartum oligogalactia.
Precaution and warning: slightly toxic. Used with cautiously for pregnant woman. (The picture is only for learning and identification the herb; the specific use of the herb please consult the herbalist or health professionals)

Common Fibraurea Stem (Huangteng)
Chinese phonetic alphabet/pin yin: huáng téng
Chinese characters simplified/traditional:黄藤/黃藤
Chinese nickname's alphabet (Nickname's Chinese characters): Hongteng(红藤)
Latin: Fibraureae Caulis (Common name: Common Fibraurea Stem)

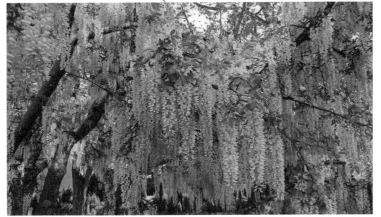

Plant: *Fibraurea recisa* Pierre.
TCM prepared in ready-to-use forms (medicinal parts): it's dried lianoid stem which harvested in autumn or winter.

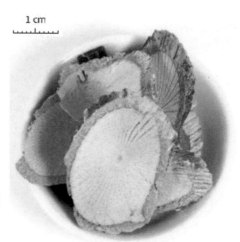

Property and flavor: cold; bitter.
Main and collateral channels: heart and
liver meridians.
Administration and dosage: 30-60 g.
Topical application in appropriate amount.
Indication: constipation, diarrhea and
dysentery, sore throat, swelling abscess
and skin infection.
It is key herb to treat acute appendicitis and
enteritis.

(The picture is only for learning and identification the herb; the specific use of the
herb please consult the herbalist or health professionals)

Malabarica Flower (Mumianhua)
Chinese phonetic alphabet/pin yin: mù mián huā
Chinese characters simplified/traditional:木棉花/木棉花
Chinese nickname's alphabet (Nickname's Chinese characters): Mumian/ Banzhihua/
Qiongzhi(木棉/斑枝花/琼枝)
Latin: Gossampini Flos (Common name: Malabarica Flower)

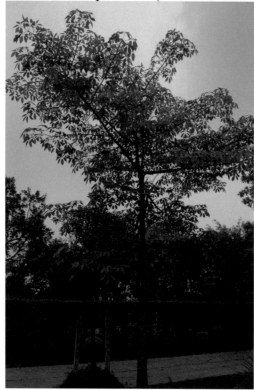

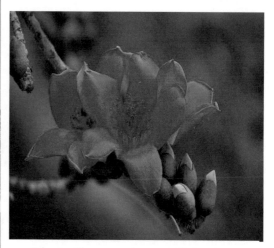

Plant: *Gossampinus malabarica*
(DC.) Merr.

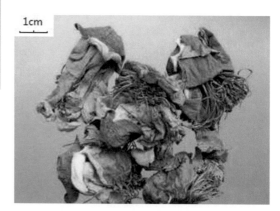

TCM prepared in ready-to-use forms
(medicinal parts): it's dried flower.
Property and flavor: cool; sweet, bland.
Main and collateral channels: large
intestine meridian.
Administration and dosage: 6-9 g.

Indication: diarrhea, dysentery and hemorrhoids.
(The picture is only for learning and identification the herb; the specific use of the herb please consult the herbalist or health professionals)

Helite (Daqingyan)
Chinese phonetic alphabet/pin yin: dà qīng yán
Chinese characters simplified/traditional:大青盐/大青鹽
Chinese nickname's alphabet (Nickname's Chinese characters): Rongyan(戎盐)
Latin: Helitum (Common name: Helite)

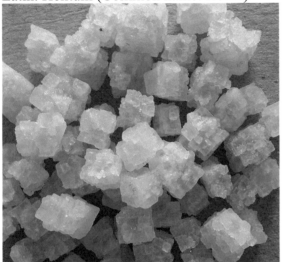

Mineral: main component NaCl
TCM prepared in ready-to-use forms (medicinal parts): it's lack salt crystal.
Property and flavor: cold; salty.
Main and collateral channels: heart, kidney and bladder meridians.
Administration and dosage: 1.2-2.5 g, used in pills or powder. Topical application in appropriate amount, for brushing teeth or dissolved in water as gargle and collyrium.

Indication: hematemesis, hematuria, swelling painful gum, gingival bleeding, red eye and dry stool.
It is taken as seasoning in some part of China.
Precaution and warning: used with caution in patients with edema pregnancy.
(The picture is only for learning and identification the herb; the specific use of the herb please consult the herbalist or health professionals)

Cottonrose Hibiscus (Mufurongye)

Chinese phonetic alphabet/pin yin: mù fú róng yè
Chinese characters simplified/traditional :木芙蓉叶/木芙蓉葉
Chinese nickname's alphabet (Nickname's Chinese characters): Jushuangye/ Tiegusan (拒霜叶/铁箍散)
Latin: Hibisci Mutabilis Folium (Common name: Cottonrose Hibiscus)

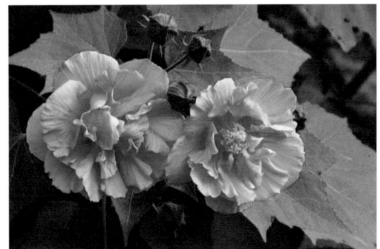

Plant: *Hibiscus mutabilis* L.

TCM prepared in ready-to-use forms (medicinal parts): it's dried leaf which harvested

in summer or autumn.
Property and flavor: neutral; pungent.
Main and collateral channels: lung and liver meridians.
Administration and dosage: 10-30 g. Topical application in appropriate amount.

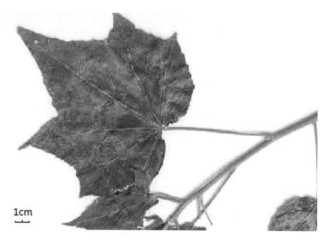

Indication: abscess, cellulitis, shingles, scalds, burns, swelling painful eyes with congestion and traumatic injuries.
(The picture is only for learning and identification the herb; the specific use of the herb please consult the herbalist or health professionals)

Ilex Chinese Leaf (Sijiqing)
Chinese phonetic alphabet/ pin yin: sì jì qīng
Chinese characters simplified/traditional: 四季青/四季青
Chinese nickname's alphabet (Nickname's Chinese characters): Hongdongqing/ Youyeshu/ Shudingzi (红冬青/油叶树/ 树顶子)
Latin: Ilicis Chinensis Folium (Common name: Ilex Chinese Leaf)

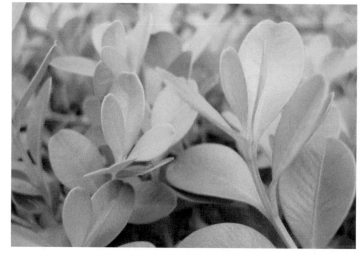

Plant: *Ilex chinensis* Sims.

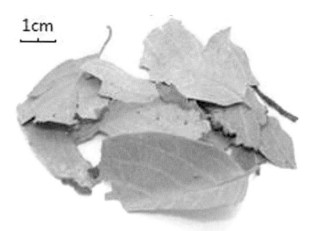

TCM prepared in ready-to-use forms (medicinal parts): it's dried leaf which harvested in autumn or winter.
Property and flavor: cold; bitter, astringent.
Main and collateral channels: lung, large intestine and gallbladder meridians.

Administration and dosage: 15-60 g. Topical application in appropriate amount, decocted it with water for topical application.

Indication: cough with heat, swelling and sore throat, dysentery, hypochondriac pain and pyretic stranguria; external used for burn, scald, skin ulcer.

It is good at treating burn and scald.

(The picture is only for learning and identification the herb; the specific use of the herb please consult the herbalist or health professionals)

Chinese Holly Leaf (Gouguye)

Chinese phonetic alphabet/pin yin: gǒu gǔ yè

Chinese characters simplified/traditional: 枸骨叶/枸骨葉

Chinese nickname's alphabet (Nickname's Chinese characters): Yangjiaoci/ Gouqingle (羊角刺/ 狗青芛)

Latin: Ilicis Cornutae Folium (Common name: Chinese Holly Leaf)

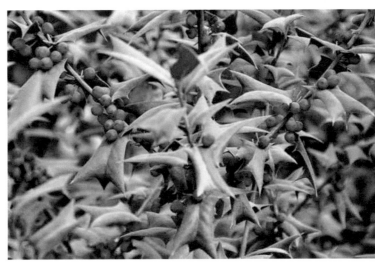

Plant: *Ilex cornuta* Lindle. ex Paxt.

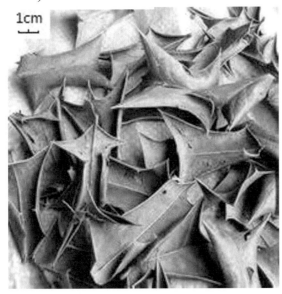

TCM prepared in ready-to-use forms (medicinal parts): it's dried leaf which harvested in autumn.

Property and flavor: cool; bitter.

Main and collateral channels: liver and kidney meridians.

Administration and dosage: 9-15 g.

Indication: phthisis, hemoptysis, fever, dizziness and vertigo.

(The picture is only for learning and identification the herb; the specific use of the herb please consult the herbalist or health professionals)

Ovateleaf Holly Bark (Jiubiying)

Chinese phonetic alphabet/pin yin: jiù bì yìng

Chinese characters simplified/traditional:救必应/救必應

Chinese nickname's alphabet (Nickname's Chinese characters): Tiedongqing/ Xiongdanmu/ Baiyinxiang/ Misuimu(铁冬青/熊胆木/白银香/米碎木)

Latin: Ilicis Rotundae Cortex (Common name: Ovateleaf Holly Bark)

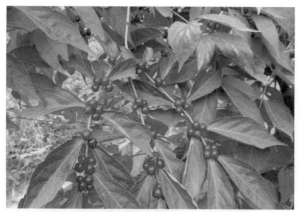

Plant: *Ilex totunda* Thunb.

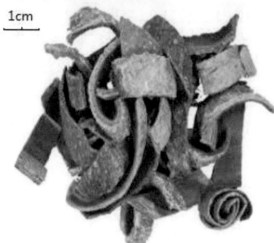

1cm

TCM prepared in ready-to-use forms (medicinal parts): it's dried bark which harvested in summer or autumn.
Property and flavor: cold; bitter.
Main and collateral channels: lung, stomach, large intestine and liver meridians.
Administration and dosage: 9-30 g. Topical application in appropriate amount, decocted it into thick decoction for topical application.
Indication: sore throat, diarrhea, dysentery, distending pain, arthralgia, eczema, sore, boil and traumatic injuries.
(The picture is only for learning and identification the herb; the specific use of the herb please consult the herbalist or health professionals)

Shorttube Lagotis Herb (Honglian)

Chinese phonetic alphabet/pin yin: hóng lián
Chinese characters simplified/traditional: 洪连/洪連
Chinese nickname's alphabet (Nickname's Chinese characters): Zanghuanglian/Tu'ercao(藏黄连/兔耳草)
Latin: Lagotidis Herba (Common name: Shorttube Lagotis Herb)

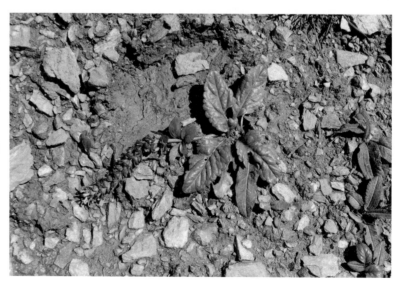

Plant: *Lagotis brevituba* Maxim.

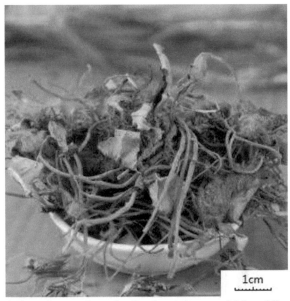

TCM prepared in ready-to-use forms (medicinal parts): it's dried whole herb which harvested in summer or autumn.
Property and flavor: cold; bitter, sweet.
Main and collateral channels: lung, heart and liver meridians.
Administration and dosage: 1-6 g.
Indication: fever, fret, thirst, cough, headache, dizziness, jaundice, menstrual irregularities, drug or food poisoning.

(The picture is only for learning and identification the herb; the specific use of the herb please consult the herbalist or health professionals)

Chinese Mahonia Stem (Gonglaomu)

Chinese phonetic alphabet/pin yin: gōng láo mù
Chinese characters simplified/traditional:功劳木/功勞木
Chinese nickname's alphabet (Nickname's Chinese characters): Shidagonglao/ Huangtianzhu/ Tuhuangbai(十大功劳/黄天竹/土黄柏)
Latin: Mahoniae Caulis (Common name: Chinese Mahonia Stem)

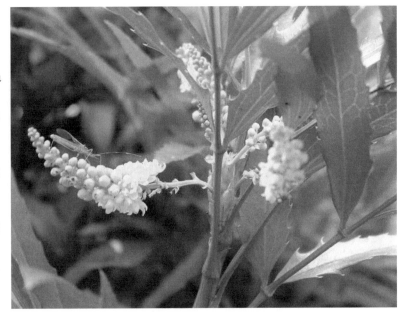

Plant: *Mahonia bealei* (Fort.) Garr. (or *Mahonia fortunei* (Lindl.) Fedde.)

TCM prepared in ready-to-use forms (medicinal parts): it's dried stem which harvested all year round.
Property and flavor: cold; bitter.
Main and collateral channels: liver, stomach and large intestine meridians.
Administration and dosage: 9-15 g. Topical application in appropriate amount.
Indication: cough, diarrhea, dysentery, jaundice, red urine, toothache, sore, boil, swelling and abscess.

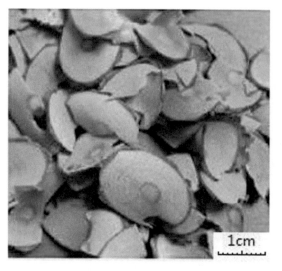

1cm

(The picture is only for learning and identification the herb; the specific use of the herb please consult the herbalist or health professionals)

Asiatic Moonseed Rhizome (Beidougen)
Chinese phonetic alphabet/pin yin: běi dòu gēn
Chinese characters simplified/traditional:北豆根/北豆根
Chinese nickname's alphabet (Nickname's Chinese characters): Huangtiaoxiang/ Yedougen/ Bianfuteng(黄条香/野豆根/蝙蝠藤)
Latin: Manispermi Rhizoma (Common name: Asiatic Moonseed Rhizome)

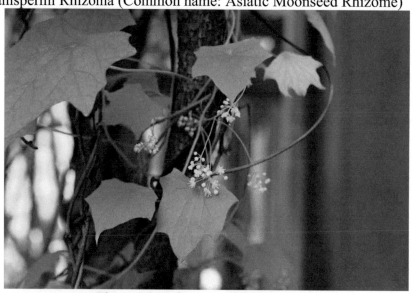

Plant: *Menispermum dauricum* DC.

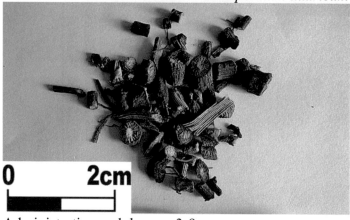

0   2cm

TCM prepared in ready-to-use forms (medicinal parts): it's dried rhizome which harvested in spring or autumn.
Property and flavor: cold; bitter.
Main and collateral channels: lung, stomach and large intestine meridians.

Administration and dosage: 3-9 g.

99

Indication: swelling and sore throat, diarrhea, dysentery, arthralgic.

Precaution and warning: slightly toxic. Incompatible with Black False Hellebore. (The picture is only for learning and identification the herb; the specific use of the herb please consult the herbalist or health professionals)

Mirabilite Preparation (Xiguashuang)

Chinese phonetic alphabet/pin yin: xī guā shuāng

Chinese characters simplified/traditional: 西瓜霜/西瓜霜

Chinese nickname's alphabet (Nickname's Chinese characters):Xiguaxiao(西瓜硝)

Latin: Mirabilitum Praeparatum (Common name: Mirabilite Preparation)

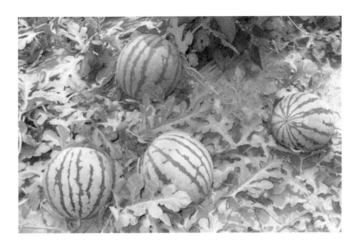

Plant: *Citrullus lanatus* (Thunb.) Mansfeld.

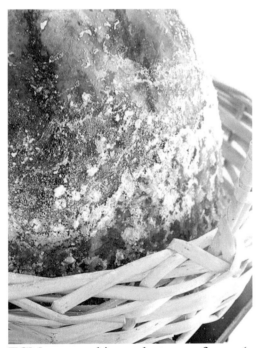

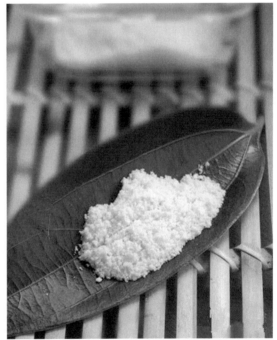

TCM prepared in ready-to-use forms (medicinal parts): it's prepared form the fruit with Sodium Sulfate.

Processing: cut the pedicle of the fresh watermelon as a top cover, removed the melon pulp and seed, filled in the Sodium Sulfate, covered the top and pegged with prod, put into the pan and covered, put in a cool and ventilated place, wait until there is precipitation of frost on the watermelon surface, the frost is the Mirabilite Preparation.

Property and flavor: cold; salty.

Main and collateral channels: lung, stomach and large intestine meridians.

Administration and dosage: 0.5-1.5 g. Topical application in appropriate amount, ground it into powder for blow application.

Indication: swelling, sore and aphtha.

(The picture is only for learning and identification the herb; the specific use of the herb please consult the herbalist or health professionals)

Acaulescent Pegaeophyton Root and Rhizome (Gaoshanlagencai)

Chinese phonetic alphabet/pin yin: gāo shān là gēn cài

Chinese characters simplified/traditional: 高山辣根菜/高山辣根菜

Chinese nickname's alphabet (Nickname's Chinese characters): Suluogabao(苏罗尕保)

Latin: Pegaeophyti Radix et Rhizoma (Common name: Acaulescent Pegaeophyton Root and Rhizome)

Plant: *Pegaeophyton scapiflorum* Marq. et Shaw.

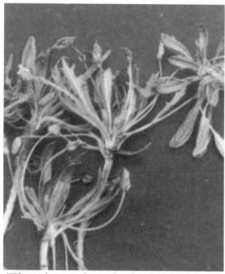

TCM prepared in ready-to-use forms (medicinal parts): it's dried root and rhizome which harvested in autumn.

Property and flavor: cold; pungent, bitter.

Main and collateral channels: lung and liver meridians.

Administration and dosage: 3-6 g, decocted or used in pills and powder. Appropriate amount for topical application, ground into powder for application.

Indication: fever, cough, hemoptysis, edema in the limb and traumatic hemorrhage.

(The picture is only for learning and identification the herb; the specific use of the herb please consult the herbalist or health professionals)

Amur Cork-tree (Guanhuangbai)

Chinese phonetic alphabet/pin yin: guān huáng bǎi

Chinese characters simplified/traditional:关黄柏/關黃柏

Chinese nickname's alphabet (Nickname's Chinese characters): Huangbo(黃檗)

Latin: Phellodendri Amurensis Cortex (Common name: Amur Cork-tree)

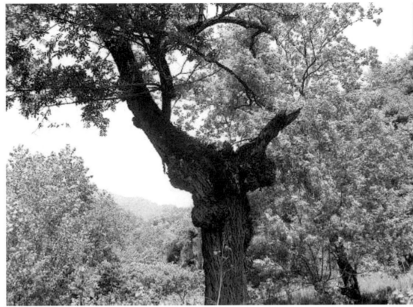

Plant: *Phellodendron amurense* Rupr.
TCM prepared in ready-to-use forms (medicinal parts): it's dried bark.
Property and flavor: cold; bitter.

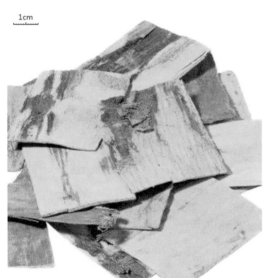

Main and collateral channels: kidney and bladder meridians.
Administration and dosage: 3-12 g. Appropriate amount for topical application.
Indication: diarrhea, dysentery, jaundice, pruritus vulvae, tinea pedis, fever, night sweating, eczema, seminal emission, sore and ulcer, swelling and toxin.

(The picture is only for learning and identification the herb; the specific use of the herb please consult the herbalist or health professionals)

Franchet Groundcherry Fruit (Jindenglong)
Chinese phonetic alphabet/pin yin: jǐn dēng lóng
Chinese characters simplified/traditional: 锦灯笼/錦燈籠
Chinese nickname's alphabet (Nickname's Chinese characters): Guniang/ Geli/ Guajindeng(菇娘/戈力/挂金灯)
Latin: Physalis Calyx seu Fructus (Common name: Franchet Groundcherry Fruit or Golden Berry)

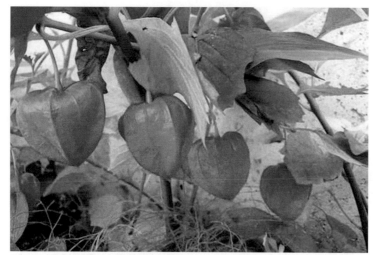

Plant: *Physalis alkekengi* L. var. *franchetii* (Mast.) Makino.

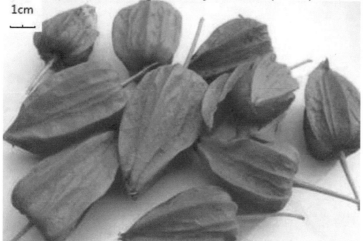

1cm

TCM prepared in ready-to-use forms (medicinal parts): it's dried calyx with fruit.
Property and flavor: cold; bitter.
Main and collateral channels: lung meridian.
Administration and dosage: 5-9 g. Appropriate amount for topical application, mashed for applying to *pars affecta*.
Indication: sore throat, loss of voice, cough, anuresis and pyretic stranguria; external use for pemphigus, eczema.
(The picture is only for learning and identification the herb; the specific use of the herb please consult the herbalist or health professionals)

Indian Quassiawood (Kumu)

Chinese phonetic alphabet/ pin yin: kǔ mù
Chinese characters simplified/traditional: 苦木/苦木
Chinese nickname's alphabet (Nickname's Chinese characters): Kushupi/ Kudanmu (苦皮树/苦胆木)
Latin: Picrasmae Ramulus et Folium (Common name: Indian Quassiawood)

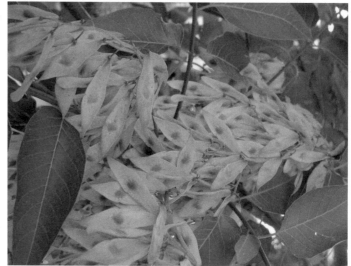

Plant: *Picrasma quassioides* (D. Don) Benn.

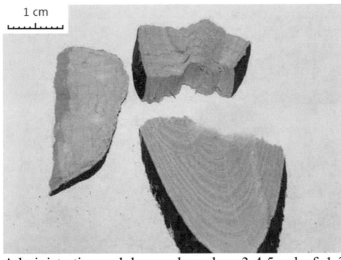

1 cm

TCM prepared in ready-to-use forms (medicinal parts): it's dried branch or leaf which harvested in summer or autumn.
Property and flavor: cold; bitter.
Main and collateral channels: lung and large intestine meridians.

Administration and dosage: branches: 3-4.5 g; leaf: 1-3 g. Appropriate amount for topical application.
Indication: anemopyretic cold, sore throat, diarrhea, dysentery, eczema, boil, insect or snake bites.
Precaution and warning: slightly toxic.
(The picture is only for learning and identification the herb; the specific use of the herb please consult the herbalist or health professionals)

Common Picria Herb (Kuxuanshen)

Chinese phonetic alphabet/
pin yin: kǔ xuán shēn
Chinese characters simplified/traditional:
苦玄参/苦玄參
Chinese nickname's alphabet (Nickname's Chin characters): Shezongguan/
Yudancao(蛇总管/鱼胆草)
Latin: Picriae Herba
(Common name: Common Picria Herb)

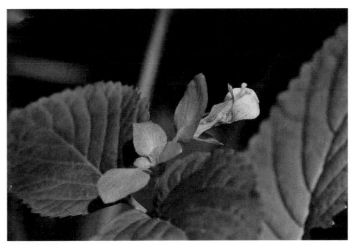

Plant: *Picria felterrae* Lour.

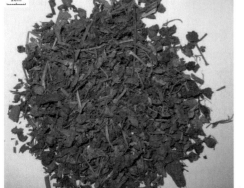

1cm

TCM prepared in ready-to-use forms (medicinal parts): it's dried herb which harvested in autumn.
Property and flavor: cold; bitter.
Main and collateral channels: lung, stomach and liver meridians.
Administration and dosage: 9-15 g.
Appropriate amount for topical application.

Indication: anemopyretic cold, swollen sore throat, mumps, dysentery, epigastrium and abdomen pain, traumatic injuries and snake bites.

(The picture is only for learning and identification the herb; the specific use of the herb please consult the herbalist or health professionals)

Polygonum Herb (Gangbangui)

Chinese phonetic alphabet/pin yin: gàng bǎn guī
Chinese characters simplified/traditional:杠板归/杠板歸
Chinese nickname's alphabet (Nickname's Chinese characters): Hebaicao/ Guanyeliao(河白草/贯叶蓼)
Latin: Polygoni Perfoliati Herba (Common name: Polygonum Herb)

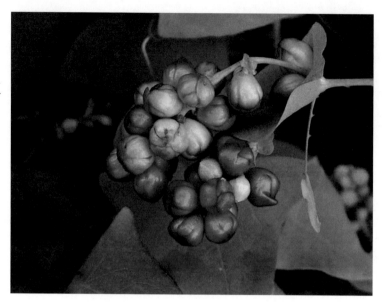

Plant: *Polygonum perfoliatum* L.

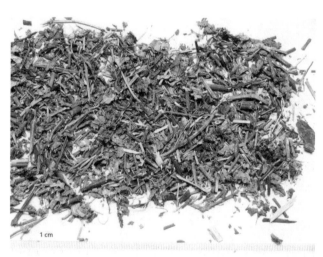

TCM prepared in ready-to-use forms (medicinal parts): it's dried aerial part which harvested in summer at flowering.
Property and flavor: mild cold; acidity.
Main and collateral channels: lung and bladder meridians.
Administration and dosage: 15-30 g. Appropriate amount for topical application. It can be decocted for fuming-washing therapy.

Indication: sore throat, cough, edema, diarrhea, dysentery, oliguria, eczema, insect or snake bites.
(The picture is only for learning and identification the herb; the specific use of the herb please consult the herbalist or health professionals)

Indigoplant Leaf (Liaodaqingye)
Chinese phonetic alphabet/pin yin: liào dà qīng yè
Chinese characters simplified/traditional:蓼大青叶/蓼大青葉
Chinese nickname's alphabet (Nickname's Chinese characters): Liaolan(蓼蓝)
Latin: Polygoni Tinctorii Folium (Common name: Indigoplant Leaf)

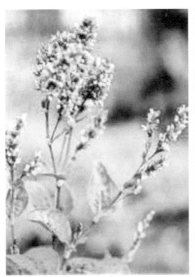
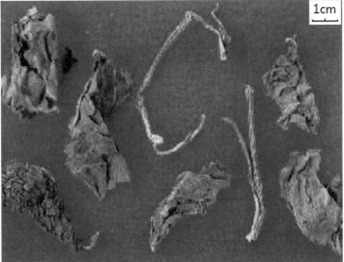

Plant: *Polygonum tinctorium* Ait.

TCM prepared in ready-to-use forms (medicinal parts): it's dried leaf which harvested in summer or autumn.

Property and flavor: cold; bitter.

Main and collateral channels: heart and stomach meridians.

Administration and dosage: 9-15 g.

Indication: fever, macula and papule eruption, cough and wheezing, mumps, erysipelas and swelling abscess.

(The picture is only for learning and identification the herb; the specific use of the herb please consult the herbalist or health professionals)

Chinese Cinquefoil (Weilingcai)

Chinese phonetic alphabet/pin yin: wěi líng cài

Chinese characters simplified/traditional:委陵菜/委陵菜

Chinese nickname's alphabet (Nickname's Chinese characters): Hamacao/ Tianqingdibai(蛤蟆草/ 天青地白)

Latin: Potenillae Chinensis Herba (Common name: Chinese Cinquefoil)

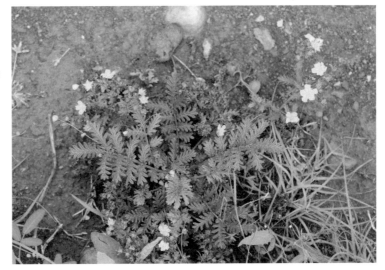

Plant: *Potentilla chinensis* Ser.

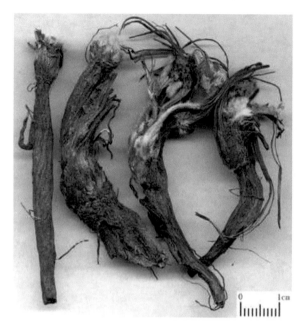

TCM prepared in ready-to-use forms (medicinal parts): it's dried root or whole herb which harvested in spring.

Property and flavor: cold; bitter.

Main and collateral channels: liver and large intestine meridians.

Administration and dosage: 9-15 g. Topical application in appropriate amount.

Indication: chronic dysentery, hemorrhoid bleeding, swelling abscess and sore, skin infection.

(The picture is only for learning and identification the herb; the specific use of the herb please consult the herbalist or health professionals)

Hooker Winghead Herb (Yishoucao)

Chinese phonetic alphabet/pin yin: yì shǒu cǎo

Chinese characters simplified/traditional :翼首草/翼首草

Chinese nickname's alphabet

(Nickname's Chinese characters):

Bangzitou/ Shizicao(棒子头/狮子草)

Latin: Pterocephali Herba (Common name: Hooker Winghead Herb)

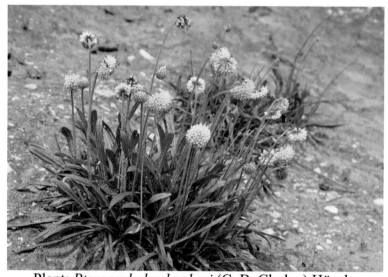

Plant: *Pterocephalus hookeri* (C. B. Clarke.) Höeck.

TCM prepared in ready-to-use forms (medicinal parts): it's dried whole grass which harvested in summer or autumn.

Property and flavor: cold; bitter.

Administration and dosage: 1-3 g.

Indication: fever and dysentery; relieve impediment.

Precaution and warning: slightly toxic.

(The picture is only for learning and identification the herb; the specific use of the herb please consult the herbalist or health professionals)

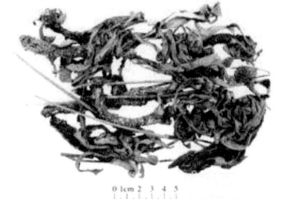

Blushred Rabdosia Herb (Donglingcao)

Chinese phonetic alphabet/pin yin: dōng líng cǎo
Chinese characters simplified/traditional: 冬凌草/冬凌草
Chinese nickname's alphabet (Nickname's Chinese characters): Shanxiangcao/ Xuehuacao/ Binglingcao(山香草/ 雪花草/冰凌草)

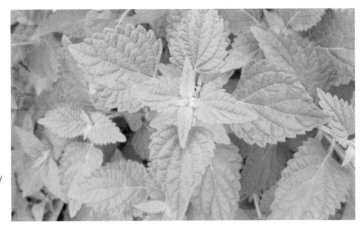

Latin: Rabdosiae Rubescentis Herba (Common name: Blushred Rabdosia Herb)
Plant: *Rabdosia rubescens* (Hemsl.)

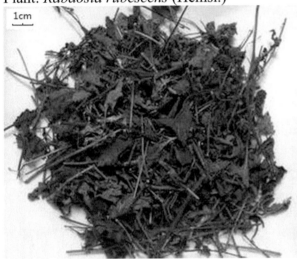

TCM prepared in ready-to-use forms (medicinal parts): it's dried aerial part which harvested in summer or autumn.
Property and flavor: mild cold; bitter, sweet.
Main and collateral channels: lung, stomach and liver meridians.
Administration and dosage: 30-60 g. Topical application in appropriate amount.

Indication: throat swelling and sore, abdominal masses, glomus, insect and snake bites.
(The picture is only for learning and identification the herb; the specific use of the herb please consult the herbalist or health professionals)

Uniflower Swisscentaury Rood (Loulu)

Chinese phonetic alphabet/pin yin: lòu lú
Chinese characters simplified/traditional:漏芦/ 漏蘆
Chinese nickname's alphabet (Nickname's Chinese characters): Langtouhua/ Yelan/ Guiyouma(狼头花/野 兰/鬼油麻)
Latin: Rhapontici Radix (Common name: Uniflower Swisscentaury Rood)

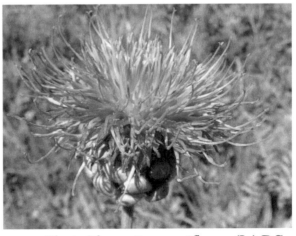

Plant: *Rhaponticum uniflorum* (L.) DC.

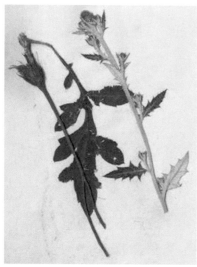 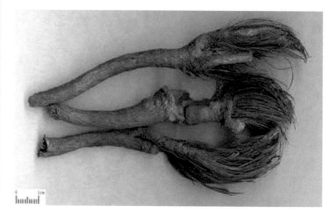

TCM prepared in ready-to-use forms (medicinal parts): it's dried root which harvested in spring or autumn.

Property and flavor: cold; bitter.

Main and collateral channels: stomach meridian.

Administration and dosage: 5-9 g.

Indication: acute mastitis, abscess, cellulitis, scrofula, sore and toxin; lactagogue. It is good at treating mastitis.

Precaution and warning: used with caution during pregnancy.

(The picture is only for learning and identification the herb; the specific use of the herb please consult the herbalist or health professionals)

Muskroot-like Semiaquilegia Root (Tiankuizi)

Chinese phonetic alphabet/pin yin: tiān kuí zǐ
Chinese characters simplified/traditional: 天葵子/天葵子
Chinese nickname's alphabet (Nickname's Chinese characters): Zibeitiankui/ Qiannianlaoshushi(紫背天葵/千年老鼠屎)
Latin: Semiaquilegiae Radix (Common name: Muskroot-like Semiaquilegia Root)

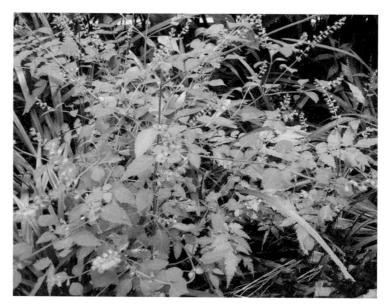

Plant: *Semiaquilegia adoxoides* (DC.) Makino.

TCM prepared in ready-to-use forms (medicinal parts): it's dried root which harvested in summer.
Property and flavor: cold; sweet, bitter.
Main and collateral channels: liver and stomach meridians.
Administration and dosage: 9-15 g.
Indication: swelling abscess, boil and sore, acute mastitis, scrofula, insect and snake bites.

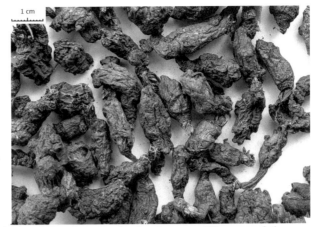

(The picture is only for learning and identification the herb; the specific use of the herb please consult the herbalist or health professionals)

Climbing Groundsel Herb (Qianliguang)

Chinese phonetic alphabet/pin yin: qiān lǐ guāng
Chinese characters simplified/traditional: 千里光/千里光
Chinese nickname's alphabet (Nickname's Chinese characters): Jiuliming/ Jiuliguang(九里明/九里光)
Latin: Senecionis Scandentis Herba (Common name: Climbing Groundsel Herb)

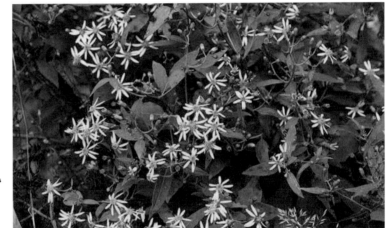

Plant: *Senecio scandenes* Buch.-Ham.

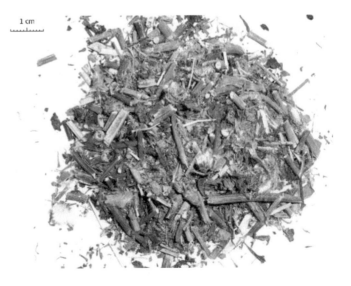

TCM prepared in ready-to-use forms (medicinal parts): it's dried aerial part which harvested all year round.
Property and flavor: cold; bitter.
Main and collateral channels: lung and liver meridians.
Administration and dosage: 15-30 g. Topical application in appropriate amount, decocted for fuming-washing therapy.

Indication: swelling abscess, sore and toxin, cold, fever, red painful eyes, eczema, diarrhea and dysentery.
(The picture is only for learning and identification the herb; the specific use of the

herb please consult the herbalist or health professionals)

Soybean Yellow Germination (Dadouhuangjuan)

Chinese phonetic alphabet/
pin yin: dà dòu huáng juǎn
Chinese characters simplified/
traditional:大豆黄卷/大豆黃卷
Chinese nickname's alphabet
(Nickname's Chinese characters):
Dadounie/ Huangjuan(大豆蘖/
黄卷)
Latin: Sojae Semen Germinatum
(Common name: Soybean
Yellow Germination)

Plant: *Glycine max* (L.) Merr.

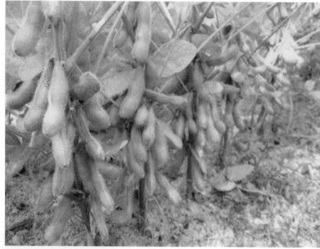

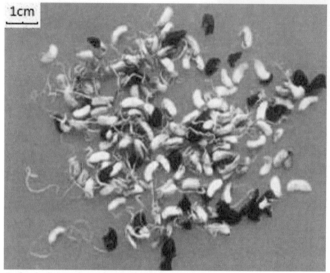

TCM prepared in ready-to-use forms (medicinal parts): it's prepared ripe seed by germination.
Processing: take the ripe seed, macerate to swollen in water, drain the water and covered with a wet textile, spray water twice a day until the sprout grow 0.5-1 cm long, take out and dry.
Property and flavor: neutral; sweet.
Main and collateral channels: spleen, stomach and lung meridians.

Administration and dosage: 9-15 g.
Indication: cold, fever, scanty sweating, oppression in the chest, epigastric stuffiness, heavy aching limbs, inhibited urination.
(The picture is only for learning and identification the herb; the specific use of the herb please consult the herbalist or health professionals)

Pig Gall Powder (Zhudanfen)

Chinese phonetic alphabet/pin yin: zhū dǎn fěn
Chinese characters simplified/traditional:猪胆粉/豬膽粉
Latin: Suis Fellis Pulvis
(Common name: Pig Gall Powder)
Animal: *Sus scrofa domestica* Brisson.

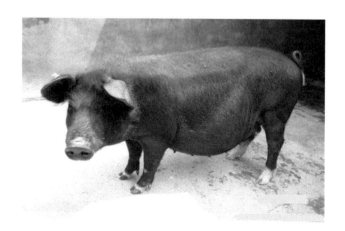

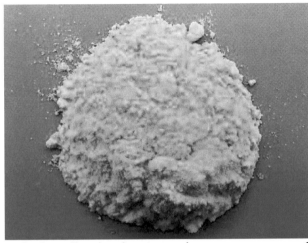

TCM prepared in ready-to-use forms (medicinal parts): it's dried bile powder.
Property and flavor: cold; bitter.
Main and collateral channels: liver, gallbladder, lung, large intestine meridians.
Administration and dosage: 0.3-0.6 g, taken with water or used in pills or powder.

Topical application in appropriate amount, ground into powder, or mixed with water for applying to the *pars affecta*.
Indication: whooping cough, asthma, febrile disease, jaundice, diarrhea, dysentery, constipation, abscess, sore and skin infection.
Attention: to protect the rare wild animals, please don't use it from wild animal.
(The picture is only for learning and identification the herb; the specific use of the herb please consult the herbalist or health professionals)

False Chinese Swertia Herb (Dangyao)

Chinese phonetic alphabet/pin yin: dāng yào
Chinese characters simplified/traditional: 当药/當藥
Chinese nickname's alphabet (Nickname's Chinese characters): Zhangyacai/Digeda(獐牙菜/地格达)
Latin: Swertiae Herba (Common name: False Chinese Swertia Herb)

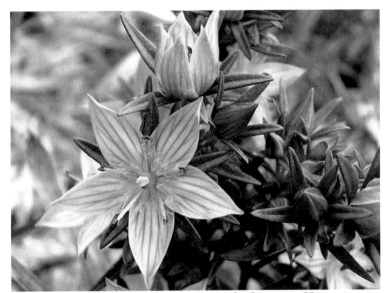

Plant: *Swertia pseudochinensis* Hara.

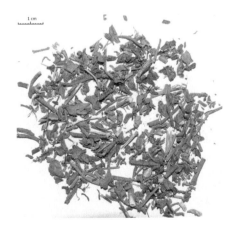

TCM prepared in ready-to-use forms (medicinal parts): it's dried herb which harvested in summer or autumn.
Property and flavor: cold; bitter.
Main and collateral channels: liver, stomach and large intestine meridians.
Administration and dosage: 6-12 g, reduce the dosage for pediatrics.
Indication: jaundice, hypochondriac pain, dysentery and anepithymia.

(The picture is only for learning and identification the herb; the specific use of the herb please consult the herbalist or health professionals)

Belleric Terminalia Fruit (Maohezi)

Chinese phonetic alphabet/pin yin: máo hē zǐ
Chinese characters simplified/traditional:毛诃子/毛訶子
Chinese nickname's alphabet (Nickname's Chinese characters): Pilile(毗黎勒)
Latin: Terminaliae Billericae Fructus (Common name: Belleric Terminalia Fruit)

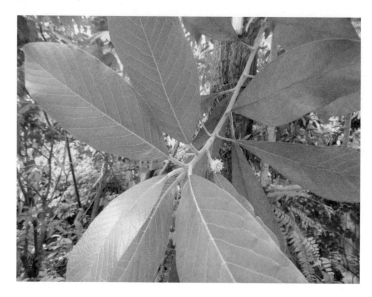

Plant: *Terminalia bellirica* (Gaertn.) Roxb.

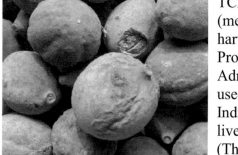

TCM prepared in ready-to-use forms (medicinal parts): it's dried ripe fruit which harvested in winter.
Property and flavor: neutral; sweet, astringent.
Administration and dosage: 3-9 g, usually used in pills or powder.
Indication: diarrhea, dysentery, weakness, liver and gallbladder diseases.
(The picture is only for learning and identification the herb; the specific use of the herb please consult the herbalist or health professionals)

Tinospora Root (Jinguolan)

Chinese phonetic alphabet/pin yin: jīn guǒ lǎn
Chinese characters simplified/traditional:金果榄/金果欖
Chinese nickname's alphabet (Nickname's Chinese characters): Qingniudan/ Jiuniudan(青牛胆/九牛胆)
Latin: Tinosporae Radix (Common name: Tinospora Root)
Plant: *Tinospora sagittata* (Olive.) Gagnep. (or *Tinospora capillipes* Gagnep.)

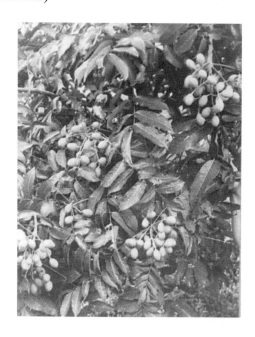

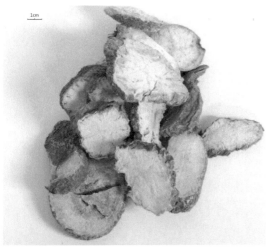

TCM prepared in ready-to-use forms (medicinal parts): it's dried root tuber which harvested in autumn or winter.

Property and flavor: cold; bitter.

Main and collateral channels: lung and large intestine meridians.

Administration and dosage: 3-9 g. Topical application in appropriate amount, ground into powder for blowing to throat, or ground with vinegar.

Indication: swollen sore throat, abscesses and cellulitis, toxin, diarrhea, dysentery, epigastrium and abdomen pain.

(The picture is only for learning and identification the herb; the specific use of the herb please consult the herbalist or health professionals)

Acute Turpinia Leaf (Shanxiangyuanye)

Chinese phonetic alphabet/pin yin: shān xiāng yuán yè

Chinese characters simplified/traditional:山香圆叶/山香圓葉

Chinese nickname's alphabet (Nickname's Chinese characters): Liangzhijian/ Qiandachui/ Qicunding(两指剑/千打锤/七寸钉)

Latin: Turpiniae Folium (Common name: Acute Turpinia Leaf)

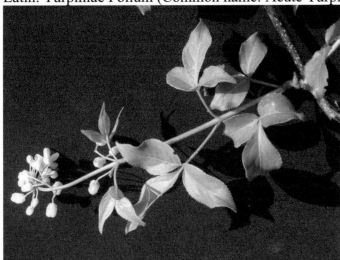

Plant: *Turpinia arguta* Seem.

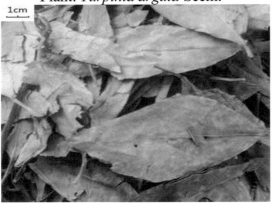

TCM prepared in ready-to-use forms (medicinal parts): it's dried leaf which harvested in summer or autumn.

Property and flavor: cold; bitter.

Main and collateral channels: lung and liver meridians.

Administration and dosage: 15-30 g. Topical application in appropriate amount.

Indication: ulcer, toxin, traumatic injuries, swelling and sore throat.

(The picture is only for learning and identification the herb; the specific use of the herb please consult the herbalist or health professionals)

Rice Bean (Chixiaodou)

Chinese phonetic alphabet/pin yin: chì xiǎo dòu
Chinese characters simplified/traditional:赤小豆/赤小豆
Chinese nickname's alphabet (Nickname's Chinese characters): Hongxiaodou(红小豆)
Latin: Vignae Semen (Common name: Rice Bean)

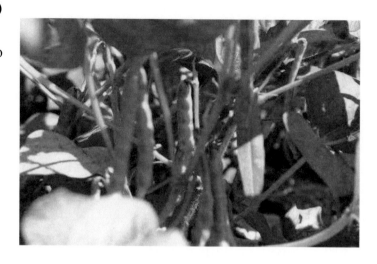

Plant: *Vigna umbellata* Ohwi. et Ohashi.
(or *Vigna angularis* Ohwi et Ohashi.)

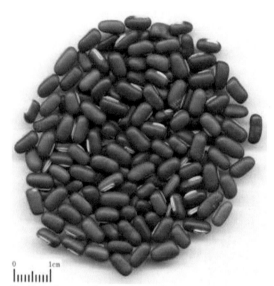

TCM prepared in ready-to-use forms (medicinal parts): it's dried mature seed which harvested in autumn.
Property and flavor: neutral; sweet, acidity.
Main and collateral channels: heart and small intestine meridians.
Administration and dosage: 9-30 g. Topical application in appropriate amount, ground into powder for applyment.

Indication: edema, jaundice, swelling abscess, sore and toxin, abdominal pain, tinea pedis and puffiness.
It is taken as food in some part of China.
(The picture is only for learning and identification the herb; the specific use of the herb please consult the herbalist or health professionals)

Mung Bean (Lyudou)
Chinese phonetic alphabet/pin yin: lǜ dòu
Chinese characters simplified/traditional:绿豆/綠豆
Chinese nickname's alphabet (Nickname's Chinese characters): Qingxiaodou(青小豆)
Latin: Radiatae Semen (Common name: Mung Bean or Green Bean)

Plant: *Vigna radiata* (Linn.) Wilczek. TCM prepared in ready-to-use forms (medicinal parts): it's dried ripe seed which harvested in autumn.

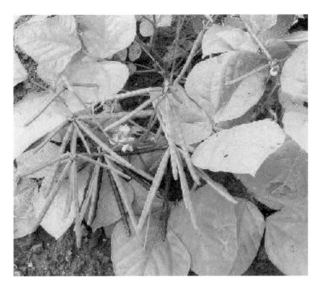

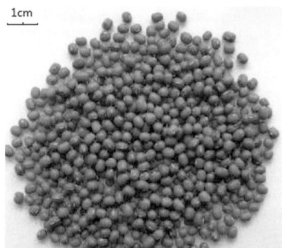

Property and flavor: cool; sweet.
Main and collateral channels: heart and stomach meridians.
Administration and dosage: 5-200 g, soaked in water first.
Indication: hyperlipidemia, heat; diuresis; anti-irritability; detoxic.

It is good at detoxifing Common Monkshood Daugher Root's, Croton Fruit's and Arsenolite's etc's poisonous.
It is taken as food in some part of China.
(The picture is only for learning and identification the herb; the specific use of the herb please consult the herbalist or health professionals)

Black Nightshade (Longkui)

Chinese phonetic alphabet/pin yin: lóng kuí
Chinese characters simplified/traditional: 龙葵/龍葵
Chinese nickname's alphabet (Nickname's Chinese characters): Yelaohu/ Yehaijiao/ Tianqiezi(野老虎/野海角/天茄子)
Latin: Solani Nigri Herba (Common name: Black Nightshade or Morel)

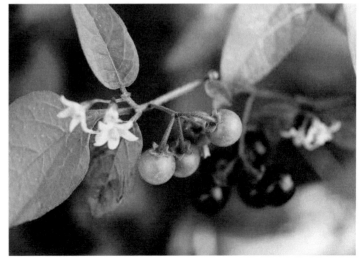

Plant: *Solanum nigrum* L. (or *Solanum nigrum* L. var *pauciflorun* Liou.)

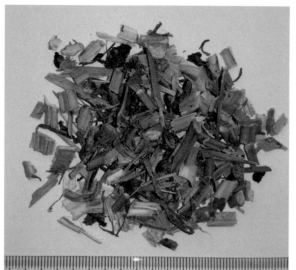

TCM prepared in ready-to-use forms (medicinal parts): it's dried whole herb which harvested in spring.
Property and flavor: cold; bitter, mild sweet.
Administration and dosage: 15-50 g for oral administration. Appropriate amount applies to *pars affecta* for topical application.
Indication: cold with fever, toothache, chronic bronchitis, diarrhea, urinary tract infection, mastitis and leucorrhea; external used for carbuncle, furuncle, pemphigus and snake bites.

Precaution and warnings: slightly toxic. Use with caution during pregnancy.
(The picture is only for learning and identification the herb; the specific use of the herb please consult the herbalist or health professionals)

Xie Xia Yao(泻下药)-purgating herbs
Xie Xia Yao is a kind of herbs which's the major functions are purgation, diuresis, detumescence.

Rhubarb (Dahuang)

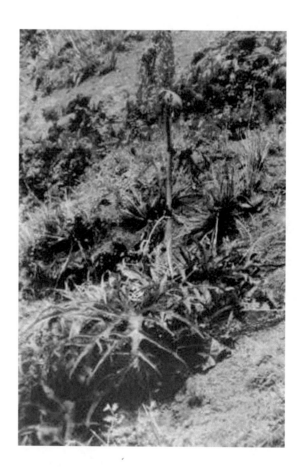

Chinese phonetic alphabet/pin yin: dà huáng
Chinese characters simplified/traditional:
大黄/大黃
Chinese nickname's alphabet (Nickname's
Chinese characters):
Jiangjun/ Huangliang/ Huoshen (将军/黄良/火参)
Latin: Rhei Radix et Rhizoma (Common name: Rhubarb)
Plant: *Rheum palmatum* L.(or *Rheum tanguticum* Maxim. ex Balf., *Rheum officinale* Baill.)

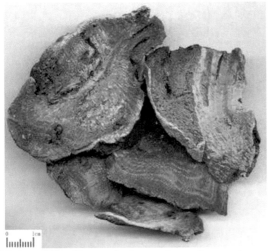

TCM prepared in ready-to-use forms (medicinal parts): it's dried root and rhizome which harvested in autumn.
Property and flavor: cold; bitter.

Main and collateral channels: spleen, stomach, large intestine, liver and pericardium meridians.
Administration and dosage: 3-15 g. It should not be decocted long for purgation (such as Rhubarb). Topical application in appropriate amount, ground into powder and apply to the locations of injuries.
Indication: constipation, abdominal pain, jaundice, bleeding from five sense organs or subcutaneous tissue, hematemesis, red eyes, sore throat, stranguria, amenrrhea, carbuncle sore, traumatic injuries and edema; external use for burn and scald.
It is key herb to treat constipation caused by heat.
Precaution and warning: use with caution in pregnant woman, or woman in menstrual period or lactation.
(The picture is only for learning and identification the herb; the specific use of the herb please consult the herbalist or health professionals)

Sodium Sulfate (Mangxiao)
Chinese phonetic alphabet/pin yin: máng xiāo
Chinese characters simplified/traditional:芒硝/芒硝
Chinese nickname's alphabet (Nickname's Chinese characters): Puxiao/ Tuxiao/ Penxiao (朴硝/土硝/盆硝)
Latin: Natrii Sulfas (Common name: Sodium Sulfate or Mirabilite)

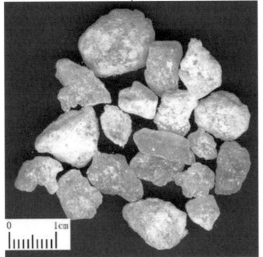

Mineral: main component $Na_2SO_4·10H_2O$
TCM prepared in ready-to-use forms (medicinal parts): it's cleaned mineral.
Property and flavor: cold; bitter, salty.
Main and collateral channels: stomach and large intestine meridians.
Administration and dosage: 6-12 g, add to prepared decoction, usually not decocted. Topical application in appropriate amount.

Indication: constipation, indigestion and abdominal pain; external use for mastitis and hemorrhoids.

It is key herb to treat constipation caused by dry and hard stool.

Precaution and warning: use with caution during pregnancy. Incompatible with Sulfur and Common Burreed Tuber.

(The picture is only for learning and identification the herb; the specific use of the herb please consult the herbalist or health professionals)

Aloes (Luhui)

Chinese phonetic alphabet/pin yin: lú huì
Chinese characters simplified/traditional:芦荟/蘆薈
Chinese nickname's alphabet (Nickname's Chinese characters): Nuhui/ Laowei(奴会/劳伟)
Latin: Aloe (Common name: Aloes)

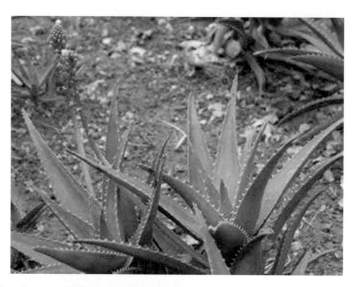

Plant: *Aloe vera* L. (or *Aloe ferox* Miller., *Aloe barbadensis* Miller.)

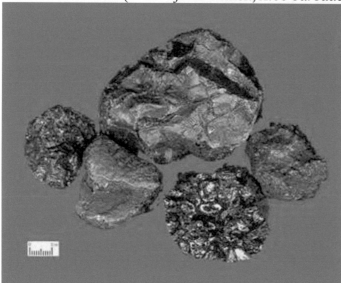

TCM prepared in ready-to-use forms (medicinal parts): it's dried extractor get form leaf juice. Property and flavor: cold; bitter. Main and collateral channels: liver, stomach and large intestine meridians.

Administration and dosage: 2-5 g, usually used in pills or powder. Topical application in appropriate amount, ground into powder and apply to the *pars affecta.*
Indication: constipation, infantile malnutrition and convulsion; external use to treat tinea, sore and scabies.

Precaution and warning: use with caution during pregnancy.

Attention: to protect the rare wild plant, please don't use the herb from wild plant.
(The picture is only for learning and identification the herb; the specific use of the herb please consult the herbalist or health professionals)

Senna Leaf (Fanxieye)

Chinese phonetic alphabet/ pin yin: fān xiè yè

Chinese characters simplified/traditional: 番泻叶/番瀉葉

Chinese nickname's alphabet (Nickname's Chinese characters): Zhannaye/ Paozhuye (旃那叶/泡竹叶)

Latin: Sennae Folium (Common name: Senna Leaf)

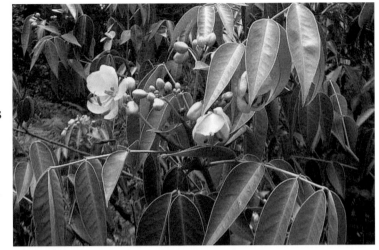

Plant: *Cassia angustifolia* Vahl. (or *Cassia acutifolia* Del.)

TCM prepared in ready-to-use forms (medicinal parts): it's dried leaf.

Property and flavor: cold; sweet, bitter.

Main and collateral channels: large intestine meridian.

Administration and dosage: 2-6 g, added when the decoction is nearly done, or soaked in boiling water.

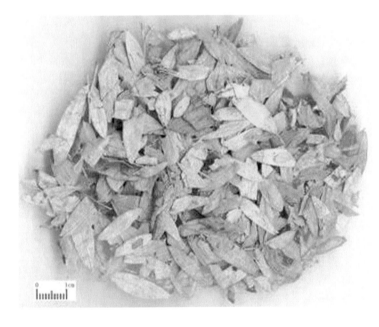

Indication: constipation, abdominal pain, edema, ventosity and stagnation.
It is commonly used in treating habitual constipation.
Precaution and warning: use with caution during pregnancy.
(The picture is only for learning and identification the herb; the specific use of the herb please consult the herbalist or health professionals)

Hemp Seed (Huomaren)

Chinese phonetic alphabet/pin yin: huǒ má rén

Chinese characters simplified/traditional:火麻仁/火麻仁

Chinese nickname's alphabet (Nickname's Chinese characters): Maziren/ Damazi(麻子仁/大麻子)

Latin: Cannabis Fructus (Common name: Hemp Seed)

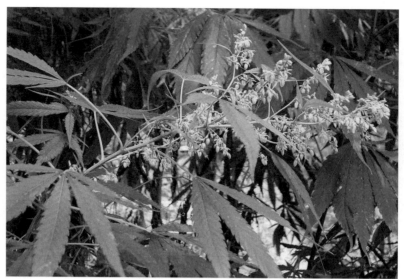

Plant: *Cannabis sativa* L.

TCM prepared in ready-to-use forms (medicinal parts): it's dried mature seed.
Property and flavor: neutral; sweet.
Main and collateral channels: spleen, stomach and large intestine meridians.
Administration and dosage: 10-15 g.
Indication: blood vacuity, liquid depletion and constipation.
It is taken as food in some part of China.
(The picture is only for learning and identification the herb; the specific use of the herb please consult the herbalist or health professionals)

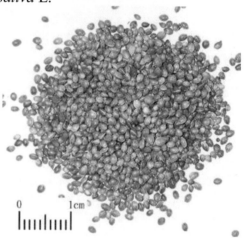

Chinese Dwarf Cherry Seed (Yuliren)

Chinese phonetic alphabet/pin yin: yù lǐ rén
Chinese characters simplified/traditional: 郁李仁/郁李仁
Chinese nickname's alphabet (Nickname's Chinese characters): Liren/ Yuli/ Shanmeizi(李仁/郁李/山梅子)
Latin: Pruni Semen (Common name: Chinese Dwarf Cherry Seed)

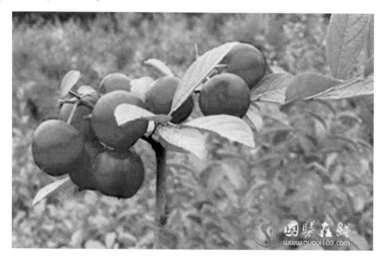

Plant: *Prunus humilis* Bunge. (or *Prunus japonica* Thunb., *Prunus pedunculata* Maxim.)

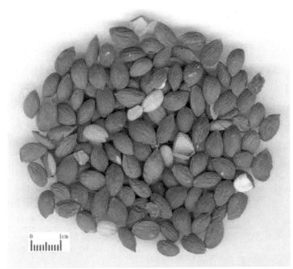

TCM prepared in ready-to-use forms (medicinal parts): it's dried mature seed.

Property and flavor: neutral; bitter, pungent and sweet.

Main and collateral channels: spleen, large intestine and small intestine meridians.

Administration and dosage: 6-10 g.

Indication: dyspepsia, abdominal distension, constipation, edema, indigestion, oliguria and tinea.

It is taken as food in some part of China.

Precaution and warning: use with caution during pregnancy.

(The picture is only for learning and identification the herb; the specific use of the herb please consult the herbalist or health professionals)

Gansui Root (Gansui)

Chinese phonetic alphabet/ pin yin: gān suì

Chinese characters simplified/traditional:甘遂/甘遂

Chinese nickname's alphabet (Nickname's Chinese characters): Zhutian/ Ganze(主田/甘泽)

Latin: Kansui Radix (Common name: Gansui Root)

Plant: *Euphorbia kansui* T. N. Liou ex S. B. Ho.

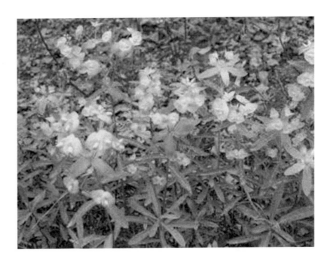

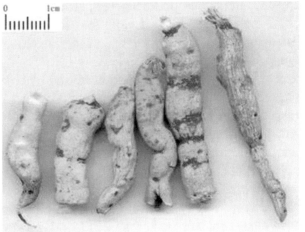

TCM prepared in ready-to-use forms (medicinal parts): it's dried root tuber which removed bark and harvested in spring or autumn.

Property and flavor: cold; bitter

Main and collateral channels: lung, kidney and large intestine meridians.

Administration and dosage: 0.5-1.5 g. usually used in pill or powder. External use in appropriate amount of unprocessed one.

Indication: edema, phlegm accumulation, cough with asthma, oliguria, sore, constipation and skin infection.

Precaution and warning: toxic. Contraindicated during pregnancy. Incompatible with Liquorice Root.

(The picture is only for learning and identification the herb; the specific use of the

herb please consult the herbalist or health professionals)

Croton Fruit (Badou)
Chinese phonetic alphabet/pin yin: bā dòu
Chinese characters simplified/traditional:巴豆/巴豆
Chinese nickname's alphabet (Nickname's Chinese characters): Jiangzi/ Mangzi(江子/芒子)
Latin: Crotonis Fructus (Common name: Croton Fruit)

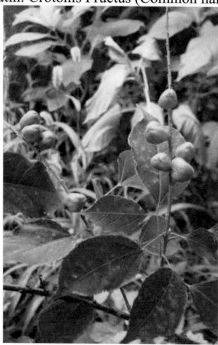

Plant: *Croton tiglium* L.

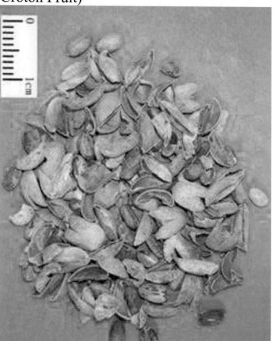

TCM prepared in ready-to-use forms (medicinal parts): it's dried mature seed.

Property and flavor: hot; pungent.
Main and collateral channels: stomach and large intestine meridians.
Administration and dosage: 0.1-0.3 g (defatted croton seed powder). Topical application in appropriate amount, ground into powder and apply to the *pars affecta,* or mashed and wrapped in cloth for rubbing the *pars affecta.*
Indication: constipation, edema, excessive phlegm; external use for sore, scarbies and tinea.
It is key herb to treat constipation caused by cold/chill (*Hanliang*).
Precaution and warning: highly toxic. Contraindicated during pregnancy. Incompatible with Pharbitis Seed.
Attachment: Defatted Croton Seed Powder: remove testa of the clean seed, pulverize into mud. Wrapped with paper then steam, squeezes deoiling, relapse several times until it is not sticky. Grinds it into powder then add starch and mix well to make its fatty oil contents between 18% and 20%.
(The picture is only for learning and identification the herb; the specific use of the herb please consult the herbalist or health professionals)

Peking Euphorbia Root (Jingdaji)

Chinese phonetic alphabet/pin yin: jīng dà jǐ
Chinese characters simplified/
traditional:京大戟/京大戟
Chinese nickname's alphabet
(Nickname's Chinese characters):
Xiamaxian/ DaJi(下马仙/大戟)
Latin: Euphorbiae Pekinensis Radix
(Common name: Peking Euphorbia Root)
Plant: *Euphorbia pekinensis* Rupr.

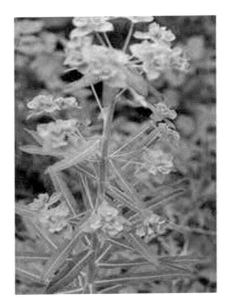

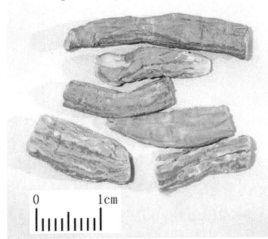

TCM prepared in ready-to-use
forms (medicinalparts): it's
dried root which harvested
in autumn or winter.
Property and flavor: cold; bitter.
Main and collateral channels: lung,
spleen and kidney meridians.

Administration and dosage: 1.5-3 g. Used in pills or powder, 1 g per time. Processed
with vinegar for oral administration. Topical application in appropriate amount,
unprocessed one is used.
Indication: edema, abdominal effusion, cough with asthma, oliguria, constipation,
sore and scrofula.
Precaution and warning: toxic. Contraindicated during pregnancy. Incompatible
with Liquorice Root.
Attention: to protect the rare wild plant, please don't use the herb from wild plant.
(The picture is only for learning and identification the herb; the specific use of the
herb please consult the herbalist or health professionals)

Knoxia Root (Hongdaji)

Chinese phonetic
alphabet/pin yin: hóng dà jǐ
Chinese characters
simplified/traditional:红大戟/
紅大戟
Chinese nickname's alphabet
(Nickname's Chinese
characters): Hongyaji/ Zidaji/
Guangdaji(红牙戟/紫大戟/广
大戟)
Latin: Knoxiae Radix
(Common name: Knoxia
Root or Red Euphorbia Root)

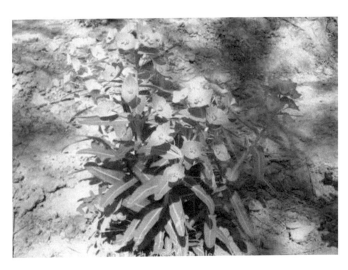

Plant: *Knoxia valerianoides* Thorel. et Pitard.

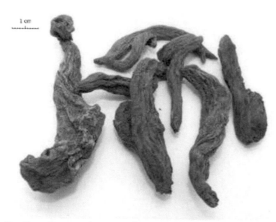

TCM prepared in ready-to-use forms (medicinal parts): it's dried root which harvested in autumn or winter.

Property and flavor: cold; bitter.

Main and collateral channels: lung, spleen and kidney meridians.

Administration and dosage: 1.5-3 g. Used in pills or powder, 1 g per time. Processed with vinegar for oral administration. Topical application in appropriate amount, unprocessed one is used.

Indication: edema, pleural effusion, coughs with asthma, anuria, constipation, carbuncle and scrofula.

Precaution and warning: slightly toxic. Contraindicated during pregnancy.

(The picture is only for learning and identification the herb; the specific use of the herb please consult the herbalist or health professionals)

Pharbitis Seed (Qianniuzi)

Chinese phonetic alphabet/pin yin: qiān niú zǐ

Chinese characters simplified/traditional:牵牛子/牽牛子

Chinese nickname's alphabet (Nickname's Chinese characters): Heichou/ Baichou/ Erchou/Labahuazi(黑丑/白丑/二丑/喇叭花子)

Latin: Pharbitidis Semen (Common name: Pharbitis Seed or Morning Glory Seed)

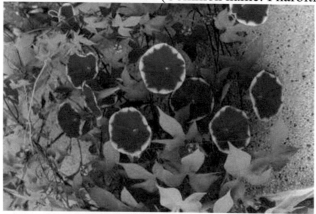

TCM prepared in ready-to-use forms (medicinal parts): it's dried ripe seed.

Property and flavor: cold; bitter.

Main and collateral channels: lung, kidney and large intestine meridians.

Administration and dosage: 3-6 g. Used in pills or powder, 1.5-3 g per time.

Indication: edema, anuria, constipation, cough, abdominal pain caused by ascaris or cestode.

Plant: *Pharbitis nil* (L.) Choisy. (or *Pharbitis pupurea* (L.) Voigt.)

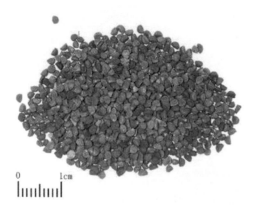

Precaution and warning: toxic. Contraindicated for pregnant woman. Incompatible with Croton Fruit and Defatted Croton Seed Powder.

(The picture is only for learning and identification the herb; the specific use of the herb please consult the herbalist or health professionals)

Lilac Daphne Flower Bud (Yuanhua)

Chinese phonetic alphabet/pin yin: yuán huā

Chinese characters simplified/traditional:芫花/芫花

Chinese nickname's alphabet (Nickname's Chinese characters): Chiyua/ Wanhua(赤芫/莞花)

Latin: Genkwa Flos (Common name: Lilac Daphne Flower Bud)

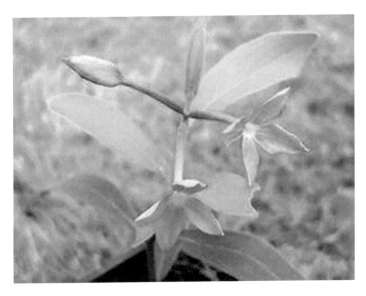

Plant: *Daphne genkwa* Sieb. et Zucc. TCM prepared in ready-to-use forms (medicinal parts): it's dried flower bud. Property and flavor: warm; bitter, pungent.

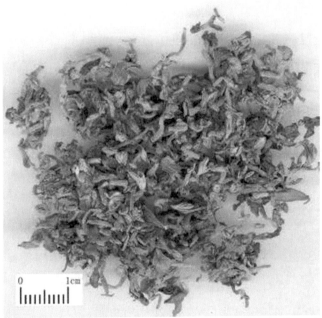

Main and collateral channels: lung, spleen and kidney meridians.
Administration and dosage: 1.5-3 g. Ground into powder for oral administration one (processed with vinegar) 0.6-0.9 g per time. Topical application in appropriate amount.

Indication: edema, hydrothorax, ascites, cough and wheezing and anuria; external use for tinea, scabies and chilblains.

Precaution and warning: toxic. Contraindicated for pregnant woman. Incompatible with Liquorice Root.

(The picture is only for learning and identification the herb; the specific use of the herb please consult the herbalist or health professionals)

Caper Euphorbia Seed (Qianjinzi)
Chinese phonetic alphabet/pin yin: qiān jīn zǐ
Chinese characters simplified/traditional:千金子/千金子
Chinese nickname's alphabet (Nickname's Chinese characters): Qianliangjin/ Xusuizi/ Lianbu(千两金/续随子/联步)
Latin: Euphorbiae Semen (Common name: Caper Euphorbia Seed or Moleplant Seed)

Plant: *Euphorbia lathyris* L.
TCM prepared in ready-to-use forms (medicinal parts): it's dried mature seed.
Property and flavor: warm; pungent.
Main and collateral channels: liver, kidney and large intestine meridians.

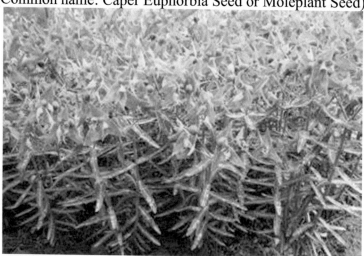

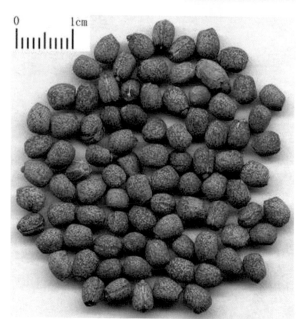

Administration and dosage: 1-2 g, removed testa and oil, usually used in pills or powder. Topical application in appropriate amount, mashed into paste for external use.
Indication: edema, excessive phlegm, abdominal distension, dyspepsia, anuria and constipation; external use for wart, scabies and tinea.

Precaution and warning: toxic. Contraindicated for pregnant woman.
Attachment: Caper Euphorbia Seed Powder: Rub off testa of clean seed, pulverize into mud. Wrapped with paper then steam, squeezes deoiling, relapse several times until it is not stick, grinds it into powder.
(The picture is only for learning and identification the herb; the specific use of the herb please consult the herbalist or health professionals)

Castor Seed (Bimazi)

Chinese phonetic alphabet/pin yin: bì má zǐ
Chinese characters simplified/traditional:蓖麻子/蓖麻子
Chinese nickname's alphabet (Nickname's Chinese characters): Bimaren/ Damazi/ Hongdamazi(蓖麻仁/大麻子/红大麻子)
Latin: Ricini Semen (Common name: Castor Seed or Castor Bean)

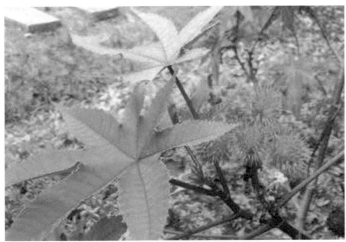

Plant: *Ricinus communis* L.

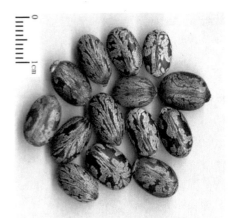

TCM prepared in ready-to-use forms (medicinal parts): it's dried mature seed.
Property and flavor: neutral; sweet, pungent.
Main and collateral channels: large intestine and lung meridians.
Administration and dosage: 2-5 g. Topical application in appropriate amount.
Indication: wart, pharyngitis, scrofula, constipation and cellulitis.
Precaution and warning: toxic.

(The picture is only for learning and identification the herb; the specific use of the herb please consult the herbalist or health professionals)

Pokeberry Root (Shanglu)

Chinese phonetic alphabet/pin yin: shāng lù
Chinese characters simplified/ traditional:商陆/商陸
Chinese nickname's alphabet (Nickname's Chinese characters): Danglu/ Shanluobo(当陆/山萝卜)
Latin: Phytolaccae Radix (Common name: Pokeberry Root)
Plant: *Phytolacca acinosa* Roxb. (or *Phytolacca americana* L.)

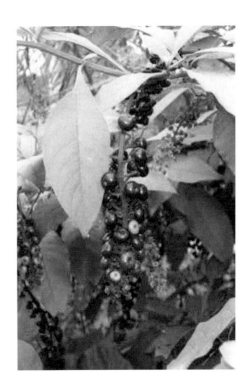

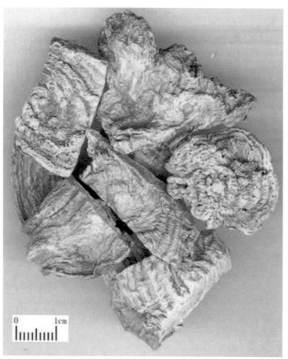

TCM prepared in ready-to-use forms (medicinal parts): it's dried root which harvested in winter.
Property and flavor: cold; bitter.
Main and collateral channels: lung, spleen, kidney and large intestine meridians.
Administration and dosage: 3-9 g. Topical application in appropriate amount. It can be decocted for fuming-washing therapy.
Indication: edema, ventosity, constipations, dysuria; external use for carbuncle sore.

Precaution and warning: toxic. Contraindicated for pregnant woman.
(The picture is only for learning and identification the herb, the specific use of the herb please consult the herbalist or health professionals)

Linseed (Yamazi)
Chinese phonetic alphabet/pin yin: yǎ má zǐ
Chinese characters simplified/traditional:亚麻子/亞麻子
Chinese nickname's alphabet (Nickname's Chinese characters): Humazi/ Bishihuma(胡麻子/壁虱胡麻)
Latin: Lini Semen (Common name: Linseed)

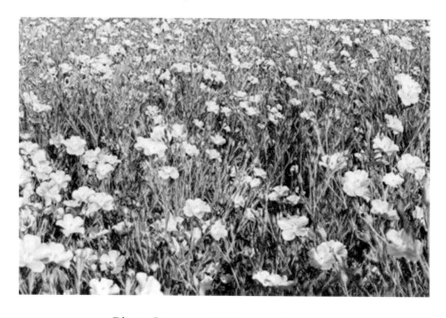

Plant: *Linum usitatissimum* L.

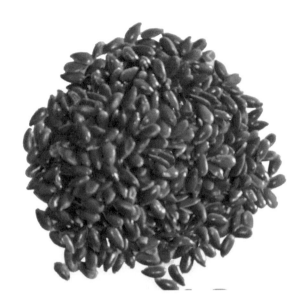

1 cm

TCM prepared in ready-to-use forms (medicinal parts): it's dried ripe seed.

Property and flavor: neutral; sweet.

Main and collateral channels: lung, kidney and large intestine meridians.

Administration and dosage: 9-15 g.

Indication: constipation caused by dryness, itch and hair loss.

Precaution and warning: contraindicated for patients with efflux diarrhea.

(The picture is only for learning and identification the herb; the specific use of the herb please consult the herbalist or health professionals)

Exsiccated Sodium Sulfate (Xuanmingfen)

Chinese phonetic alphabet/pin yin: xuán míng fěn

Chinese characters simplified/traditional:玄明粉/玄明粉

Chinese nickname's alphabet (Nickname's Chinese characters): Bailongfen(白龙粉)

Latin: Natrii Sulfas Exsiccatus (Common name: Exsiccated Sodium Sulfate)

Mineral: main component Na_2SO_4

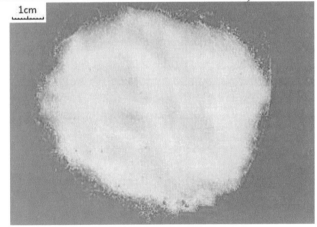

1cm

TCM prepared in ready-to-use forms (medicinal parts): it's cleaned mineral.

Property and flavor: cold; bitter, salty.

Main and collateral channels: stomach and large intestine meridians.

Administration and dosage: 3-9 g, dissolved in prepared decoction.Topical application in appropriate amount.

Indication: heat, constipation, distention and abdomenal pain; external use for swelling, sore, abscess and eryipelas.

Precaution and warning: contraindicated in pregnancy. Incompatible with Sulfur and Common Burreed Tuber.

(The picture is only for learning and identification the herb; the specific use of the herb please consult the herbalist or health professionals)

Raisin Tree Seed (Zhijuzi)

Chinese phonetic alphabet/pin yin: zhǐ jǔ zǐ
Chinese characters simplified/traditional: 枳椇子/枳椇子
Chinese nickname's alphabet (Nickname's Chinese characters): Mumi/ Guaizaozi (木蜜/拐枣子)
Latin: Hoveniae Fructus (Common name: Raisin Tree Seed or Hovenia Fruit)

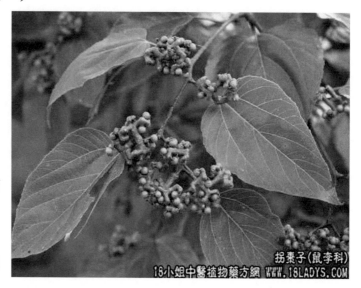

Plant: *Hovenia dulcis* Thunnb. (or *Hovenia acerba* Lindl., *Hovenia trichocarpa* Chun et Tsiang)

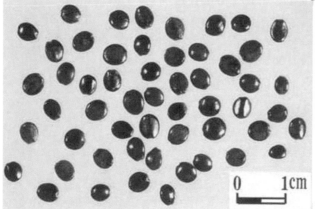

TCM prepared in ready-to-use forms (medicinal parts): it's dried fruit (with Inflorescence axis).
Property and flavor: neutral; sweet.
Main and collateral channels: stomach meridian.
Administration and dosage: 6-15 g.

Indication: irritability, thirst, vomiting, difficulty in urination and defecation; alleviate a hangover.
It is taken as food in some part of China.
(The picture is only for learning and identification the herb; the specific use of the herb please consult the herbalist or health professionals)

Qu Feng Shi Yao(祛风湿药)-antirheumatic herbs

Qu Feng Shi Yao is a kind of herbs which's the major functions are acesodyne, anti-inflammatory, antiallergic; some of them can sedate, and treat convulsion, rheumatic, arthralgia, apoplexy and tetanus.

Doubleteeth Pubescent Angelica Root (Duhuo)

Chinese phonetic alphabet/pin yin: dú huó
Chinese characters simplified/traditional:独活/獨活
Chinese nickname's alphabet (Nickname's Chinese characters): Changshengcao/ Duhua(长生草/独滑)

Latin: Angelicae Pubescentis Radix (Common name: Doubleteeth Pubescent Angelica Root)

Plant: *Angelica pubescens* Maxim.f. *biserrata* Shan. et Yuan.
TCM prepared in ready-to-use forms (medicinal parts): it's dried root which harvested in spring or autumn.

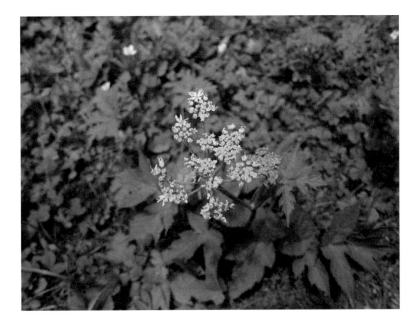

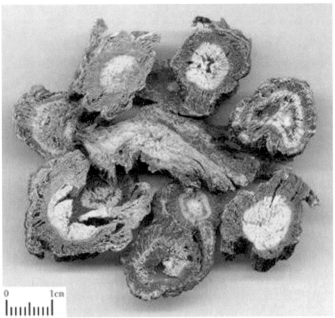

Property and flavor: mild warm; pungent, bitter.
Main and collateral channels: kidney and bladder meridians.
Administration and dosage: 3-10 g.

Indication: rheumatic, arthralgia, headache, pain in the loins and knee.
It is good at treating chronic painful *bi* disorder.
(The picture is only for learning and identification the herb; the specific use of the herb please consult the herbalist or health professionals)

Chinese Clematis Root (Weilingxian)
Chinese phonetic alphabet/pin yin: wēi líng xiān
Chinese characters simplified/traditional:威灵仙/威靈仙
Chinese nickname's alphabet (Nickname's Chinese characters): Lingxian/ Tiepatou(灵仙/铁耙头)
Latin: Clematidis Rhizoma et Radix (Common name: Chinese Clematis Root)

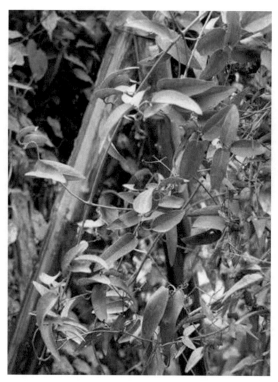

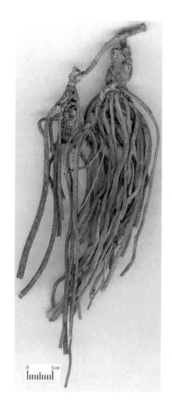

Plant: *Clematis chinensis* Osbeck. (or *Clematis hexapetala* Pall., *Clematis manshurica* Rupr.)

TCM prepared in ready-to-use forms (medicinal parts): it's dried root which harvested in autumn.

Property and flavor: warm; pungent, salty.

Main and collateral channels: bladder meridian.

Administration and dosage: 6-10 g.

Indication: painful *bi* disorder, rheumatic, arthralgia, numbness of limbs, spasm, hypertonicity of the sinew and vessels.

It is key herb to treat numbness or pain in limbs and spasm.

(The picture is only for learning and identification the herb; the specific use of the herb please consult the herbalist or health professionals)

Fourstamen Stephania Root (Fangji)

Chinese phonetic alphabet/pin yin: fáng jǐ
Chinese characters simplified/traditional:防己/防己
Chinese nickname's alphabet (Nickname's Chinese characters): Mufangji(木防己)
Latin: Stephaniae Tetrandrae Radix (Common name: Fourstamen Stephania Root)

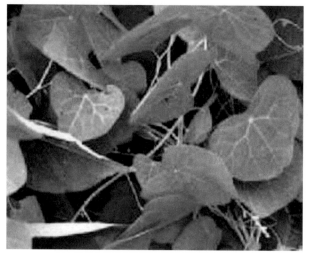

Plant: *Stephania tetrandra* S. Moore.

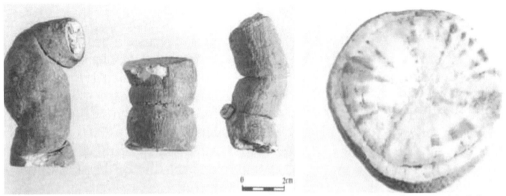

TCM prepared in ready-to-use forms (medicinal parts): it's dried root which harvested in spring or autumn.

Property and flavor: cold; bitter.

Main and collateral channels: bladder and lung meridians.

Administration and dosage: 5-10 g.

Indication: painful *bi* disorder, edema, beriberi, dysuria, eczema, sore and toxin. It is key herb to treat joint pain and swelling.

(The picture is only for learning and identification the herb; the specific use of the herb please consult the herbalist or health professionals)

Largeleaf Gentian Root (Qinjiao)

Chinese phonetic alphabet/pin yin: qín jiāo

Chinese characters simplified/traditional:秦艽/秦艽

Chinese nickname's alphabet (Nickname's Chinese characters): Dayelongdan/Qinzhua(大叶龙胆/秦爪)

Latin: Gentianae Macrophyllae Radix (Common name: Largeleaf Gentian Root)

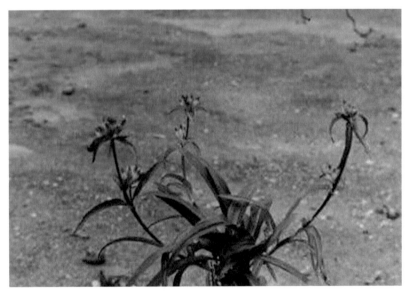

Plant: *Gentiana macrophylla* Pall. (or *Gentiana straminea* Maxim.,*Gentiana crassicaulis* Duthie ex Burk., *Gentiana dahurica* Fisch.)

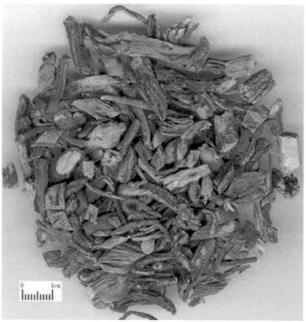

TCM prepared in ready-to-use forms (medicinal parts): it's dried root which harvested in spring or autumn.
Property and flavor: neutral; bitter, pungent.
Main and collateral channels: stomach, liver and gallbladder meridians.
Administration and dosage: 3-10 g.

Indication: painful *bi* disorder, rheumatism, arthralgia, hypertonicity of sinew and vessels, spasm, joint pain, fever, jaundice and infantile malnutrition.
It is commonly used in treating painful *bi* disorder with the heat.
(The picture is only for learning and identification the herb; the specific use of the herb please consult the herbalist or health professionals)

Paniculate Swallowwort Root (Xuchangqing)
Chinese phonetic alphabet/pin yin: xú cháng qīng
Chinese characters simplified/traditional:徐长卿/徐長卿
Chinese nickname's alphabet (Nickname's Chinese characters): Liaodiaozhu/Xiaoyaozhu(寮刁竹/逍遥竹)
Latin: Cynanchi Paniculati Radix et Rhizoma (Common name: Paniculate Swallowwort Root)

Plant:
Cynanchum paniculatum (Bunge.) Kitagawa.
TCM prepared in ready-to-use forms (medicinal parts): it's dried root and rhizome which harvested in autumn.

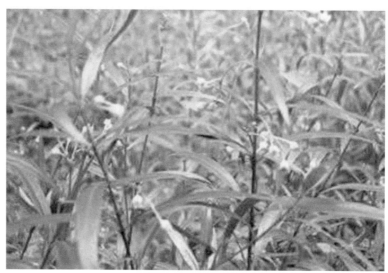

Property and flavor: warm; pungent.
Main and collateral channels: liver and stomach meridians.
Administration and dosage: 3-12 g, added when the decoction is nearly done.
Indication: painful *bi* disorder, ventosity, stomachache, toothache, loins pain, traumatic injury, urticaria, eczema and rubella.

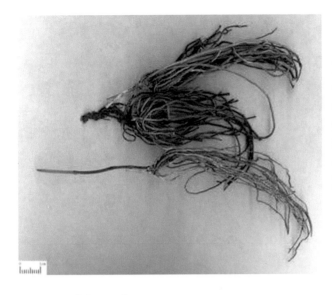

It is key herb to treat rheumatic arthritis and pain in limbs.
(The picture is only for learning and identification the herb; the specific use of the herb please consult the herbalist or health professionals)

Papaya (Mugua)

Chinese phonetic alphabet/pin yin: mù guā
Chinese characters simplified/traditional:木瓜/木瓜
Chinese nickname's alphabet (Nickname's Chinese characters): Mingzha/ Tiejiaoli(楔楂/铁脚梨)
Latin: Chaenomelis Fructus (Common name: Papaya or Common Floweringqince Fruit)

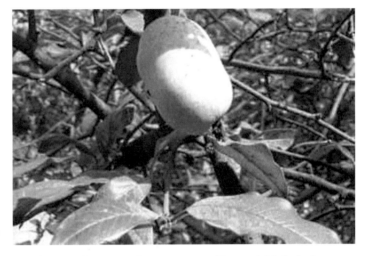

Plant: *Chaenomeles speciosa* (Sweet) Nakai. (or *Chaenomeles sinensis* (Thouin.) Koehne.)

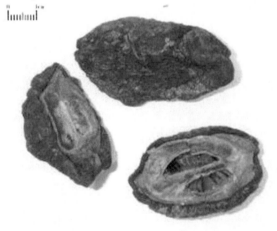

TCM prepared in ready-to-use forms (medicinal parts): it's dried nearly ripe fruit.
Property and flavor: warm; acidity.
Main and collateral channels: liver and spleen meridians.
Administration and dosage: 6-9 g.
Indication: joint pain, vomiting, beriberi and edema, tinea, pain and hypertonicity of the sinews.
It is key herb to treat numbness or pain in limbs, spasm, diarrhea and vomiting.

It is taken as food in some part of China.
(The picture is only for learning and identification the herb; the specific use of the herb please consult the herbalist or health professionals)

Chinese Taxillus Herb (Sangjisheng)

Chinese phonetic alphabet/ pin yin: sāng jì shēng

Chinese characters simplified/traditional:桑寄生/桑寄生

Chinese nickname's alphabet (Nickname's Chinese characters): Guangjisheng/ Sangshangjisheng (广寄生/桑上寄生)

Latin: Taxilli Herba (Common name: Chinese Taxillus Herb or Parasitic Loranthus Herb)

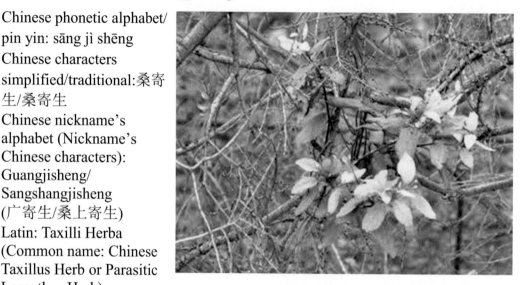

Plant: *Taxillus chinensis* (DC.) Danser. (or *Taxillus sutchuenensis* (Lecomte.) Danser.)

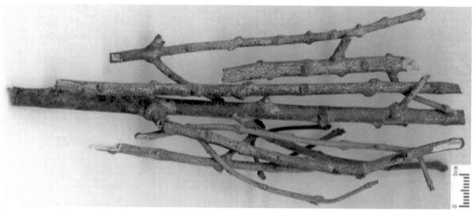

TCM prepared in ready-to-use forms (medicinal parts): it's dried stem and branch with leaves which harvested in winter.

Property and flavor: neutral; bitter, sweet.

Main and collateral channels: liver and kidney meridians.

Administration and dosage: 9-15 g.

Indication: painful *bi* disorder, soreness and weakness of waist and knees, muscles weakness, messive hemorrhage after pregnancy, fetal irritability, dizziness, vertigo and hypertension.

It is key herb to treat soreness and weakness of waist and knees, threatened abortion. (The picture is only for learning and identification the herb; the specific use of the herb please consult the herbalist or health professionals)

Slenderstyle Acanthopanax Bark (Wujiapi)

Chinese phonetic alphabet/pin yin: wǔ jiā pí

Chinese characters simplified/traditional:五加皮/五加皮

Chinese nickname's alphabet (Nickname's Chinese characters): Nanwujiapi/ Wugupi(南五加皮/五谷皮)

Latin: Acanthopanacis Cortex (Common name: Slenderstyle Acanthopanax Bark)

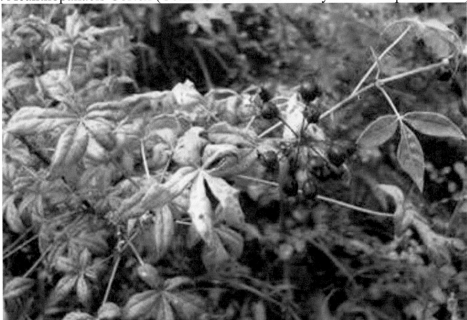

Plant: *Acanthopanax gracilistylus* W. W. Smith.

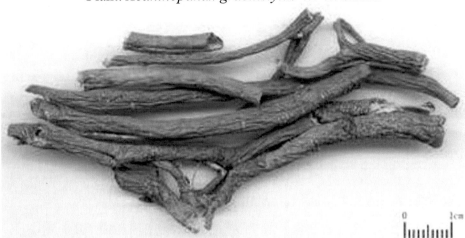

TCM prepared in ready-to-use forms (medicinal parts): it's dried root bark which harvested in summer or winter.

Property and flavor: warm; pungent and bitter.

Main and collateral channels: liver and kidney meridians.

Administration and dosage: 5-10 g.

Indication: weakness, body virtual fatigue, edema and tinea pedis.

It is key herb to treat rheumatic arthralgia, weakness of the muscles and bones .

(The picture is only for learning and identification the herb; the specific use of the herb please consult the herbalist or health professionals)

Long-nosed Pit Viper (Qishe)

Chinese phonetic alphabet/pin yin: qí shé

Chinese characters simplified/traditional:蕲蛇/蕲蛇

Chinese nickname's alphabet (Nickname's Chinese characters): Baihuashe/Wubushe (白花蛇/五步蛇)

Latin: Agkistrodon (Common name: Long-nosed Pit Viper)

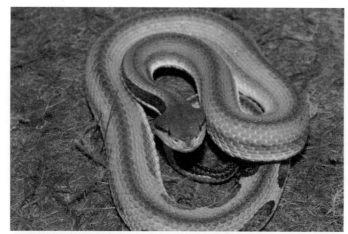

Animal: *Agkisrodon acutus* (Güenther).

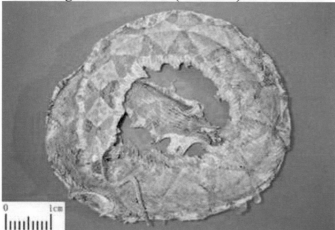

TCM prepared in ready-to-use forms (medicinal parts): it's dried the whole body except the entrails/visceral. Property and flavor: warm; sweet, salty. Main and collateral channels: liver meridian. Administration and dosage: 3-9 g. Ground into powder for oral administration: 1-1.5 g per time, 2-3 times a day. Indication: numbness spasm, stroke, hemiplegia, apoplexy, convulsive spasm, tetanus, leprosy. It is commonly used in treating convulsive, spasm and hemiplegic. **Precaution and warning**: toxic.

Attention: To protect the rare wild animals, please don't use it from wild animal. (The picture is only for learning and identification the herb; the specific use of the herb please consult the herbalist or health professionals)

Coin-like White-banded Snake (Jinqianbaihuashe)

Chinese phonetic alphabet/pin yin: jīn qián bái huā shé
Chinese characters simplified/traditional:金钱白花蛇/金錢白花蛇
Chinese nickname's alphabet (Nickname's Chinese characters): Yinhuanshe(银环蛇)
Latin: Bungarus Parvus (Common name: Coin-like White-banded Snake)

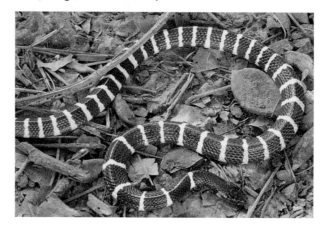

Animal: *Bungarus multicinctus* Blyth.

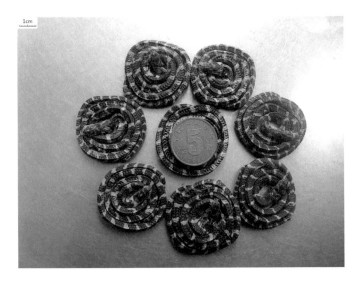

TCM prepared in ready-to-use forms (medicinal parts): it's dried body.
Property and flavor: warm; sweet, salty.
Main and collateral channels: liver meridian.
Administration and dosage: 2-5 g. It can be ground into powder for oral administration: 1-1.5 g.
Indication: numbness, spasm, hemiplegia, convulsions, tetanus, leprosy, scabies and tinea.

Precaution and warning: toxic.
Attention: to protect the rare wild animal, don't use it from wild animal.
(The picture is only for learning and identification the herb; the specific use of the herb please consult the herbalist or health professionals)

Siegesbeckia Herb (Xixiancao)

Chinese phonetic alphabet/pin yin: xī xiān cǎo
Chinese characters simplified/traditional:豨莶草/豨薟草
Chinese nickname's alphabet (Nickname's Chinese characters): Zhucao/ Feizhucao/ Zhanbuzha(珠草/肥猪草/粘不扎)
Latin: Siegesbeckiae Herba (Common name: Siegesbeckia Herb)

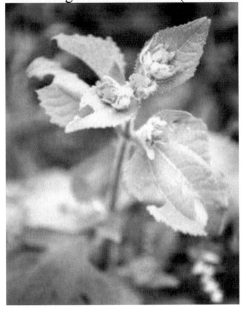

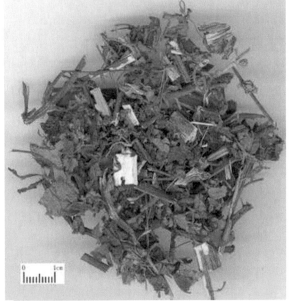

Plant: *Siegesbeckia orientalis* L. (or *Siegesbeckia pubescens* Makino., *Siegesbeckia glabrescens* Makino.)

TCM prepared in ready-to-use forms (medicinal parts): it's dried above-ground part which harvested in summer or autumn.

Property and flavor: cold; bitter, pungent.
Main and collateral channels: liver and kidney meridians.
Administration and dosage: 9-12 g.

Indication: painful *bi* disorder, muscle weakness, soreness and weakness of waist and knees, paralysis, hemiplegia, rubella, eczema and numbness of limbs.
(The picture is only for learning and identification the herb; the specific use of the herb please consult the herbalist or health professionals)

Chinese Starjasmine Stem (Luoshiteng)

Chinese phonetic alphabet/pin yin: luò shí téng
Chinese characters simplified/traditional: 络石藤/絡石藤
Chinese nickname's alphabet (Nickname's Chinese characters): Shiling/ Mingshi/ Yunhua(石鲮/明石/云花)
Latin: Trachelospermi Caulis et Folium (Common name: Chinese Starjasmine Stem)

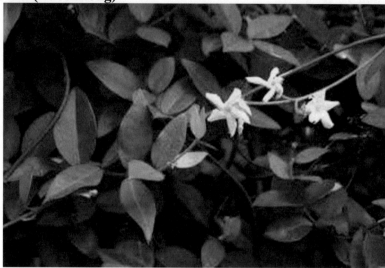
Plant: *Trachelospermum jasminoides* (Lindl.) Lem.

TCM prepared in ready-to-use forms (medicinal parts): it's dried lianoid stem with leaf which harvested in winter.
Property and flavor: mild cold; bitter.
Main and collateral channels: heart, liver and kidney meridians.
Administration and dosage: 6-12 g.
Indication: fever, spastic muscles, waist and knee pain, sore throat, swollen, traumatic injury.

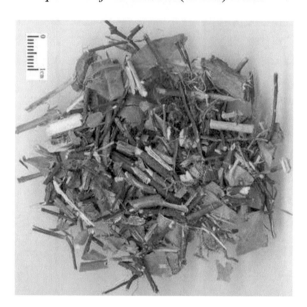

(The picture is only for learning and identification the herb; the specific use of the herb please consult the herbalist or health professionals)

Mulberry Twig (Sangzhi)

Chinese phonetic alphabet/pin yin: sāng zhī
Chinese characters simplified/traditional:桑枝/桑枝
Chinese nickname's alphabet (Nickname's Chinese characters): Sangtiao(桑条)
Latin: Mori Ramulus (Common name: Mulberry Twig)

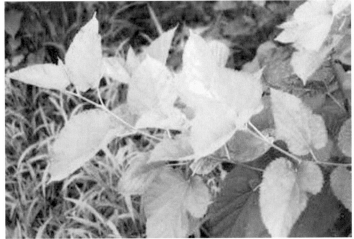

Plant: *Morus alba* L.

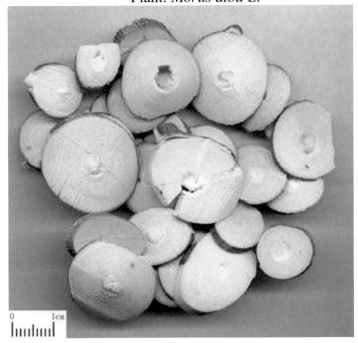

TCM prepared in ready-to-use forms (medicinal parts): it's dried twig which harvested from March to July.

Property and flavor: neutral; mild bitter. Main and collateral channels: liver meridian.

Administration and dosage: 9-15 g. Indication: rheumatic, arthralgia, joint pain and numbness of limbs.

(The picture is only for learning and identification the herb; the specific use of the herb please consult the herbalist or health professionals)

Kadsura Pepper Stem (Haifengteng)

Chinese phonetic alphabet/pin yin: hǎi fēng téng
Chinese characters simplified/traditional: 海风藤/海風藤
Chinese nickname's alphabet (Nickname's Chinese characters): Payanxiang/Bayanxiang(爬岩香/巴岩香)
Latin: Piperis Kadsurae Caulis (Common name: Kadsura Pepper Stem)

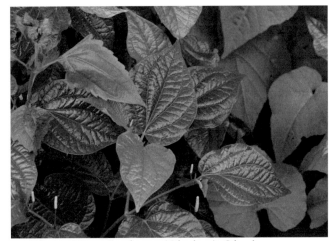

Plant: *Piper kadsura* (Choisy.) Ohwi.

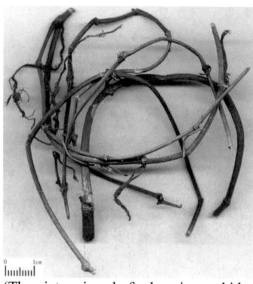

TCM prepared in ready-to-use forms (medicinal parts): it's dried cane which harvested in summer or autumn.
Property and flavor: mild warm; bitter, pungent.
Main and collateral channels: liver meridian.
Administration and dosage: 6-12 g.
Indication: rheumatic and arthralgia, limb pain, tendons spasm, flex unfavorable and hypertonicity of the sinew and vessels.
It is commonly used in treating joint pain and stiffness.

(The picture is only for learning and identification the herb; the specific use of the herb please consult the herbalist or health professionals)

Common Monkshood Mother Root (Chuanwu)

Chinese phonetic alphabet/pin yin: chuān wū
Chinese characters simplified/traditional:
川乌/川烏
Chinese nickname's alphabet (Nickname's Chinese characters): E'erhua/ Tiehua/ Chuanwutou(鹅儿花/ 铁花/川乌头)
Latin: Aconiti Radix (Common name: Common Monkshood Mother Root or Monkshood Grows in Sichuan Province)

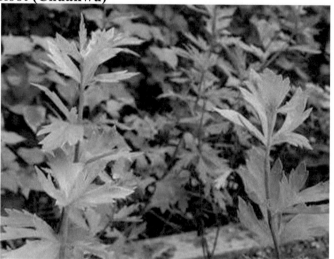

Plant: *Aconitum carmichaeli* Debx.

TCM prepared in ready-to-use forms (medicinal parts): it's dried root tuber which harvested in June, July or August.
Property and flavor: hot; pungent, bitter.
Main and collateral channels: heart, liver, kidney and spleen meridians.
Administration and dosage: generally, use the prepared one.
Indication: rheumatic, arthralgia, joint pain, cold pain in the heart; anaesthesia.

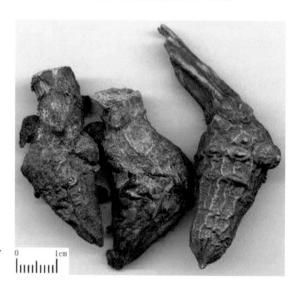

It is commonly used in treating rheumatic arthritis and rheumatoid arthritis.

Precaution and warning: highly toxic. Unprocessed one should be used cautiously for oral administration. Contraindicated for pregnant woman. Incompatible with Pinellia Tuber, Snakegourd Fruit, Snakegourd seed, Snakegourd peel, Snakegourd Root, Tendrilleaf Fritillary Bulb, Thunberg Fritillary Bulb, Ussuri Fritillary Bulb, Sinkiang Fritillary Bulb, Hubei Fritillary Bulb, Japanese Ampelopsis Root and Common Bletilla Tuber.

(The picture is only for learning and identification the herb; the specific use of the herb please consult the herbalist or health professionals)

Prepared Common Monkshood Mother Root (Zhichuanwu)

Chinese phonetic alphabet/
pin yin: zhì chuān wū

Chinese characters simplified/
traditional:制川乌/制川烏

Latin: Aconiti Radix Cocta
(Common name: Prepared
Common Monkshood Mother
Root)

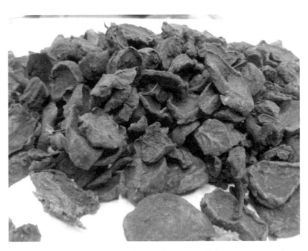

Drug: it is processed Common
Monkshood Mother Root
TCM prepared in ready-to-use
forms (medicinal parts)

Processing: chop Common
Monkshood Mother Root in
suitable size. Soak it in water
until there is no dry core, then boil in the water until there is no white core and testes becomes slight numb, take out, 60% dry in air, cut into slices and dry thoroughly.

Property and flavor: hot; pungent, bitter.

Main and collateral channels: heart, liver, kidney and spleen meridians.

Administration and dosage: 1.5-3 g. It should be decocted first for a long time.

Indication: joint pain, pain in heart and abdomen, colic pain; it can be applied for anesthesia.

Precaution and warning: toxic. Contraindicated for pregnant woman. Incompatible with Pinellia Tuber, Snakegourd Fruit, Snakegourd seed, Snakegourd peel, Snakegourd Root, Tendrilleaf Fritilary Bulb, Thunberg Fritillary Bulb, Ussuri Fritillary Bulb, Sinkiang Fritillary Bulb, Hubei Fritillary Bulb, Japanese Ampelopsis Root and Common Bletilla Tuber.

(The picture is only for learning and identification the herb; the specific use of the herb please consult the herbalist or health professionals)

Tripterygium Herb (Leigongteng)

Chinese phonetic alphabet/pin yin: léi gōng téng

Chinese characters simplified/traditional:雷公藤/雷公藤

Chinese nickname's alphabet (Nickname's Chinese characters): Huangtenggen/ Huangtengcao/Hongzigen(黄藤根/黄藤草/红紫根)

Latin: Tripterygii Radix et Rhizoma (Common name: Tripterygium Herb)

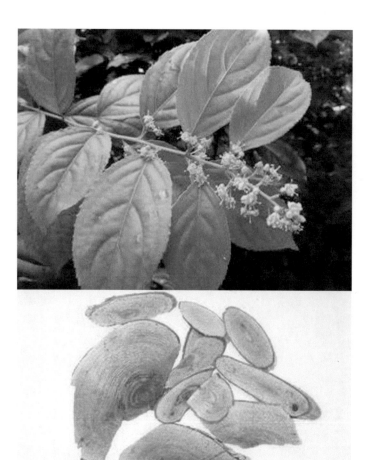

Plant: *Tripterygium wilfordii* Hook. f.
TCM prepared in ready-to-use forms (medicinal parts): it's dried root and stem removed bark which harvested in autumn.
Property and flavor: cool; bitter, pungent.
Main and collateral channels: liver and kidney meridians.
Administration and dosage: 10-25 g (expel the root bark); It should be decocted first.
Or used in powder or capsule: 0.5-1.5. Topical application in appropriate amount.

Indication: rheumatic, arthralgia, skin itch and leprosy; promote blood circulation; dredge collaterals; reduce swelling and relieve pain.
It is commonly used in treating rheumatic arthritis and rheumatoid arthritis.
Precaution and warning: highly toxic. Contraindicated for pregnant woman.
(The picture is only for learning and identification the herb; the specific use of the herb please consult the herbalist or health professionals)

Chinese Silkvine Root-bark (Xiangjiapi)
Chinese phonetic alphabet/pin yin:xiāng jiā pí
Chinese characters simplified/traditional:香加皮/香加皮
Chinese nickname's alphabet (Nickname's Chinese characters): Beiwujiapi/

Yangtaoshao/ Gangliupi(北五加皮/羊桃梢/杠柳皮)
Latin: Periplocae Cortex
(Common name: Chinese Silkvine Root-bark)
Plant: *Periploca sepium* Bge.
TCM prepared in ready-to-use forms (medicinal parts): it's dried root bark which harvested in spring or autumn.

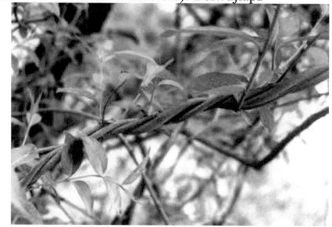

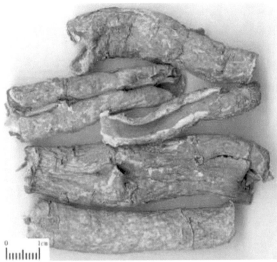

Property and flavor: warm; pungent, bitter.
Main and collateral channels: liver, kidney and heart meridians.
Administration and dosage: 3-6 g.
Indication: soreness and weakness of waist and knees, palpitations, shortness of breath, edema of lower limbs.
Precaution and warning: toxic. Avoid over-dosage.

(The picture is only for learning and identification the herb; the specific use of the herb please consult the herbalist or health professionals)

Obscured Homalomena Rhizome (Qiannianjian)

Chinese phonetic alphabet/pin yin: qiān nián jiàn
Chinese characters simplified/traditional: 千年健/千年健
Chinese nickname's alphabet (Nickname's Chinese characters): Yibaozhen/ Qiannianjian(一包针/ 千年见)
Latin: Homalomenae Rhizoma (Common name: Obscured Homalomena Rhizome)

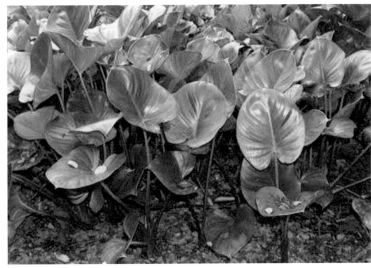

Plant: *Homalomena occulta* (Lour.) Schott.

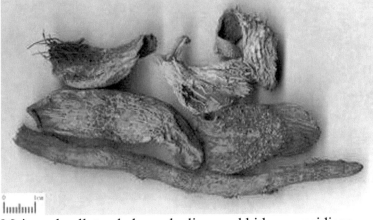

TCM prepared in ready-to-use forms (medicinal parts): it's dried rhizome which harvested in spring or autumn.
Property and flavor: warm; bitter, pungent.

Main and collateral channels: liver and kidney meridians.

Administration and dosage: 5-10 g.

Indication: rheumatic, arthralgia, cold waist and knee pain, numbness of limb and spasm.

(The picture is only for learning and identification the herb; the specific use of the herb please consult the herbalist or health professionals)

Harlequin Glorybower Leaf and Twig (Chouwutong)

Chinese phonetic alphabet/pin yin: chòu wú tóng

Chinese characters simplified/traditional: 臭梧桐/臭梧桐

Chinese nickname's alphabet (Nickname's Chinese characters): Choutong/ Bajiaowutong/ Haizhouchangshan (臭桐/八角梧桐/ 海州常山)

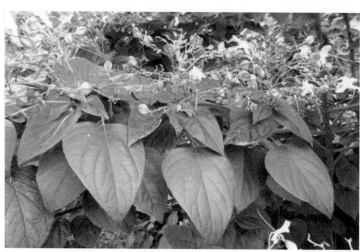

Plant: *Clerodendrum trichotomum* Thunb.

Latin: Clerodendri Trichotomi Folium et Ramulus (Common name: Harlequin Glorybower Leaf and Twig)

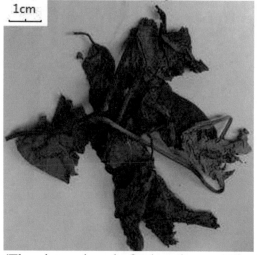

TCM prepared in ready-to-use forms (medicinal parts): it's dried leaf and twig which harvested in summer.

Property and flavor: cold; bitter, pungent.

Main and collateral channels: liver meridian.

Administration and dosage: 5-15 g. The herb should not be boiled for a long time.

Topical application in appropriate amount, its decoction can be used for wash therapy.

Indication: rheumatism and numbness of limbs; reduce blood pressure; external used for eczema.

(The picture is only for learning and identification the herb; the specific use of the herb please consult the herbalist or health professionals)

Orientvine Stem (Qingfengteng)

Chinese phonetic alphabet/pin yin: qīng fēng téng

Chinese characters simplified/traditional:青风藤/青風藤

Chinese nickname's alphabet (Nickname's Chinese characters): Qingteng/ Xunfengteng/ Dianfangji/ Daqingmuxiang(青藤/寻风藤/滇防己/大青木香)

Latin: Sinomenii Caulis (Common name: Orientvine Stem)

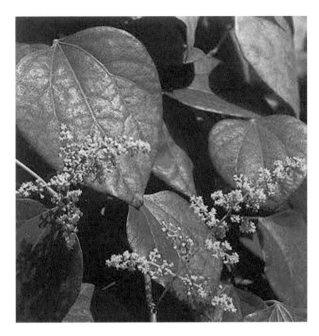

Plant: *Sinomenium acutum* (Thunb.) Rehd. et Wils. (or *Sinomenium acutum* (Thunb.) Rehd. et Wils. var. *cinereum* Rehd. et Wils.)

TCM prepared in ready-to-use forms (medicinal parts): it's dried lianoid stem which harvested in autumn or winter.

Property and flavor: neutral; bitter, pungent.

Main and collateral channels: liver and spleen meridians.

Administration and dosage: 6-12 g.

Indication: painful *bi* disorder, swelling of joints, paralysis and itching. (The picture is only for learning and identification the herb; the specific use of the herb please consult the herbalist or health professionals)

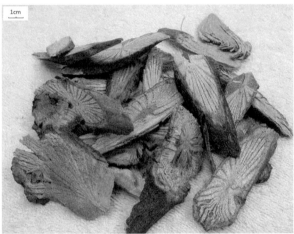

Luffa Vegetable Sponge (Sigualuo)

Chinese phonetic alphabet/ pin yin: sī guā luò
Chinese characters simplified/ traditional:丝瓜络/絲瓜絡
Chinese nickname's alphabet (Nickname's Chinese characters): Siguawang/ Siguake/ Gualuo(丝瓜网/丝瓜壳/瓜络)
Latin: Luffae Fructus Retinervus (Common name: Luffa Vegetable Sponge or Loofah Vegetable Sponge)
Plant: *Luffa cylindrica* (L.) Roem.

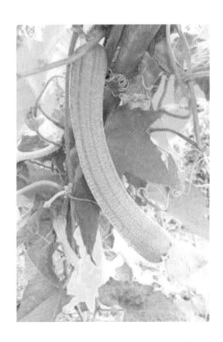

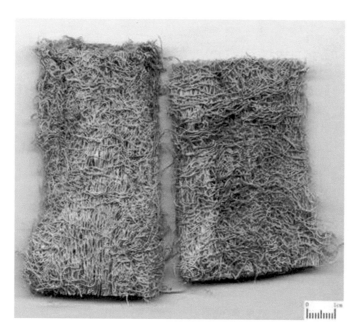

TCM prepared in ready-to-use forms (medicinal parts): it's dried ripe fruit collaterals/ vascular bundles.
Property and flavor: neutral; sweet.
Main and collateral channels: lung, stomach and liver meridians.
Administration and dosage: 5-12 g.
Indication: rheumatism, arthralgia, spasm, agalactia and acute mastitis; lactagogue.

(The picture is only for learning and identification the herb; the specific use of the herb please consult the herbalist or health professionals)

Common Clubmoss Herb (Shenjincao)

Chinese phonetic alphabet/pin yin: shēn jīn cǎo
Chinese characters simplified/traditional:伸筋草/伸筋草
Chinese nickname's alphabet (Nickname's Chinese characters): Shisong/ Shizicao/ Niuweicai(石松/狮子草/牛尾菜)
Latin: Lycopodii Herba (Common name: Common Clubmoss Herb)

TCM prepared in ready-to-use forms (medicinal parts): it's dried whole herb which harvested in summer or autumn.
Property and flavor: warm; mild bitter, pungent.
Main and collateral channels: liver, spleen and kidney meridians.
Administration and dosage: 3-12 g.

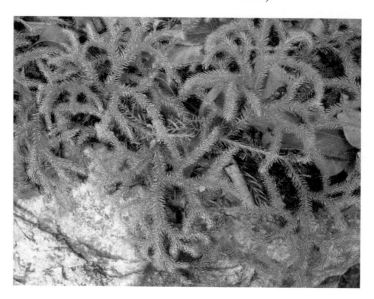

Plant: *Lycopodium japonicum* Thunb.

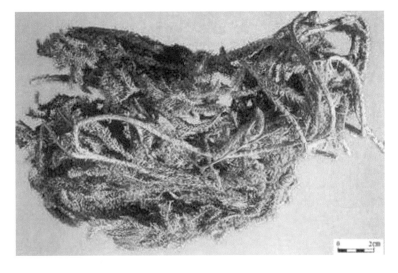

Indication: joint pain, poor flexion and extension. (The picture is only for learning and identification the herb; the specific use of the herb please consult the herbalist or health professionals)

Pyrola Herb (Luxiancao)

Chinese phonetic alphabet/pin yin: lù xián cǎo

Chinese characters simplified/traditional:鹿衔草/鹿銜草

Chinese nickname's alphabet (Nickname's Chinese characters): Luticao/ Xiaoqinwangcao/ Poxuedan(鹿蹄草/小秦王草/破血丹)

Latin: Pyrolae Herba (Common name: Pyrola Herb)

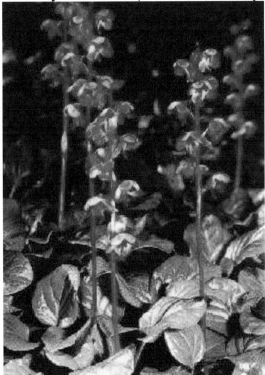

Plant: *Pyrola calliantha* H. Andres. (or *Pyrola decorata* H. Andres.)

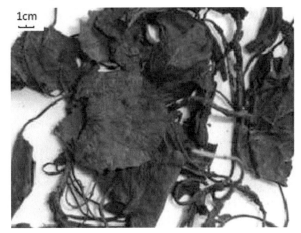

TCM prepared in ready-to-use forms (medicinal parts): it's dried whole herb which harvested in November or December.

Property and flavor: warm; sweet, bitter.

Main and collateral channels: liver and kidney meridians.

Administration and dosage: 9-15 g.

Indication: painful *bi* disorder, weakness in loins and knees, menorrhagia and chronic cough.

(The picture is only for learning and identification the herb; the specific use of the herb please consult the herbalist or health professionals)

Black-tail Snake (Wushaoshe)

Chinese phonetic alphabet/pin yin: wū shāo shé

Chinese characters simplified/traditional: 乌梢蛇/烏梢蛇

Chinese nickname's alphabet (Nickname's Chinese characters): Wushe/ Wufengshe (乌蛇/乌风蛇)

Latin: Zaocys (Common name: Black-tail Snake)

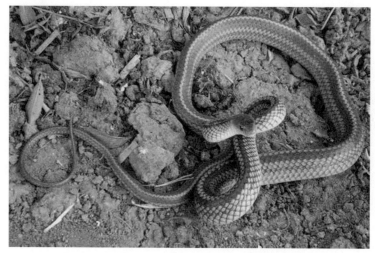
Animal: *Zoacys dhumnades* (Cantor.)

TCM prepared in ready-to-use forms (medicinal parts): it's dried the whole body except the entrails/visceral get in summer or autumn.

Property and flavor: neutral; sweet.

Main and collateral channels: liver meridian.

Administration and dosage: 6-12 g.

Indication: numbness, spasm, stroke hemiplegia, apoplexy, convulsion, tetanus, leprosy, mange, scrofula, scabies and tinea.

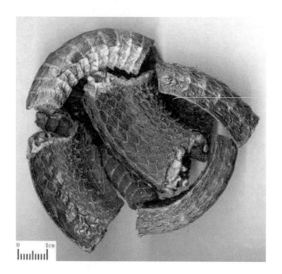

It is taken as food in some part of China.

Attention:

to protect the rare wild animals, please don't use it from wild animal.

(The picture is only for learning and identification the herb; the specific use of the herb please consult the herbalist or health professionals)

Beautiful Sweetgum Fruit (Lulutong)

Chinese phonetic alphabet/pin yin: lù lù tōng

Chinese characters simplified/traditional:路路通/路路通

Chinese nickname's alphabet (Nickname's Chinese characters): Fengxiangguo/ Jiukongzi/ Langmu(枫香果/九孔子/狼目)

Latin: Liquidambaris Fructus (Common name: Beautiful Sweetgum Fruit)

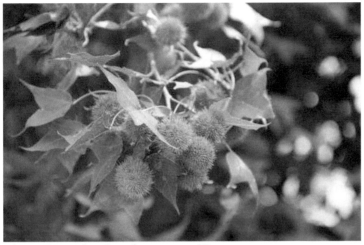

Plant: *Liquidambar formosana* Hance.

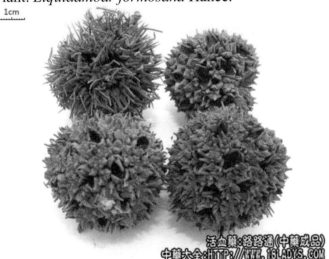

1cm

活血藥:路路通(中藥成品)
中藥大全:HTTP://WWW.16LADYS.COM

TCM prepared in ready-to-use forms (medicinal parts): it's dried mature infructescence.
Property and flavor: neutral; bitter.
Main and collateral channels: liver and kidney meridians.
Administration and dosage: 5-10 g.
Indication: arthralgia, joint pain, numbness, spasm, edema, swelling and amenorrhea; lactagogue.
(The picture is only for learning and identification the herb; the specific use of the herb please consult the herbalist or health professionals)

Nippon Yam Rhizome (Chuanshanlong)

Chinese phonetic alphabet/ pin yin: chuān shān lóng
Chinese characters simplified/ traditional:穿山龙/穿山龍
Chinese nickname's alphabet (Nickname's Chinese characters): Chuandilong/ Jinganggu(穿地龙/金刚骨)
Latin: Dioscoreae Nipponicae Rhizoma (Common name: Nippon Yam Rhizome or Japanese Yam Rhizome)
Plant: *Dioscorea nipponica* Makino.

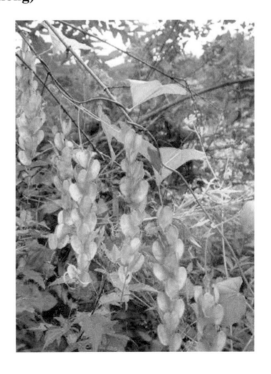

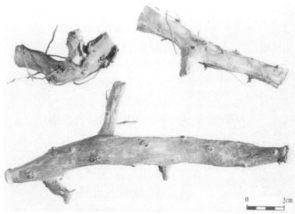

TCM prepared in ready-to-use forms (medicinal parts): it's dried rhizome which harvested in spring or autumn.
Property and flavor: warm; bitter, sweet.
Main and collateral channels: lung, liver and kidney meridians.
Administration and dosage: 9-15 g; or used in wine or liquor preparation.

Indication: joint sprain, lumbago and leg pain, numbness and pain, traumatic injuries, phlegm and cough.
Precaution and warning: it may lead to allergic reaction.
(The picture is only for learning and identification the herb; the specific use of the herb please consult the herbalist or health professionals)

Short-pedicel Aconite Root (Xueshangyizhihao)
Chinese phonetic alphabet/pin yin: xuě shàng yì zhī hāo
Chinese characters simplified/traditional:雪上一枝蒿/雪上一支蒿
Chinese nickname's alphabet (Nickname's Chinese characters): Tiebangchui/Sanzhuanban(铁棒槌/三转半)
Latin: Aconiti Brachypodi Radix (Common name: Short-pedicel Aconite Root or Short-pedicel Monkshood Root)

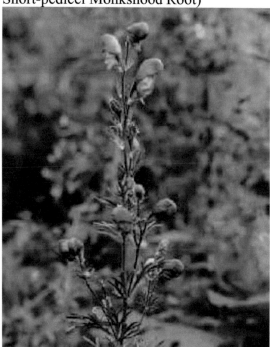
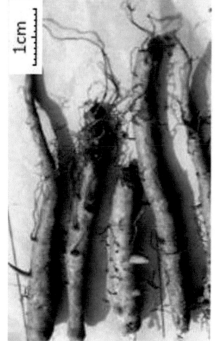

Plant: *Aconitum brachypodum* Diels. (or *Aconitum szechenyianum* Gay.)
TCM prepared in ready-to-use forms (medicinal parts): it's dried tuber root which harvested in summer.
Property and flavor: warm; bitter, pungent.
Main and collateral channels: liver meridian.
Administration and dosage: less than 0.02g for oral administration. Generally, for external use, topical application in appropriate amount. Soaked it in wine or alcohol

for days, then rubbed on the *pars affecta*.

Indication: traumatic injury, rheumatic, arthralgia, sore throat, snake bites. It is good at easing the pain.

Precaution and warning: highly toxin, Contraindicated during pregnancy. Incompatible with Pinellia Tuber, Snakegourd Fruit, Snakegourd seed, Snakegourd peel, Snakegourd Root, Tendrilleaf Fritillary Bulb, Thunberg Fritillary Bulb, Ussuri Fritillary Bulb, Sinkiang Fritillary Bulb, Hubei Fritillary Bulb, Japanese Ampelopsis Root and Common Bletilla Tuber.

(The picture is only for learning and identification the herb; the specific use of the herb please consult the herbalist or health professionals)

Silkworm Sand (Cansha)

Chinese phonetic alphabet/pin yin: cán shā

Chinese characters simplified/traditional:蚕砂/蠶沙

Chinese nickname's alphabet (Nickname's Chinese characters): Canshi/ Wancansha/ Yuancansha(蚕屎/晚蚕砂/原蚕砂)

Latin: Bombycis Faeces seu Bombycis Excrementum (Common name: Silkworm Sand or Silkworm Excrement)

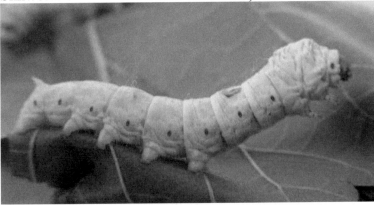

Animal: *Bombyx mori* Linnaeus.

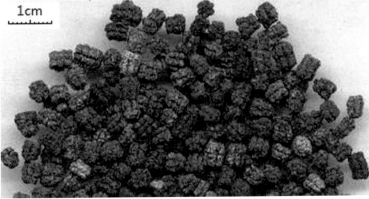

TCM prepared in ready-to-use forms (medicinal parts): it's dried excreta of silkworm.

Property and flavor: warm; pungent, sweet.

Main and collateral channels: stomach, spleen and liver meridians.

Administration and dosage: 15-40 g.

Indication: paralysis, numbness, rubella itching, abdominal pain, diarrhea, amenorrhea, metrorrhagia and eczema.

(The picture is only for learning and identification the herb; the specific use of the herb please consult the herbalist or health professionals)

Shinyleaf Prickyash Root (Liangmianzhen)

Chinese phonetic alphabet/pin yin: liǎng miàn zhēn

Chinese characters simplified/traditional:两面针/兩面針

Chinese nickname's alphabet (Nickname's Chinese characters): Rudijinniu/ Shuangmianci(入地金牛/双面刺)

Latin: Zanthoxyli Radix (Common name: Shinyleaf Prickyash Root or Nitidine)

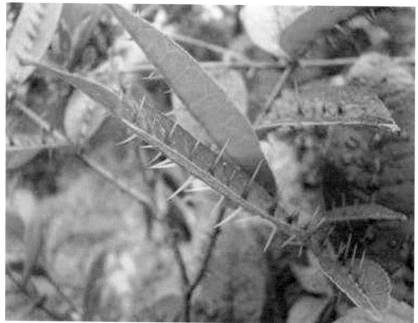

Plant: *Zanthoxylum nitidum* (Roxb.) DC.

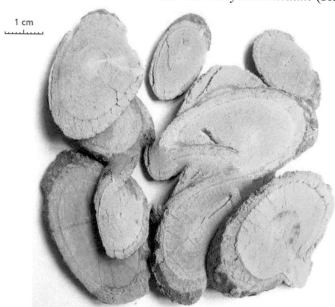

1 cm

TCM prepared in ready-to-use forms (medicinal parts): it's dried root which harvested all year round.
Property and flavor: neutral; bitter, pungent.
Main and collateral channels: liver and stomach meridians.
Administration and dosage: 5-10 g. Topical application in appropriate amount, ground into powder for applyment or decocted for bathing.

Indication: painful *bi* disorder, traumatic injuries, stomachache, toothache and bite wound of viper; external use for bums and scald.
Precaution and warning: slightly toxic. Over-dosage is inadvisable, avoid taken with sour tastes food.
(The picture is only for learning and identification the herb; the specific use of the herb please consult the herbalist or health professionals)

Kusnezoff Monkshood Root (Caowu)
Chinese phonetic alphabet/pin yin: cǎo wū
Chinese characters simplified/traditional:草乌/草烏
Chinese nickname's alphabet (Nickname's Chinese characters): Wutou/ Dubaicao/ Yaoyanghao(乌头/独白草/药羊蒿)
Latin: Aconiti Kusnezoffii Radix (Common name: Kusnezoff Monkshood Root)

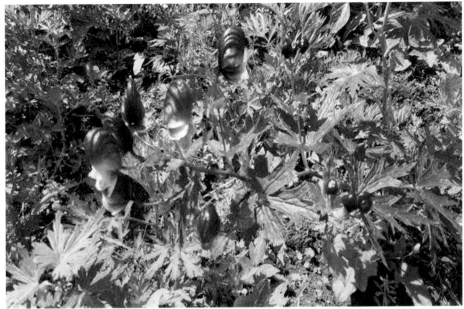

Plant: *Aconitum kusnezoffii* Reichb.

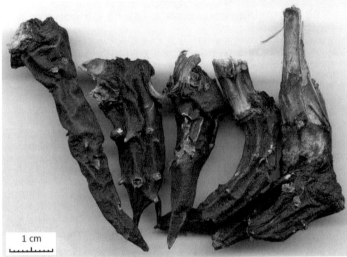

1 cm

TCM prepared in ready-to-use forms (medicinal parts): it's dried tuber root which harvested in autumn.

Property and flavor: hot; pungent and bitter.

Main and collateral channels: heart, liver, kidney and spleen meridians.

Administration and dosage: it is prepared before application, generally.

Indication: joint pain, chest and abdominal pain caused by chill (*Fenghan*) cold; sedative.

Precaution and warning: highly toxic. Unprepared one should be used cautiously for oral administration. Contraindicated for pregnant woman. Incompatible with Pinellia Tuber, Snakegourd Fruit, Snakegourd seed, Snakegourd peel, Snakegourd Root, Tendrilleaf Fritilary Bulb, Thunberg Fritillary Bulb, Ussuri Fritillary Bulb, Sinkiang Fritillary Bulb, Hubei Fritillary Bulb, Japanese Ampelopsis Root and Common Bletilla Tuber.

(The picture is only for learning and identification the herb; the specific use of the herb please consult the herbalist or health professionals)

Prepared Kusnezoff Monkshood Root (Zhicaowu)
Chinese phonetic alphabet/pin yin: zhì cǎo wū
Chinese characters simplified/traditional:制草乌/制草烏
Latin: Aconiti Kusnezoffii Radix Cocta (Common name: Prepared Kusnezoff Monkshood Root)
Drug: it is processed Kusnezoff Monkshood Root (plant: see Kusnezoff Monkshood Root)

TCM prepared in ready-to-use forms (medicinal parts) Processing: chop Kusnezoff Monkshood Root in suitable size. Soak it in water until there is no dry core, then boil in the water until there is no white core and testes becomes slight numb, dry in air appropriately, cut into slices, dry thoroughly.

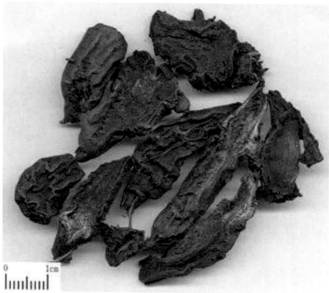

Administration and dosage: 1.5-3 g. It should be decocted first for a long time.
Indication: joint pain, pain in heart and abdomen, colic pain; it can be applied for anesthesia.

Precaution and warning: toxic. Contraindicated for pregnant woman. Incompatible with Pinellia Tuber, Snakegourd Fruit, Snakegourd seed, Snakegourd peel, Snakegourd Root, Tendrilleaf Fritilary Bulb, Thunberg Fritillary Bulb, Ussuri Fritillary Bulb, Sinkiang Fritillary Bulb, Hubei Fritillary Bulb, Japanese Ampelopsis Root and Common Bletilla Tuber.

(The picture is only for learning and identification the herb; the specific use of the herb please consult the herbalist or health professionals)

Radde Anemone Rhizome (Liangtoujian)
Chinese phonetic alphabet/pin yin: liǎng tóu jiān
Chinese characters simplified/traditional:两头尖/兩頭尖
Chinese nickname's alphabet (Nickname's Chinese characters): Zhujiexiangfu/Caowuhui(竹节香附/草乌喙)
Latin: Anemones Raddeanae Rhizoma (Common name: Radde Anemone Rhizome)

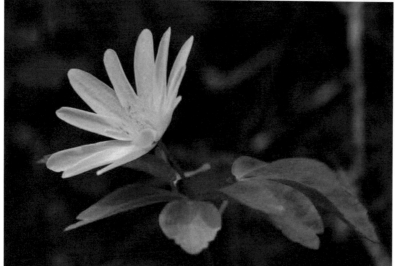

Plant: *Anemone raddeana* Regel.
TCM prepared in ready-to-use forms (medicinal parts): it's dried rhizome which harvested in summer.

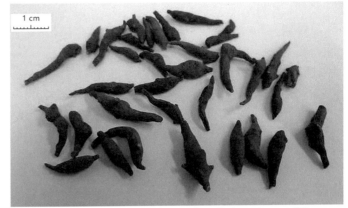

Property and flavor: hot; pungent.
Main and collateral channels: spleen meridian.
Administration and dosage: 1-3 g. Topical application in appropriate amount.

Indication: painful *bi* disorder, limbs spasm, bone and joint pain, diabrotic swelling and abscess.
Precaution and warning: toxic. Contraindicated during pregnancy.
(The picture is only for learning and identification the herb; the specific use of the herb please consult the herbalist or health professionals)

Belladonna Herb (Dianqiecao)
Chinese phonetic alphabet/ pin yin: diān qié cǎo
Chinese characters simplified/ traditional:颠茄草/顛茄草
Chinese nickname's alphabet (Nickname's Chinese characters): Meinvchao/ Bieladuonacao/ Dianqie(美女草/别拉多娜草/颠茄)
Latin: Belladonnae Herba (Common name: Belladonna Herb)
Plant: *Atropa belladonna* L.

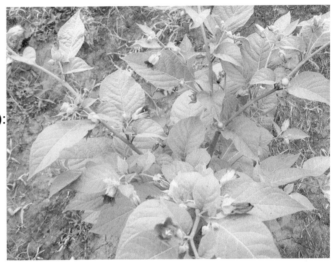

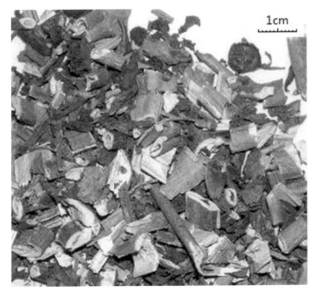

TCM prepared in ready-to-use forms (medicinal parts): it's dried whole herb which harvested from flowering to fruiting.
Property and flavor: cold; sweet.
Main and collateral channels: liver and kidney meridians.
Administration and dosage: 6-12 g.
Indication: excessive gastric acid, pain caused by gastric spasm, night sweating and excessive bronchial secretion; anticholinergic.
Precaution and warning: contraindicated in patients with glaucoma.

(The picture is only for learning and identification the herb; the specific use of the herb please consult the herbalist or health professionals)

Decumbent Corydalis Rhizome (Xiatianwu)

Chinese phonetic alphabet/pin yin: xià tiān wú
Chinese characters simplified/traditional: 夏天无/夏天無
Chinese nickname's alphabet (Nickname's Chinese characters): Fushengzijin/ Yilijindan/ Luoshuizhu(伏生紫菫/一粒金丹/落水珠)

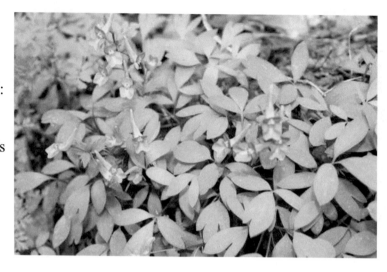

Latin: Corydalis Decumbentis Rhizoma (Common name: Decumbent Corydalis Rhizome)
Plant: *Corydalis decumbens* (Thunb.) Pers.

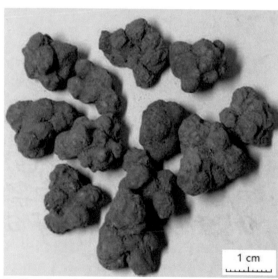

1 cm

TCM prepared in ready-to-use forms (medicinal parts): it's dried tuber which harvested in spring.
Property and flavor: warm; bitter, mild pungent.
Main and collateral channels: liver meridian.
Administration and dosage: 6-12 g, ground into powder for 3 times oral administration.

Indication: hemiplegic, headache, traumatic injuries, painful *bi* disorder, lower back and leg pain.
(The picture is only for learning and identification the herb; the specific use of the herb please consult the herbalist or health professionals)

Entada Seed (Ketengzi)

Chinese phonetic alphabet/pin yin: kē téng zǐ
Chinese characters simplified/traditional:榼藤子/榼藤子
Chinese nickname's alphabet (Nickname's Chinese characters): Xiangdou/ Yanjingdou(象豆/眼镜豆)
Latin: Entadae Semen (Common name: Entada Seed)

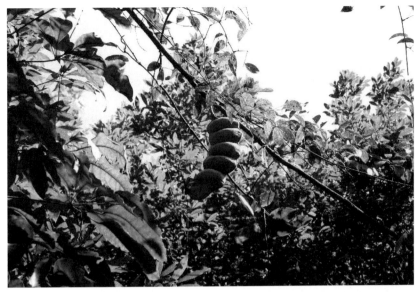

Plant: *Entada phaseoloides* (Linn.) Merr. TCM prepared in ready-to-use forms (medicinal parts): it's dried ripe seed. Property and flavor: cool; mild bitter.

Main and collateral channels: liver, spleen, stomach and kidney meridians.
Administration and dosage: 10-15 g.
Indication: deficiency of blood, pale complexion, lack of strength of limbs, pain in the epigastria and abdomen, indigestion, joints pain, frigidity and jaundice.

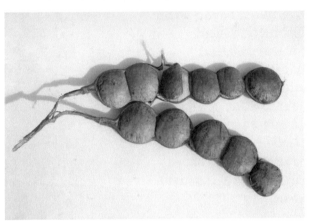

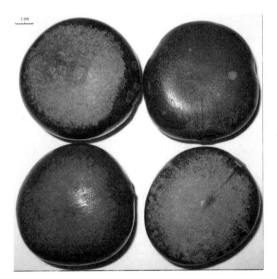

Precaution and warning: slightly toxic. Unprocessed administration is inadvisable.
Attachment: its processing: stir-bake until cooked, remove the peel.
(The picture is only for learning and identification the herb; the specific use of the herb please consult the herbalist or health professionals)

Shortscape Fleabane Herb (Dengzhanhua)
Chinese phonetic alphabet/pin yin: dēng zhǎn huā
Chinese characters simplified/traditional:灯盏花/燈盞花
Chinese nickname's alphabet (Nickname's Chinese characters): Dengzhanxixin(灯盏细辛)
Latin: Erigerontis Herba (Common name: Shortscape Fleabane Herb)

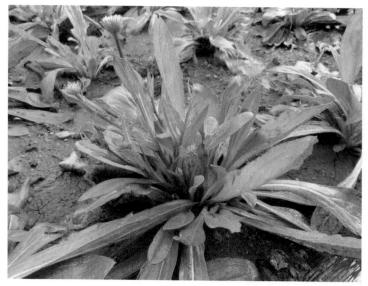

Plant: *Erigeron breviscapus* (Vant.) Hand.-Mazz.
TCM prepared in ready-to-use forms (medicinal parts): it's dried whole grass which harvested in summer or autumn.

Property and flavor: warm; mild bitter, pungent.
Main and collateral channels: liver and heart meridians.
Administration and dosage: 9-15 g, used in decoction or ground into powder added to steaming egg. Topical application in appropriate amount.

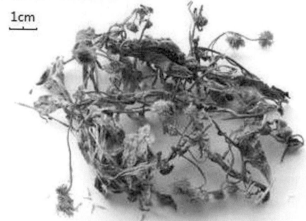

1cm

Indication: hemiplegia, heart pain, headache, painful *bi* disorders, toothache and traumatic and injuries.
(The picture is only for learning and identification the herb; the specific use of the herb please consult the herbalist or health professionals)

Common Heron's Bill Herb (Laoguancao)

Chinese phonetic alphabet/pin yin: lāo guān cǎo
Chinese characters simplified/traditional:老鹳草/老鸛草
Chinese nickname's alphabet (Nickname's Chinese characters): Laoguanzui/Laoyazui(老鹳嘴/老鸦嘴)
Latin: Erodii Herba seu Geranii Herba (Common name: Common Heron's Bill Herb or Wilford Granesbill Herb)

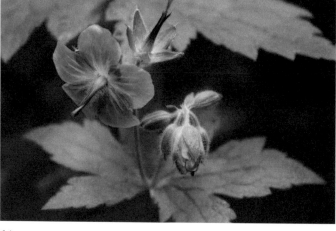

Plant: *Erodium stephanianum* Willd. (or *Geranium wilfordii* Maxim., *Geranium carolinianum* L.)

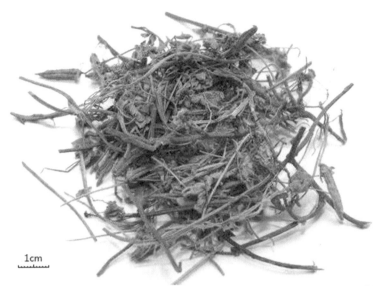

TCM prepared in ready-to-use forms (medicinal parts): it's dried whole herb which harvested in summer or autumn. Property and flavor: neutral; bitter, pungent.

Main and collateral channels: liver, kidney and spleen meridians.
Administration and dosage: 9-15 g.
Indication: numbness, spasm, sore pain in sinew and bone, painful *bi* disorder, diarrhea and dysentery.
(The picture is only for learning and identification the herb; the specific use of the herb please consult the herbalist or health professionals)

Obtuseleaf Erycibe Stem (Dinggongteng)
Chinese phonetic alphabet/pin yin: dīng gōng téng
Chinese characters simplified/traditional:丁公藤/丁公藤
Chinese nickname's alphabet (Nickname's Chinese characters) :Malazi/ Baogongteng(麻辣子/包公藤)
Latin: Erycibes Caulis (Common name: Obtuseleaf Erycibe Stem)

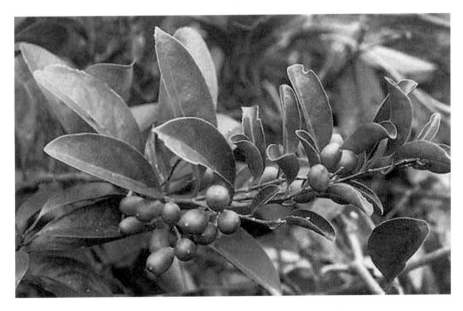

Plant: *Erycibe obtusfolia* Benth. (or *Erycibe schmidtii* Craib.)

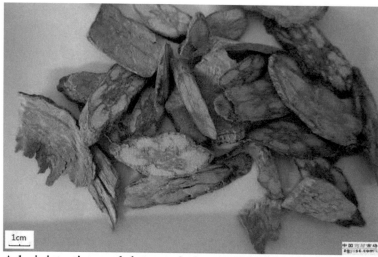

TCM prepared in ready-to-use forms (medicinal parts): it's dried lianoid stem which harvested all year round.
Property and flavor: warm; pungent.
Main and collateral channels: liver, spleen and stomach meridians.

Administration and dosage: 3-6 g, used in wine or liquor preparation for oral administration or for topical application.

Indication: painful *bi* disorder, hemiphlegia, traumatic injuries, swelling and pain.

Precaution and warning: slightly toxic. This is drastic diaphoretic medicine and should be used with caution in person who is weak constitution. Contraindicated for pregnant woman.

(The picture is only for learning and identification the herb; the specific use of the herb please consult the herbalist or health professionals)

Ginkgo Leaf (Yinxingye)

Chinese phonetic alphabet/pin yin: yín xìng yè
Chinese characters simplified/traditional:银杏叶/銀杏葉
Chinese nickname's alphabet (Nickname's Chinese characters): Baiguoye/ Gongsunshuiye(白果叶/ 公孙树叶)
Latin: Ginkgo Folium (Common name: Ginkgo Leaf)

Plant: *Ginkgo biloba* L.

TCM prepared in ready-to-use forms (medicinal parts): it's dried leaf which harvested in autumn.
Property and flavor: neutral; sweet, bitter and astringent.
Main and collateral channels: heart and lung meridians.
Administration and dosage: 9-12 g.
Indication: heart pain, hemiplegic, cough, wheezing and hyperlipoidemia.

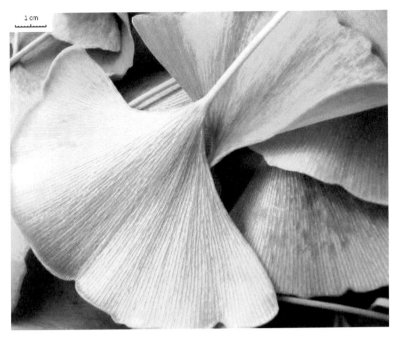

Difengpi Bark (Difengpi)

Chinese phonetic alphabet/pin yin: dì fēng pí

Chinese characters simplified/traditional:地枫皮/地楓皮

Chinese nickname's alphabet (Nickname's Chinese characters): Zhuidifeng/ Zuandifeng(追地风/钻地风)

Latin: Illicii Cortex (Common name: Difengpi Bark)

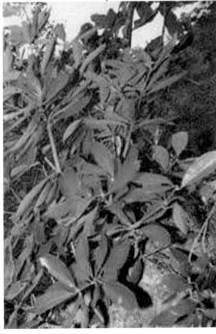

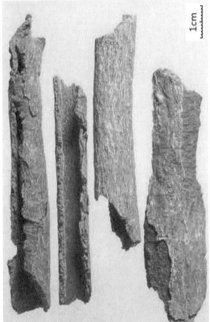

Plant: *Illicium difengpi* K. I. B. et K. I. M.

TCM prepared in ready-to-use forms (medicinal parts): it's dried stem bark which harvested in autumn.

Property and flavor: warm; mild pungent, astringent.

Main and collateral channels: bladder and kidney meridians.

Administration and dosage: 6-9 g.

Indication: arthralgia, lumbago by overstrain and injury.

Precaution and warning: slightly toxic.

Attention: to protect the rare wild plant, please don't use the herb from wild plant. (The picture is only for learning and identification the herb; the specific use of the herb please consult the herbalist or health professionals)

Honeysuckle Stem (Rendongteng)

Chinese phonetic alphabet/pin yin: rěn dōng téng
Chinese characters simplified/traditional:忍冬藤/忍冬藤
Chinese nickname's alphabet (Nickname's Chinese characters): Dabili/ Shuiyangteng/ Qianjinteng(大薜荔/水杨藤/千金藤)

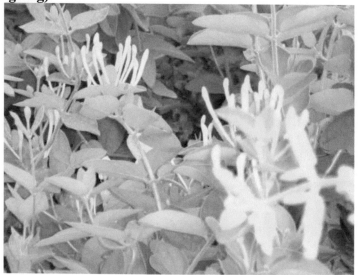

Latin: Lonicerae Japonicae Caulis (Common name:Honeysuckle Stem)
Plant: *Lonicera japonica* Thunb.

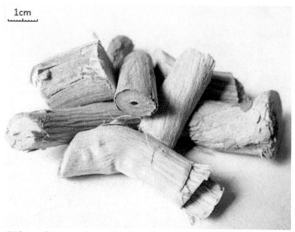

TCM prepared in ready-to-use forms (medicinal parts): it's dried stem and branch which harvested in autumn or winter.
Property and flavor: cold; sweet.
Main and collateral channels: lung and stomach meridians.
Administration and dosage: 9-30 g.
Indication: fever, dysentery with blood, swelling abscess, sore, ulcer, arthralgia, joint swelling and pain.

(The picture is only for learning and identification the herb; the specific use of the herb please consult the herbalist or health professionals)

Fewflower Lysionotus Herb (Shidiaolan)
Chinese phonetic alphabet/pin yin: shí diào lán
Chinese characters simplified/traditional:石吊兰/石吊蘭
Chinese nickname's alphabet (Nickname's Chinese characters): Heiwugu/ Shijiangdou(黑乌骨/石豇豆)
Latin: Lysionoti Herba (Common name: Fewflower Lysionotus Herb)
TCM prepared in ready-to-use forms (medicinal parts): it's dried aerial part which harvested in summer or autumn.
Property and flavor: warm; bitter.
Main and collateral channels: lung meridian.

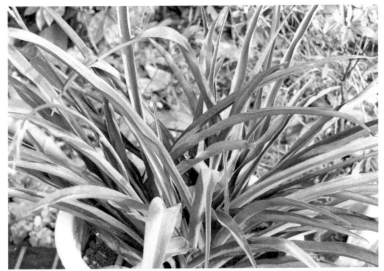

Plant: *Lysionotus pauciflorus* Maxim.

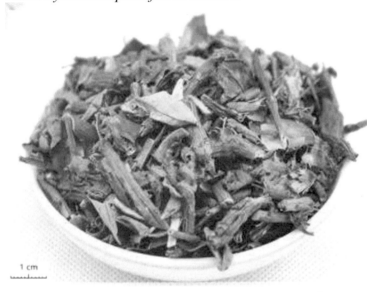

1 cm

Administration and dosage: 9-15 g. Topical application in appropriate amount, mashed for applying or decocted for rinsing.

Indication: cough, excessive phlegm, scrofula, phlegm nodule, painful *bi* disorder, dysmenorrheal, traumatic injuries.

(The picture is only for learning and identification the herb; the specific use of the herb please consult the herbalist or health professionals)

Tabularformed Pine Node (Yousongjie)

Chinese phonetic alphabet/pin yin: yóu sōng jié
Chinese characters simplified/traditional: 油松节/油松節
Chinese nickname's alphabet (Nickname's Chinese characters): Songjie(松节)
Latin: Pini Lignum Nodi (Common name: Tabularformed Pine Node)

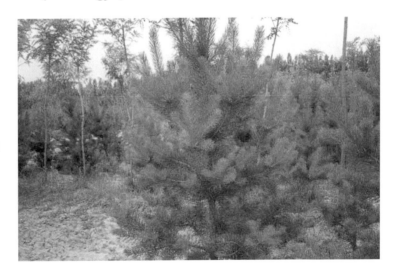

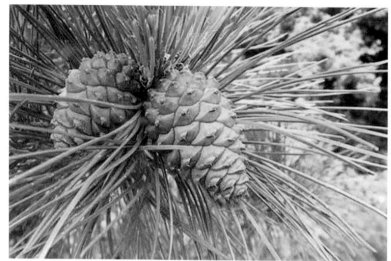

Plant: *Pinus tabulieformis* Carr. (or *Pinus massoniana* Lamb.)

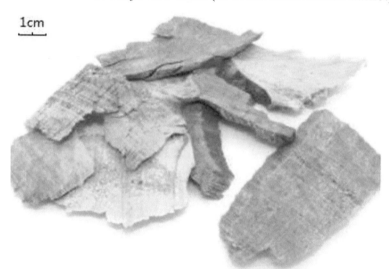

1cm

TCM prepared in ready-to-use forms (medicinal parts): it's dried tuberculate or branched node which harvested all year round.

Property and flavor: warm; bitter, pungent. Main and collateral channels: liver and kidney meridians. Administration and dosage: 9-15 g. Indication: joint pain, cramp, hypertonicity of the sinews and traumatic injuries. It is commonly used in treating chronic painful *bi* disorder.

Precaution and warning: used with caution in patients with red patches skin or scaly disease.

(The picture is only for learning and identification the herb; the specific use of the herb please consult the herbalist or health professionals)

Tuniclike Psammosilene Root (Jintiesuo)

Chinese phonetic alphabet/ pin yin: jīn tiě suǒ
Chinese characters simplified/ traditional:金铁锁/金鐵鎖
Chinese nickname's alphabet (Nickname's Chinese characters): Kunmingshashen/ Dudingzi(昆明沙参/独钉子)
Latin: Psammosilenes Radix (Common name: Tuniclike Psammosilene Root)
Plant:*Psammosilene tunicoides* W. C. Wu et C. Y. Wu.

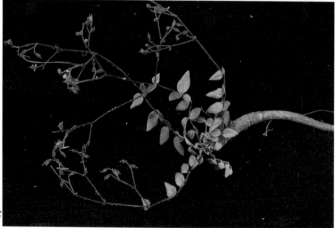

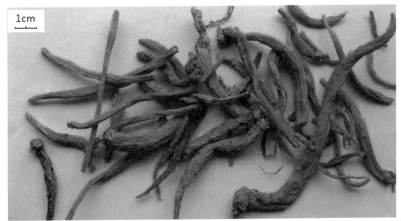

TCM prepared in ready-to-use forms (medicinal parts): it's dried root which harvested in autumn.

Property and flavor: warm; bitter, pungent.

Main and collateral channels: liver meridian.

Administration and dosage: 0.1-0.3 g, usually used in pill or powder. Topical application in appropriate amount.

Indication: painful *bi* disorder, traumatic injuries, traumatic hemorrhage; external use for insect or snake bites.

Precaution and warning: slightly toxic. Used with caution during pregnancy.

Attention: to protect the rare wild plant, please don't use the herb from wild plant. (The picture is only for learning and identification the herb; the specific use of the herb please consult the herbalist or health professionals)

Yellow Azalea Flower (Naoyanghua)

Chinese phonetic alphabet/
pin yin: nào yáng huā
Chinese characters
simplified/
traditional:闹羊花/
鬧羊花
Chinese nickname's
alphabet
(Nickname's Chinese
characters):
Yangzhizhu/
Huanghuadujuan
(羊踯躅/黄花杜鹃)
Latin: Rhododendri
Mollis Flos
(Common name:
Yellow Azalea
Flower)

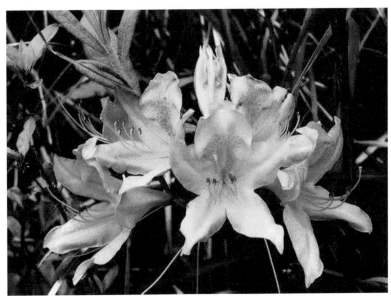

Plant: *Rhododendron molle* G. Don.

TCM prepared in ready-to-use forms (medicinal parts): it's dried flower at the flowering.

Property and flavor: warm; pungent.

Main and collateral channels: liver meridian.

Administration and dosage: 0.6-1.5 g, soaked in wine or liquor, or used in pills and powder. Topical application in appropriate amount, decocted for bathing.

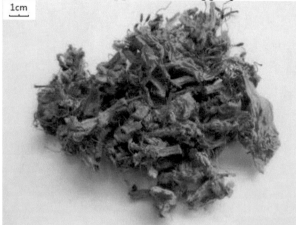

Indication: painful *bi* disorder, migraine, headache, traumatic injuries and stubborn tinea.
Precaution and warning: highly toxic. Over dosage or long-term administration is inadvisable. Use cautiously in people with weak constitution and pregnant woman. (The picture is only for learning and identification the herb; the specific use of the herb please consult the herbalist or health professionals)

Glabrous Sarcandra Herb (Zhongjiefeng)

Chinese phonetic alphabet/ pin yin: zhǒng jié fēng
Chinese characters simplified/ traditional:肿节风/腫節風
Chinese nickname's alphabet (Nickname's Chinese characters):
Jiujiecha/ Jiujiefeng/ Jiegulian (九节茶/九节风/接骨莲)
Latin: Sarcandrae Herba (Common name: Glabrous Sarcandra Herb)
Plant: *Sarcandra glabra* (Thunb.) Nakai.

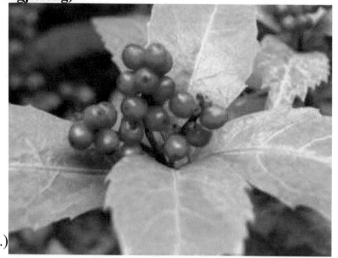

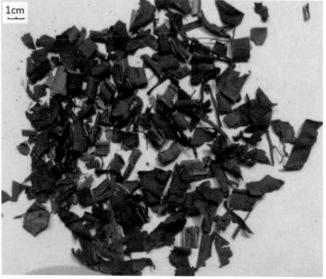

TCM prepared in ready-to-use forms (medicinal parts): it's dried whole herb which harvested in summer or autumn.
Property and flavor: neutral; bitter, pungent.
Main and collateral channels: heart and liver meridians.
Administration and dosage: 9-30 g.

Indication: macula and papule eruption, painful *bi* disorder, numbness of limbs and traumatic injuries.
(The picture is only for learning and identification the herb; the specific use of the herb please consult the herbalist or health professionals)

Snake Slough (Shetui)
Chinese phonetic alphabet/pin yin: shé tuì
Chinese characters simplified/traditional:蛇蜕/蛇蜕
Chinese nickname's alphabet (Nickname's Chinese characters): Shepi/ Shetui(蛇皮/
蛇退)
Latin: Serpentis Periostracum (Common name: Snake Slough)

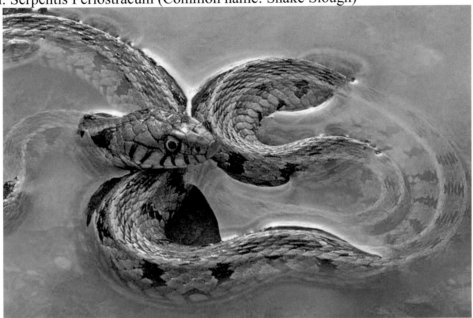

Animal: *Elaphe taeniura* Cope. (or *Elaphe carinata* (Guenther.),
Zaocys dhumnades (Cantor.))

TCM prepared in
ready-to-use forms
(medicinal parts): it's
dried epidermal
membrane.
Property and flavor:
neutral; salty, sweet.
Main and collateral
channels: liver meridian.
Administration and
dosage: 2-3 g. Ground
into powder for oral
administration: 0.3-0.6 g.

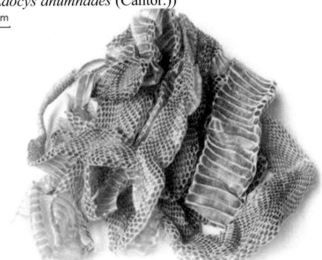

Indication: infantile convulsion, spasms and convulsions, nebula, disperse swelling
and itching of skin.
(The picture is only for learning and identification the herb; the specific use of the
herb please consult the herbalist or health professionals)

Wild Papaya (Yemugua)
Chinese phonetic alphabet/pin yin: yě mù guā
Chinese characters simplified/traditional:野木瓜/野木瓜
Chinese nickname's alphabet (Nickname's Chinese characters): Tiejiaohaitang/
Chuanmugua(铁脚海棠/川木瓜)

Latin: Stauntoniae Caulis et Folium (Common name: Wild Papaya)

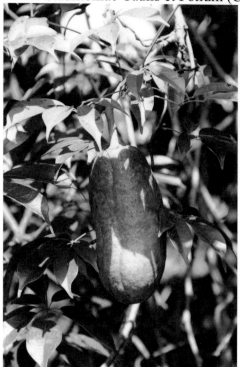

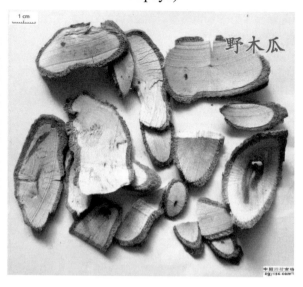

TCM prepared in ready-to-use forms (medicinal parts): it's young (floliferous) branch which harvested all year around.

Plant: *Stauntonia chinese* DC.
Property and flavor: neutral; mild bitter.
Main and collateral channels: liver and stomach meridians.
Administration and dosage: 9-15 g.
Indication: painful *bi* disorder, lower back and leg pain, headache, toothache, dysmenorrheal and traumatic injuries.
(The picture is only for learning and identification the herb; the specific use of the herb please consult the herbalist or health professionals)

Coloured Mistletoe Herb (Hujisheng)
Chinese phonetic alphabet/
pin yin: hǔ jì shēng
Chinese characters simplified/
traditional:槲寄生/槲寄生
Chinese nickname's alphabet
(Nickname's Chinese
characters): Beijisheng/
Liujisheng(北寄生/
柳寄生)
Latin: Visci Herba (Common
name: Coloured Mistletoe Herb)
Plant: *Viscum colouratum*
(Komar.) Nakai.

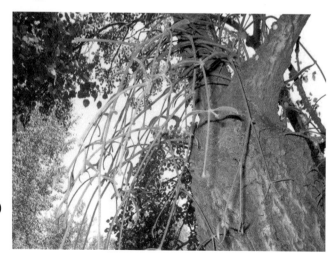

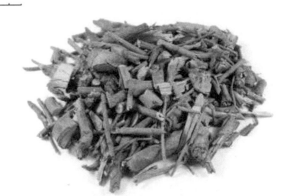

1cm

TCM prepared in ready-to-use forms (medicinal parts): it's dried stem and branch with leaf which harvested from winter to spring.

Property and flavor: neutral; bitter.

Main and collateral channels: liver and kidney meridians.

Administration and dosage: 9-15 g.

Indication: painful *bi* disorder, soreness and weakness in the waist and knees, lack of strength of sinews and bones, menstrual flooding and spotting, turbid and thick menstruation, vaginal bleeding during pregnancy, threatened miscarriage, dizziness and vertigo.

(The picture is only for learning and identification the herb; the specific use of the herb please consult the herbalist or health professionals)

Erythrina Bark (Haitongpi)

Chinese phonetic alphabet/ pin yin: hǎi tóng pí

Chinese characters simplified/ traditional:海桐皮/海桐皮

Chinese nickname's alphabet (Nickname's Chinese characters): Citongpi(刺桐皮)

Latin: Erythrinae Cortex (Common name: Erythrina Bark or Oriental Variegata Coralbean Bark)

Plant: *Erythrina variegata* L. var. *orientalis* (L.) Merr. (or *Bombys mori* L.)

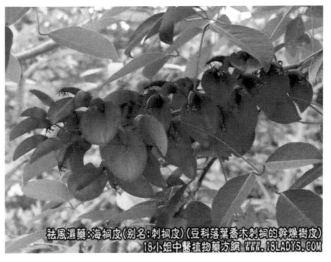

祛風濕藥:海桐皮(別名:刺桐皮)(豆科落葉喬木刺桐的幹燥樹皮)
18小姐中醫植物藥方網 WWW.18LADYS.COM

1cm

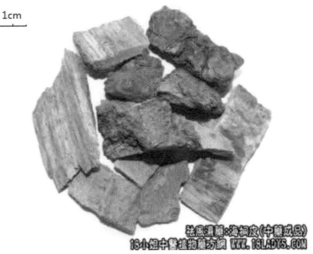

祛風濕藥:海桐皮(中藥成品)
18小姐中醫植物藥方網 WWW.18LADYS.COM

TCM prepared in ready-to-use forms (medicinal parts): it's dried thorny bark which harvested in summer.

Property and flavor: neutral; bitter, pungent.

Main and collateral channels: liver and spleen meridians.

Administration and dosage: 6-12 g. appropriate amount for topical application.

Indication: treat rheumatic, joint pain, spasm of the limbs and lower back and knee pain. External used for scabies and eczema.

It is commonly used in treating joint pain of low limbs.
(The picture is only for learning and identification the herb; the specific use of the herb please consult the herbalist or health professionals)

Hairy Birthwort Herb (Xungufeng)

Chinese phonetic alphabet/ pin yin: xún gǔ fēng
Chinese characters simplified/traditional: 寻骨风/尋骨風
Chinese nickname's alphabet (Nickname's Chinese characters): Baimianfeng/ Huangmuxiang (白面风/黄木香)
Latin: Aristolochiae Mollissimae Herba (Common name: Hairy Birthwort Herb)

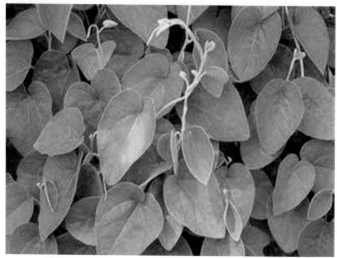

Plant: *Aristcolochia mollissima* Hance.

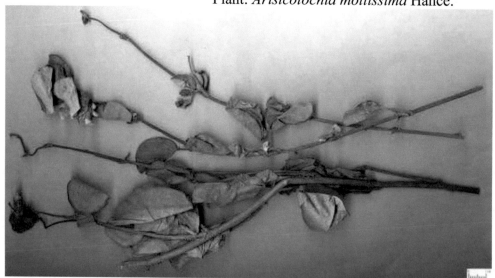

TCM prepared in ready-to-use forms (medicinal parts): it's dried whole herb which harvested in summer or autumn.
Property and flavor: neutral; bitter, pungent.
Main and collateral channels: liver meridian.
Administration and dosage: 10-15 g.
Indication: joint pain, numbness of the limbs, tendon and muscle spasms and pain form external injury.
(The picture is only for learning and identification the herb; the specific use of the herb please consult the herbalist or health professionals)

Hua Shi Yao(化湿药)-dampness~transforming herbs

Hua Shi Yao is a kind of herbs which's the major functions are to treat abdominal distension, nausea, diarrhea.

Atractylodes Rhizome (Cangzhu)

Chinese phonetic alphabet/
pin yin: cāng zhù
Chinese characters
simplified/traditional:
苍术/蒼朮
Chinese nickname's alphabet
(Nickname's Chinese
characters): Chizhu/
Qiangtoucai
(赤术/枪头菜)
Latin: Atractylodis Rhizoma
(Common name:
Atractylodes Rhizome)

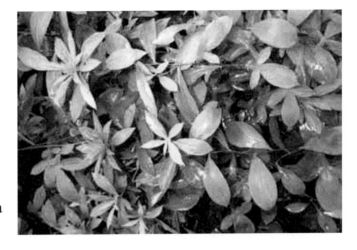

Plant: *Atractylodes lancea* (Thunb.) DC.
(or *Atractylodes chinensis* (DC.) Koidz.)

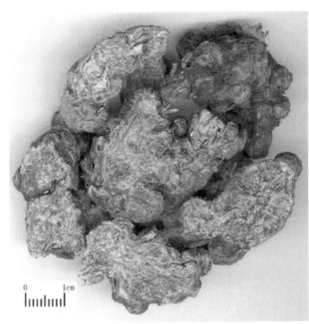

TCM prepared in ready-to-use forms (medicinal parts): it's dried rhizome which harvested in spring or autumn.
Property and flavor: warm; pungent, bitter.
Main and collateral channels: spleen, stomach and liver meridians.
Administration and dosage: 3-9 g.
Indication: abdominal distention, diarrhea, edema, beriberi, painful *bi* disorder, chill (*Fenghan*) cold, nyctalopia and blurred vision.

It is key herb to treat dizziness, fatigue and abdominal distension.
(The picture is only for learning and identification the herb; the specific use of the herb please consult the herbalist or health professionals)

Officinal Magnolia Bark (Houpo)
Chinese phonetic alphabet/pin yin: hòu pò
Chinese characters simplified/traditional:厚朴/厚樸
Chinese nickname's alphabet (Nickname's Chinese characters): Houpi/ Chongpi/
Chuanpo(厚皮/重皮/川朴)
Latin: Magnoliae Officinalis Cortex (Common name: Officinal Magnolia Bark)
Plant: *Magnolia officinalis* Rehd. et Wils. (or *Magnolia officinalis* Rehd. et Wils. var. *biloba* Rehd. et Wils.)

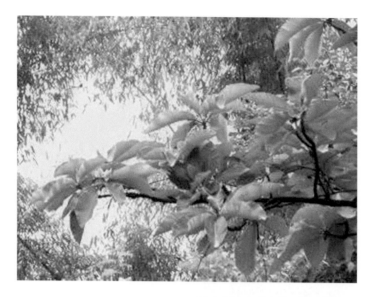

TCM prepared in ready-to-use forms (medicinal parts): it's dried stem bark which harvested from April to June. Property and flavor: warm; bitter, pungent. Main and collateral channels: spleen, stomach, lung and large intestine meridians.

Administration and dosage: 3-10 g.
Indication: diarrhea, dyspepsia, vomiting, constipation, abdominal distension, profuse sputum and cough.
It is key herb to remove food retention and flatulence.

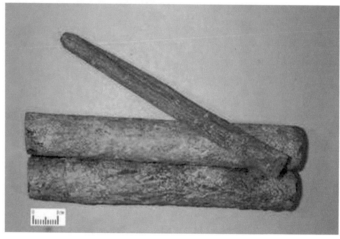

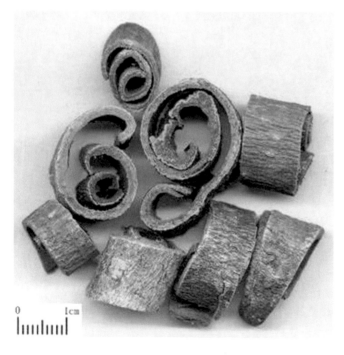

Attention:
to protect the rare wil d plant, please don't use the herb from wild plant.
(The picture is only for learning and identification the herb; the specific use of the herb please consult the herbalist or health professionals)

Cablin Patchouli Herb (Guanghuoxiang)

Chinese phonetic alphabet/pin yin: guǎng huò xiāng
Chinese characters simplified/traditional: 广藿香/廣藿香
Chinese nickname's alphabet (Nickname's Chinese characters): Huoxiang/ Dayebohe/ Shanhuixiang(藿香/大叶薄荷/山茴香)
Latin: Pogostemonis Herba (Common name: Cablin Patchouli Herb)

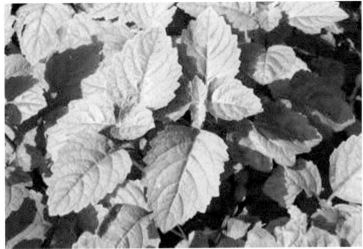
Plant: *Pogostemon cablin* (Blanco.) Benth.

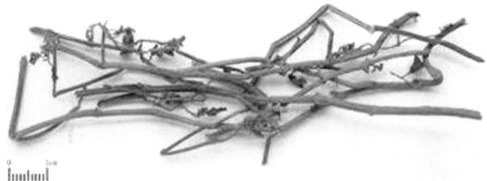

TCM prepared in ready-to-use forms (medicinal parts): it's dried above-ground part harvested when it is lush foliage.
Property and flavor: mild warm; pungent.
Main and collateral channels: spleen, stomach and liver meridians.
Administration and dosage: 3-10 g. It should not be decocted long for the herb.
Indication: abdominal distension, vomit, diarrhea, fever, fatigue, heatstroke, abdominal pain and headache.
It is key herb to treat poor appetite, vomiting, abdominal fullness and distention.
It is taken as seasoning in some part of China.
(The picture is only for learning and identification the herb; the specific use of the herb please consult the herbalist or health professionals)

Villous Amomum Fruit (Sharen)

Chinese phonetic alphabet/pin yin: shā rén
Chinese characters simplified/traditional:砂仁/砂仁
Chinese nickname's alphabet (Nickname's Chinese characters): Suosharen/ Xiaodoukou(缩砂仁/小豆蔻)
Latin: Amomi Fructus (Common name: Villous Amomum Fruit)

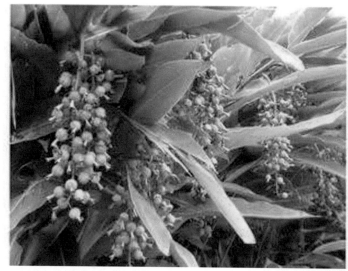

Plant: *Amomum villosum* Lour. (or *Amomum longiligulare* T. L. Wu, *Amomum villosum* Lour. var. *xanthioides* T. L. Wu et Senjen.)
TCM prepared in ready-to-use forms (medicinal parts): it's dried mature fruit.
Property and flavor: warm; pungent.

Main and collateral channels: spleen, stomach and kidney meridians.
Administration and dosage: 3-6 g, added when the decoction is nearly done.
Indication: abdominal distension, vomit, diarrhea, dyspepsia and threatened miscarriage.

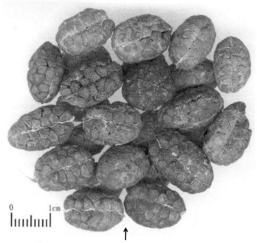

Amomum longiligulare T. L. Wu

It is key herb to treat abdominal fullness and distention and improve the digestion.
It is taken as seasoning in some part of China.
Attention:
to protect the rare wild plant, please don't use the herb from wild plant.
(The picture is only for learning and identification the herb; the specific use of the herb please consult the herbalist or health professionals)

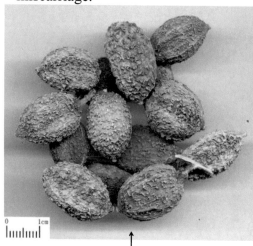

Amomum villosum Lour.

Round Cardamon Fruit (Baidoukou)
Chinese phonetic alphabet/pin yin: bái dòu kòu
Chinese characters simplified/traditional:白豆蔻/白豆蔻
Chinese nickname's alphabet (Nickname's Chinese characters): Duogu/ Qiaokou/ Baikou/ Doukou(多骨/壳蔻/白蔻/豆蔻)
Latin: Amomi Fructus Rotundus (Common name: Round Cardamon Fruit or Amomum Cardamon)
Plant: *Amomum kravanh* Pierre. ex Gagnep. (or *Amomum compactum* Soland.ex Maton.)

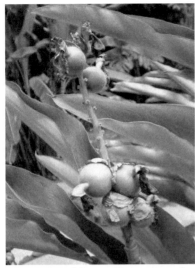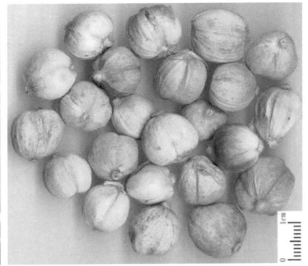

TCM prepared in ready-to-use forms (medicinal parts): it's dried mature fruit.

Property and flavor: warn; pungent.

Main and collateral channels: lung, spleen and stomach meridians.

Administration and dosage: 3-6 g, added when the decoction is nearly done.

Indication: abdominal distension, vomit, diarrhea, dyspepsia and indigestion.

It is taken as seasoning in some part of China.

(The picture is only for learning and identification the herb; the specific use of the herb please consult the herbalist or health professionals)

Fortune Eupatorium Herb (Peilan)

Chinese phonetic alphabet/pin yin: pèi lán

Chinese characters simplified/traditional: 佩兰/佩蘭

Chinese nickname's alphabet (Nickname's Chinese characters): Lancao/ Shuixiang(兰草/水香)

Latin: Eupatorii Herba (Common name: Fortune Eupatorium Herb)

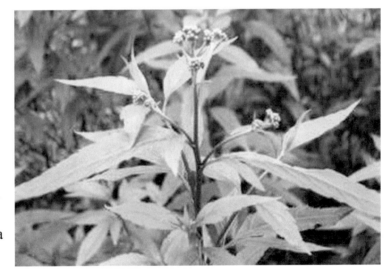

Plant: *Eupatorium fortunei* Turcz.

TCM prepared in ready-to-use forms (medicinal parts): it's dried aerial part which harvested in summer or autumn.

Property and flavor: neutral; pungent.

Main and collateral channels: spleen, stomach and lung meridians.

Administration and dosage: 3-10 g.

178

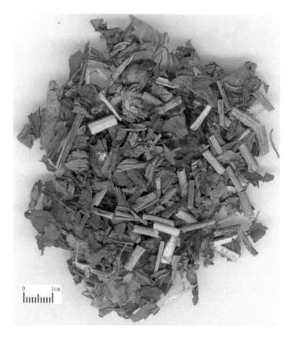

Indication: abdominal distension, vomit, diarrhea, heatstroke, fetid breath, abdominal pain, headache and fatigue.
(The picture is only for learning and identification the herb; the specific use of the herb please consult the herbalist or health professionals)

Katsumada Galangal Seed (Caodoukou)

Chinese phonetic alphabet/pin yin: cǎo dòu kòu
Chinese characters simplified/traditional: 草豆蔻/草豆蔻
Chinese nickname's alphabet (Nickname's Chinese characters): Caokou(草蔻)
Latin: Alpiniae Katsumadai Semen (Common name: Katsumada Galangal Seed)

1cm

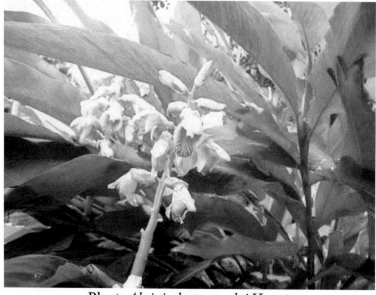

Plant: *Alpinia katsumadai* Hayata.

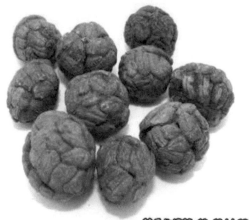

TCM prepared in ready-to-use forms (medicinal parts): it's dried mature seed.
Property and flavor: warm; pungent.
Main and collateral channels: spleen and stomach meridians.
Administration and dosage: 3-6 g.

芳香化湿药:草 蔻(中药成品)
16小姐中鬶植物藥方網 WWW.16LADYS.COM

179

Indication: abdominal distension, vomit, dyspepsia, abdominal pain and cold/chill (*Hanliang*) pain.

It is taken as seasoning in some part of China.

(The picture is only for learning and identification the herb; the specific use of the herb please consult the herbalist or health professionals)

Caoguo (Caoguo)

Chinese phonetic alphabet/pin yin: cǎo guǒ

Chinese characters simplified/traditional:草果/草果

Chinese nickname's alphabet (Nickname's Chinese characters): Caoguozi/ Caoguoren(草果子/草果仁)

Latin: Tsaoko Fructus (Common name: Caoguo)

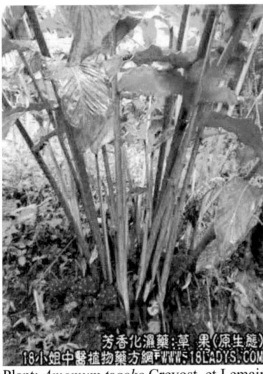

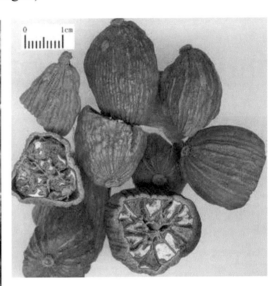

TCM prepared in ready-to-use forms (medicinal parts): it's dried mature fruit.
Property and flavor: warm; pungent.

Plant: *Amomum tsaoko* Crevost. et Lemaire.

Main and collateral channels: spleen and stomach meridians.

Administration and dosage: 3-6 g.

Indication: abdominal distension, vomit, dyspepsia, abdominal pain, malaria and pestilence fever.

It is taken as seasoning in some part of China.

(The picture is only for learning and identification the herb; the specific use of the herb please consult the herbalist or health professionals)

Barberry Rood (Sankezhen)

Chinese phonetic alphabet/pin yin: sān kē zhēn

Chinese characters simplified/traditional:三颗针/三顆針

Chinese nickname's alphabet (Nickname's Chinese characters): Gounaizi/ Suanculiu(狗奶子/酸醋溜)

Latin: Berberidis Radix (Common name: Barberry Rood)

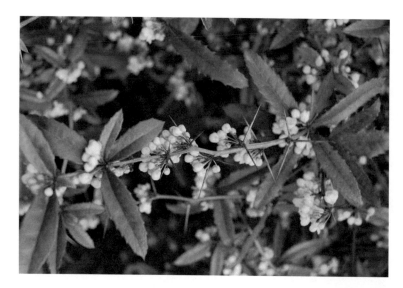

Plant: *Berberis soulieana* Schneid. (or *Berberis wilsonae* Hemsl., *Berberis poiretii* Schneid., *Berberis vernae* Schneid.)

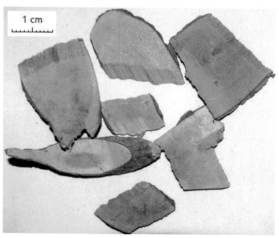

TCM prepared in ready-to-use forms (medicinal parts): it's dried root which harvested in autumn or spring.
Property and flavor: cold; bitter.
Main and collateral channels: liver, stomach and large intestine meridians.
Administration and dosage: 9-15 g.
Indication: dysentery, jaundice, eczema, sore throat, red eye, otitis, swelling abscess, skin infections and sodoku.

Precaution and warning: toxic.
(The picture is only for learning and identification the herb; the specific use of the herb please consult the herbalist or health professionals)

Li Shui Shen Shi Yao(利水渗湿药)-diuretics for eliminating dampness
Li Shui Shen Shi Yao is a kind of herbs which's the major functions are diuresis, detumescence; some of them also have function of cholagogic.

Indian Bread (Fuling)

Chinese phonetic alphabet/pin yin: fú líng
Chinese characters simplified/traditional:茯苓/茯苓
Chinese nickname's alphabet (Nickname's Chinese characters): Fulingge/ Yunling/ Songshu(茯苓个/云苓/松薯)
Latin: Poria (Common name: Indian Bread)

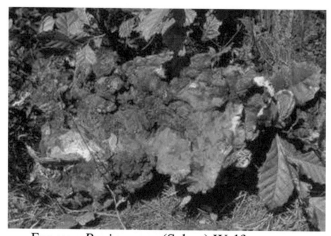

Fungus: *Poria cocos* (Schw.) Wolf.

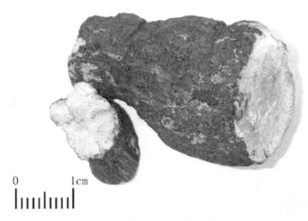

0   1cm

TCM prepared in ready-to-use forms (medicinal parts): it's dried sclerotium which harvested between July and September.
Property and flavor: neutral; sweet, bland.
Main and collateral channels: heart, lung, spleen and kidney meridians.

Administration and dosage: 10-15 g.
Indication: edema, oliguria, phlegm, diarrhea, insomnia and palpitation; appetizers, relieve uneasiness of mind and body tranquilization.
It is key herb to induce diuresis to alleviate edema.
It is taken as food in some part of China.
(The picture is only for learning and identification the herb; the specific use of the herb please consult the herbalist or health professionals)

Coix Seed (Yiyiren)
Chinese phonetic alphabet/pin yin:
yì yǐ rén
Chinese characters simplified/traditional:
薏苡仁/薏苡仁
Chinese nickname's alphabet (Nickname's Chinese characters):
Yimi(薏米)
Latin: Coicis Semen (Common name: Coix Seed)

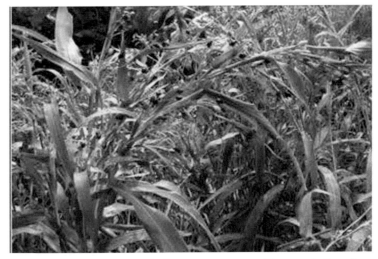

Plant: *Coix lacrymajobi* L. var. *mayuen* (Roman.) Stapf.

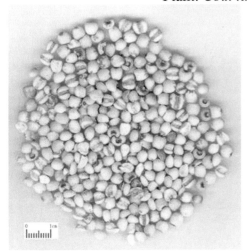

TCM prepared in ready-to-use forms (medicinal parts): it's dried mature kernel.
Property and flavor: cool; sweet, bland.
Main and collateral channels: stomach, lung and spleen meridians.
Administration and dosage: 9-30 g.
Indication: edema, beriberi, dysuria, spasm, diarrhea, lung abscess, appendicitis and flat wart.
It is taken as food in some part of China.
Precaution and warning: use with caution during pregnancy.

(The picture is only for learning and identification the herb; the specific use of the herb please consult the herbalist or health professionals)

Oriental Waterplantain Rhizome (Zexie)

Chinese phonetic alphabet/pin yin: zé xiè
Chinese characters simplified/traditional: 泽泻/澤瀉
Chinese nickname's alphabet (Nickname's Chinese characters): Shuize/ Ruyihua(水泽/如意花)
Latin: Alismatis Rhizoma (Common name: Oriental Waterplantain Rhizome)

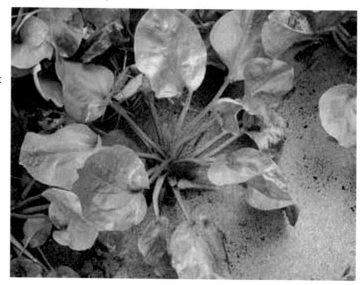

Plant: *Alisma orientale* (Sam.) Juzep. (or *Alisma plantago-aquatica* Linn.)

TCM prepared in ready-to-use forms (medicinal parts): it's dried stem tuber which harvested in winter.
Property and flavor: cold; sweet and bland.
Main and collateral channels: kidney and bladder meridians.
Administration and dosage: 6-10 g.
Indication: diarrhea, edema, phlegm, dizziness, pyretic strangury and hyperlipidemia; diuresis.

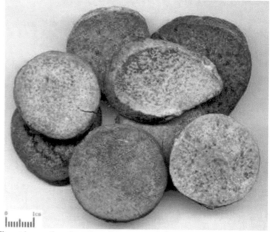

(The picture is only for learning and identification the herb; the specific use of the herb please consult the herbalist or health professionals)

Plantain Seed (Cheqianzi)

Chinese phonetic alphabet/ pin yin: chē qián zǐ
Chinese characters simplified/traditional:车前子/車前子
Chinese nickname's alphabet (Nickname's Chinese characters): Cheqianshi/ Niumecaozi(车前实/牛么草子)
Latin: Plantaginis Semen (Common name: Plantain Seed)

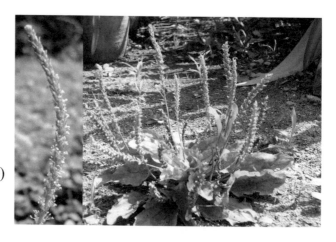

Plant: *Plantago asiatica* L. (or *Plantago depressa* Willd.)

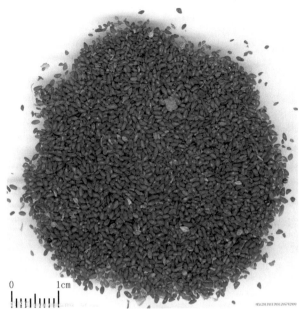

TCM prepared in ready-to-use forms (medicinal parts): it's dried mature seed.
Property and flavor: cold; sweet.
Main and collateral channels: liver, kidney, lung and small intestine meridians.
Administration and dosage: 9-15 g, wrap-boiling.
Indication: dysuria, edema, abdominal distension, pyretic strangury, red eyes, profuse sputum and cough.
It is commonly used in inducing diuresis.

(The picture is only for learning and identification the herb; the specific use of the herb please consult the herbalist or health professionals)

Talc (Huashi)

Chinese phonetic alphabet/pin yin: huá shí

Chinese characters simplified/traditional:滑石/滑石

Chinese nickname's alphabet (Nickname's Chinese characters): Yeshi/ Tuoshi/ Gongshi/(液石/脱石/共石)

Latin: Talcum (Common name: Talc)

Mineral: main component $Mg_3(Si_4O_{10})(OH)_2$

TCM prepared in ready-to-use forms (medicinal parts): it's clean mineral (powder).
Property and flavor: cold; sweet, bland.
Main and collateral channels: bladder, lung and stomach meridians.
Administration and dosage: 10-20 g. It should be decocted first. Appropriate amount for topical application, ground into powder and apply to *pars affecta.*

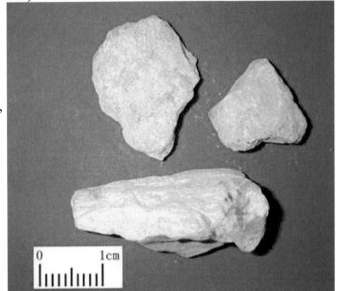

Indication: pyretic strangury, urolithiasis and diarrhea; external use for eczemas, dampness sore and heat rash.
It is key herb to treat eczema and miliaria.
(The picture is only for learning and identification the herb; the specific use of the herb please consult the herbalist or health professionals)

Akebia Stem (Mutong)

Chinese phonetic alphabet/ pin yin: mù tōng

Chinese characters simplified/ traditional:木通/木通

Chinese nickname's alphabet (Nickname's Chinese characters): Fuzhi/ Dingweng(附支/丁翁)

Latin: Akebiae Caulis (Common name: Akebiae Stem)

Plant: *Akebia quinata* (Thunb.) Decne. (or *Akebia trifoliata* (Thumb.) Koidz., *Akebia trifoliata* (Thumb.) Koidz. var. *australis* (Diels.) Rehd.)

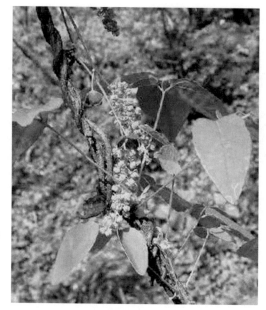

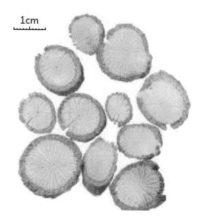

TCM prepared in ready-to-use forms (medicinal parts): it's dried lianoid stem which harvested in autumn.

Property and flavor: cold; bitter.

Main and collateral channels: heart, small intestine and bladder meridians.

Administration and dosage: 3-6 g.

Indication: aphtha, hematuria, edema, pyretic strangury, leucorrhea, arthralgia and amenorrhea; lactagogue.

It is key herb to treat vexation and urine red.

(The picture is only for learning and identification the herb; the specific use of the herb please consult the herbalist or health professionals)

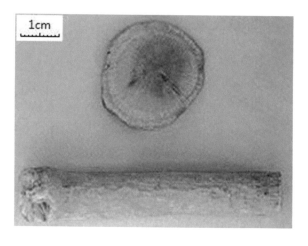

Armand Clematis Stem (Chuanmutong)

Chinese phonetic alphabet/pin yin: chuān mù tōng

Chinese characters simplified/traditional:川木通/川木通

Chinese nickname's alphabet (Nickname's Chinese characters): Huaimutong/ Xiaomutong(淮木通/小木通)

Latin: Clematidis Armandii Caulis (Common name: Armand Clematis Stem)

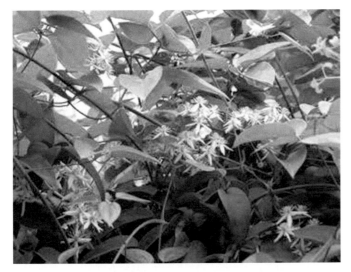

Plant: *Clematis armandii* Franch. (or *Clematis montana* Buch.-Ham.)

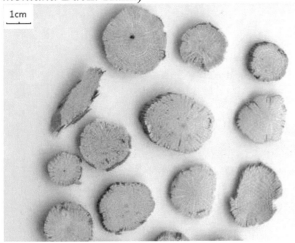

TCM prepared in ready-to-use forms (medicinal parts): it's dried lianod stem which harvested in spring or autumn.
Property and flavor: cold; bitter.
Main and collateral channels: heart, small intestine and bladder meridians.
Administration and dosage: 3-6 g.
Indication: stranguria, edema, vexation, mouth and tongue sore, amenorrhea, arthralgin; lactagogue.
(The picture is only for learning and identification the herb; the specific use of the herb please consult the herbalist or health professionals)

Christina Loosestrife (Jinqiancao)

Chinese phonetic alphabet/pin yin: jīn qián cǎo
Chinese characters simplified/traditional: 金钱草/金錢草
Chinese nickname's alphabet (Nickname's Chinese characters): Luodijinqian(落地金钱)
Latin: Lysimachiae Herba (Common name: Christina Loosestrife)

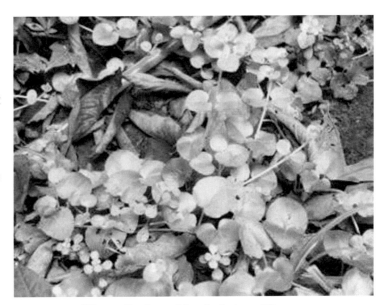

Plant: *Lysimachia christinae* Hance.

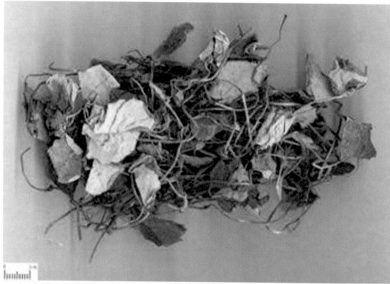

TCM prepared in ready-to-use forms (medicinal parts): it's dried whole herb which harvest in summer or autumn.
Property and flavor: mild cold; sweet and salty.
Main and collateral channels: liver, gallbladder, kidney and bladder meridians.

Administration and dosage: 15-60 g.
Indication: pyretic strangury, urolithiasis, dysuria and pain, jaundice, carbuncle, insect and snake bites.
It is key herb to treat urolithiasis.
(The picture is only for learning and identification the herb; the specific use of the herb please consult the herbalist or health professionals)

Virgate Wormwood Herb (Yinchen)
Chinese phonetic alphabet/pin yin: yīn chén
Chinese characters simplified/traditional:茵陈/茵陳
Chinese nickname's alphabet (Nickname's Chinese characters): Mianyinchen/ Ronghao/ Maxian(绵茵陈/绒蒿/马先)
Latin: Artemisiae Scopariae Herba (Common name: Virgate Wormwood Herb)

Plant: *Artemisia scoparia* Waldst. et Kit. (or *Artemisia capillaris* Thunb.)

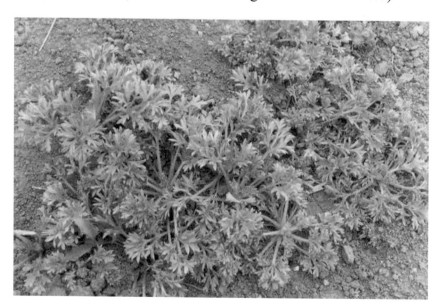

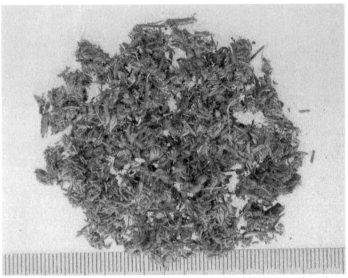

TCM prepared in ready-to-use forms (medicinal parts): it's dried whole herb which harvest in spring.
Property and flavor: mild cold; bitter, pungent.
Main and collateral channels: spleen, stomach, liver and gallbladder meridians.

Administration and dosage: 6-15 g. Topical application in appropriate amount. It can be decocted for fuming-washing therapy.

Indication: jaundice, dysuria, skin itching, hepatitis.

It is key herb to treat jaundice.

(The picture is only for learning and identification the herb; the specific use of the herb please consult the herbalist or health professionals)

Chuling (Zhuling)

Chinese phonetic alphabet/pin yin: zhū líng
Chinese characters simplified/traditional:猪苓/猪苓
Chinese nickname's alphabet (Nickname's Chinese characters): Zhufuling/ Zhulingzhi(猪茯苓/猪灵芝)
Latin: Polyporus (Common name: Chuling or Grifola)

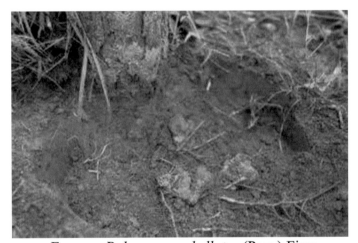

Fungus: *Polyporus umbellatus* (Pers.) Fires.

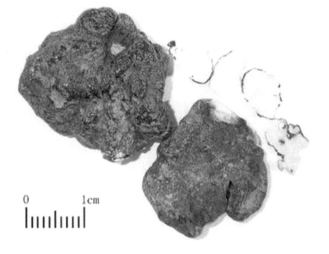

TCM prepared in ready-to-use forms (medicinal parts): it's dried sclerotium which harvested in spring or winter.
Property and flavor: neutral; sweet, bland.
Main and collateral channels: kidney and bladder meridians.
Administration and dosage: 6-12 g.

Indication: diarrhea, edema, leucorrhea with turbid and abnormal vaginal discharge; diuresis.
(The picture is only for learning and identification the herb; the specific use of the herb please consult the herbalist or health professionals)

Ricepaperplant Pith (Tongcao)

Chinese phonetic alphabet/pin yin: tōng cǎo

Chinese characters simplified/traditional: 通草/通草

Chinese nickname's alphabet (Nickname's Chinese characters): Baitongcao/ Tonghua/ Datongcao(白通草/ 通花/大通草)

Latin: Tetrapanacis Medulla (Common name: Ricepaperplant Pith)

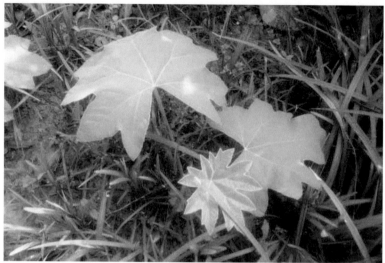

Plant: *Tetrapanax papyriferus* (Hook.) K. Koch.

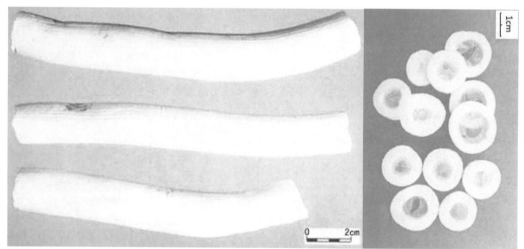

TCM prepared in ready-to-use forms (medicinal parts): it's dried stem pith which harvested in autumn.
Property and flavor: mild cold; sweet, bland.
Main and collateral channels: lung and stomach meridians.
Administration and dosage: 3-5 g.
Indication: hot and humid urine, gonorrhea, urine astringent and pain, edema, oliguria; lactagogue.
Precaution and warning: use with caution during pregnancy.
(The picture is only for learning and identification the herb; the specific use of the herb please consult the herbalist or health professionals)

Hypoglaucous Collett Yam Rhizome (Bixie)

Chinese phonetic alphabet/
pin yin: bì xiè
Chinese characters simplified/
traditional:萆薢/萆薢
Chinese nickname's alphabet
(Nickname's Chinese characters):
Fenbixie/ Mianbixie(绵萆薢/
粉萆薢)
Latin: Dioscoreae Hypoglaucae
Rhizoma seu Dioscoreae
Spongiosae Rhizoma (Common
name: Hypoglaucous Collett Yam
Rhizome or Sevenlobed Yam
Rhizome)
Plant: *Dioscorea hypoglauca* Palibin.
(or *Dioscorea spongiosa* J. Q. Xi, M.
Mizuno et W., *Dioscorea futschauensis*
Uline ex R. Kunth., *Dioscorea
septemloba* Thunbt.)

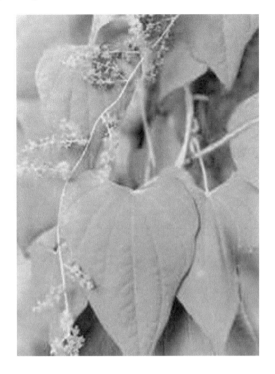

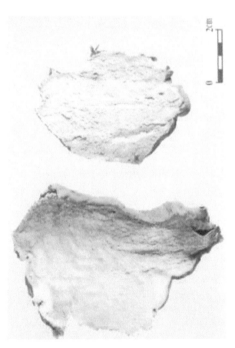

TCM prepared in ready-to-use forms
(medicinal parts): it's dried rhizome and root
which harvested in autumn or winter.
Property and flavor: neutral; bitter.
Main and collateral channels: kidney and
stomach meridians.
Administration and dosage: 9-15 g.
Indication: turbid urine, leucorrhea
excessive, sodoku, painful *bi* disorder,
inhibited joint, aching lower back and knees.
It is key herb to treat stranguria which is
marked by chyluria.
(The picture is only for learning and
identification the herb; the specific use of
the herb please consult the herbalist or
health professionals)

Shearer's Pyrrosia Leaf (Shiwei)

Chinese phonetic alphabet/pin yin: shí wěi
Chinese characters simplified/traditional:石韦/石韋
Chinese nickname's alphabet (Nickname's Chinese characters): Shipi(石皮)
Latin: Pyrrosiae Folium (Common name: Shearer's Pyrrosia Leaf)

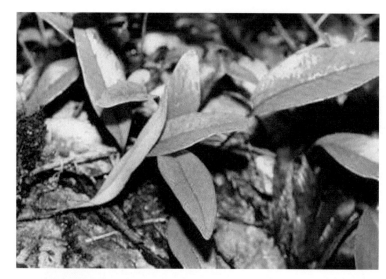

Plant: *Pyrrosia lingua* (Thunb.) Farwell. (or *Pyrrosia sheareri* (Bak.) Ching., *Pyrrosia petiolosa* (Christ.) Ching.)

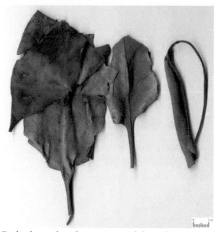

TCM prepared in ready-to-use forms (medicinal parts): it's dried leaf which harvested all year round.
Property and flavor: mild cold; bitter, sweet.
Main and collateral channels: lung and bladder meridians.
Administration and dosage: 6-12 g.
Indication: pyretic strangury, hematuria, urolithiasis, dysuria, hematemesis, cough with asthma, menstrual flooding and spotting.

It is key herb to treat bloody stranguria.
(The picture is only for learning and identification the herb; the specific use of the herb please consult the herbalist or health professionals)

Japanese Climbing Fern Spore (Haijinsha)

Chinese phonetic alphabet/pin yin: hǎi jīn shā
Chinese characters simplified/traditional: 海金沙/海金沙
Chinese nickname's alphabet (Nickname's Chinese characters): Jinshateng/ Zuozhuanteng(金沙藤/左转藤)

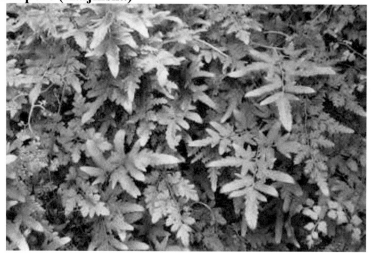

Latin: Lygodii Spora (Common name: Japanese Climbing Fern Spore)
Plant: *Lygodium japonicum* (Thunb.) Sw.

TCM prepared in ready-to-use forms (medicinal parts): it's dried mature spore.
Property and flavor: cold; sweet, salty.
Main and collateral channels: bladder and small intestine meridians.
Administration and dosage: 6-15 g, wrap-boiling.
Indication: pyretic strangury, urolithiasis, hematuria, turbid urine, urethral acerbity pain.
It is key herb to treat pain and difficulty in micturition.

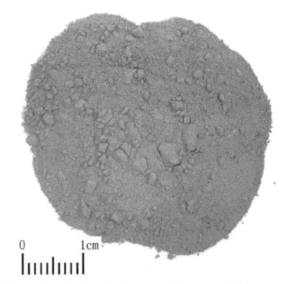

(The picture is only for learning and identification the herb; the specific use of the herb please consult the herbalist or health professionals)

Lilac Pink Herb (Qumai)

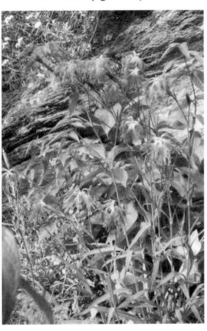

Chinese phonetic alphabet/pin yin: qú mài
Chinese characters simplified/ traditional:瞿麦/瞿麥
Chinese nickname's alphabet (Nickname's Chinese characters): Jujumai(巨句麦)
Latin: Dianthi Herba (Common name: Lilac Pink Herb)
Plant: *Dianthus superbus* L. (or *Dianthus chinensis* L.)

TCM prepared in ready-to-use forms (medicinal parts): it's dried aerial part which harvested at flowering.
Property and flavor: cold; bitter.
Main and collateral channels: small intestine and heart meridians.
Administration and dosage: 9-15 g.
Indication: pyretic strangury, urolithiasis, hematuria, dysuria, urethral acerbity pain, menstrual block.

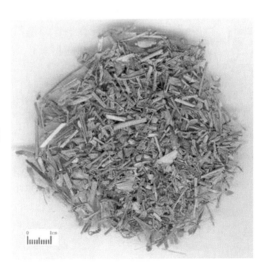

(The picture is only for learning and identification the herb; the specific use of the herb please consult the herbalist or health professionals)

Common Knotgrass Herb (Bianxu)

Chinese phonetic alphabet/pin yin: biǎn xù
Chinese characters simplified/traditional:萹蓄/萹蓄
Chinese nickname's alphabet (Nickname's Chinese characters): Bianzhu(萹竹)
Latin: Polygoni Avicularis Herba (Common name: Common Knotgrass Herb)

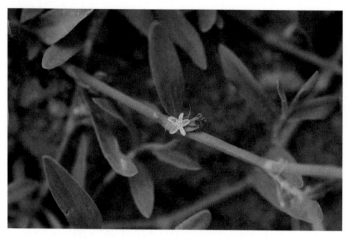

Plant: *Polygonum aviculare* L.

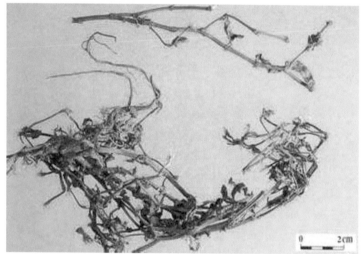

TCM prepared in ready-to-use forms (medicinal parts): it's dried aerial part which harvested in summer.
Property and flavor: mild cold; bitter.
Main and collateral channels: bladder meridian.

Administration and dosage: 9-15 g. Appropriate amount for topical application, decocted for bathing of the *pars affecta*.
Indication: urethral acerbity pain, pyretic stranguria, eczema, pruritus vulvae, colpitis and abnormal vaginal discharge; diuresis.
(The picture is only for learning and identification the herb; the specific use of the herb please consult the herbalist or health professionals)

Belvedere Fruit (Difuzi)
Chinese phonetic alphabet/pin yin: dì fū zǐ
Chinese characters simplified/traditional:地肤子/地膚子
Chinese nickname's alphabet (Nickname's Chinese characters): Dikui/ Dimai(地葵/地麦)
Latin: Kochiae Fructus (Common name: Belvedere Fruit)

Plant: *Kochia scoparia* (L.) Schrad.
TCM prepared in ready-to-use forms (medicinal parts): it's dried mature fruit.
Property and flavor: cold; bitter, pungent.

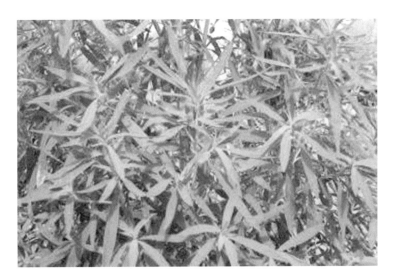

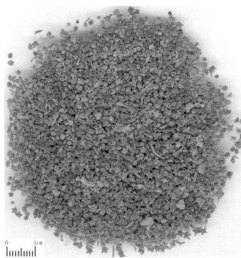

Main and collateral channels: kidney and bladder meridians.
Administration and dosage: 9-15 g. Topical application in appropriate amount. It can be decocted for fuming-washing therapy.
Indication: painful urination, vulvae leucorrhea, rubella, eczema, pudendal itching and skin pruritus.

(The picture is only for learning and identification the herb; the specific use of the herb please consult the herbalist or health professionals)

Common Rush (Dengxincao)

Chinese phonetic alphabet/pin yin: dēng xīn cǎo
Chinese characters simplified/traditional:灯心草/燈心草
Chinese nickname's alphabet (Nickname's Chinese characters): Yangcao/Shuidengxin(秧草/水灯心)
Latin: Junci Medulla (Common name: Common Rush or Bog Rush)

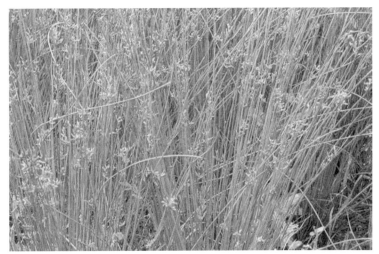

Plant: *Juncus effusus* L.

194

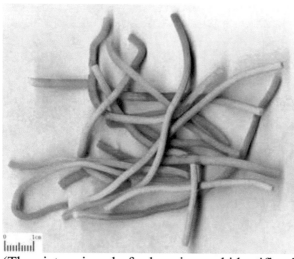

TCM prepared in ready-to-use forms (medicinal parts): it's dried stem pith which harvested in summer or winter.

Property and flavor: mild cold; sweet, bland.

Main and collateral channels: heart, lung and small intestine meridians.

Administration and dosage: 1-3 g.

Indication: fret insomnia, urethral acerbity pain, oliguria, aphtha, mouth and tongue sore.

(The picture is only for learning and identification the herb; the specific use of the herb please consult the herbalist or health professionals)

Cluster Mallow Fruit(Dongkuizi)

Chinese phonetic alphabet/pin yin: dōng kuí zǐ

Chinese characters simplified/traditional:冬葵子/冬葵子

Chinese nickname's alphabet (Nickname's Chinese characters): Kuizi/ Kuicaizi/ Dongkuiguo(葵子/葵菜子/冬葵果)

Latin: Malvae Fructus (Common name: Cluster Mallow Fruit)

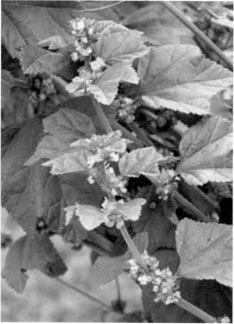
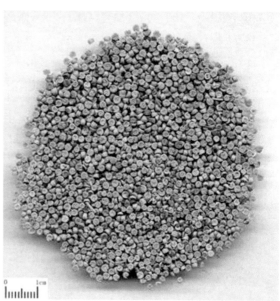

Plant: *Malva verticillata* L. (or *Malva crispa* Linn.)

TCM prepared in ready-to-use forms (medicinal parts): it's dried mature seed.

Property and flavor: cool; sweet, astringent.

Administration and dosage: 3-9 g.

Indication: edema, mastitis, constipation and annuria; lactagogue.

(The picture is only for learning and identification the herb; the specific use of the herb please consult the herbalist or health professionals)

Longtube Ground Ivy Herb (Lianqiancao)

Chinese phonetic alphabet/
pin yin: lián qián cǎo
Chinese characters simplified/traditional:
连钱草/連錢草
Chinese nickname's alphabet (Nickname's Chinese characters):
Huoxuedan(活血丹)
Latin: Glechomae Herba (Common name: Longtube Ground Ivy Herb)

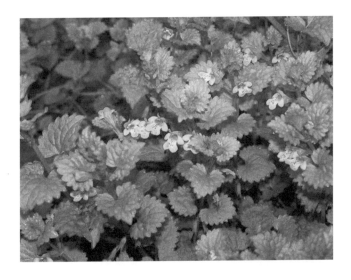

Plant: *Glechoma longituba* (Nakai.) Kupr.

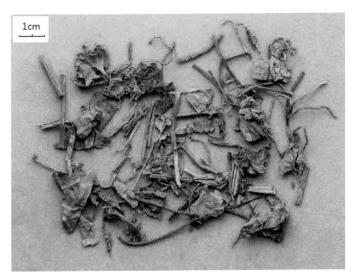

TCM prepared in ready-to-use forms (medicinal parts): it's dried aerial part which harvested in April or May.
Property and flavor: mild cold; mild bitter, pungent.
Main and collateral channels: liver, kidney and bladder meridians.

Administration and dosage: 15-30 g. Topical application in appropriate amount. It can be decocted for bathing.
Indication: pyretic strangury, urolithiasis, jaundice, edema, sore and traumatic injury.
(The picture is only for learning and identification the herb; the specific use of the herb please consult the herbalist or health professionals)

Chinese Waxgourd Peel (Dongguapi)

Chinese phonetic alphabet/pin yin: dōng guā pí
Chinese characters simplified/traditional:冬瓜皮/冬瓜皮
Chinese nickname's alphabet (Nickname's Chinese characters): Baiguapi(白瓜皮)
Latin: Benincasae Exocarpium (Common name: Chinese Waxgourd Peel or Wax Gourd Skin)

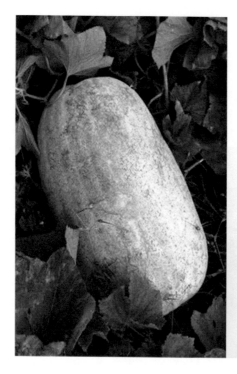
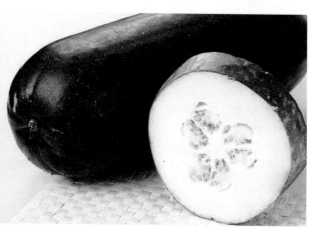

Plant: *Benincasa hispida*
(Thunb.) Cogn.

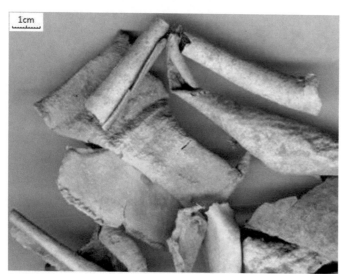

TCM prepared in ready-to-use forms (medicinal parts): it's dried ripe fruit exocarp.
Property and flavor: cool; sweet.
Main and collateral channels: spleen and small intestine meridians.
Administration and dosage: 9-30 g.

Indication: edema, puffiness, dysuria, thirsty, urinate short red.
(The picture is only for learning and identification the herb; the specific use of the herb please consult the herbalist or health professionals)

Areca Peel (Dafupi)
Chinese phonetic alphabet/pin yin: dà fù pí
Chinese characters simplified/traditional:大腹皮/大腹皮
Chinese nickname's alphabet (Nickname's Chinese characters): Binglangpi(槟榔皮)
Latin: Arecae Pericarpium (Common name: Areca Peel or The Shell of Areca Nut)

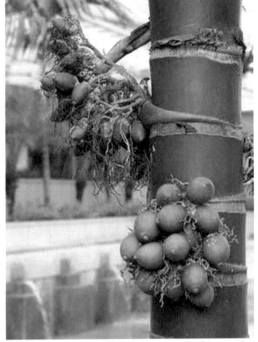

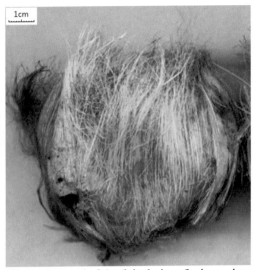

Plant: *Areca catechu* L.

TCM prepared in ready-to-use forms (medicinal parts): it's dried ripe fruit pericarp.
Property and flavor: mild warm; pungent.
Main and collateral channels: spleen, stomach, large intestine and small intestine meridians.
Administration and dosage: 5-10 g.
Indication: abdominal distension, edema, beriberi, dysuria.
(The picture is only for learning and identification the herb; the specific use of the herb please consult the herbalist or health professionals)

Corn Silk (Yumixu)

Chinese phonetic alphabet/pin yin: yù mǐ xū
Chinese characters simplified/traditional: 玉米须/玉米鬚
Chinese nickname's alphabet (Nickname's Chinese characters): Baoguxu(包谷须)
Latin: Maize Stigma seu Zeae Maydis Stylus (Common name: Corn Silk)

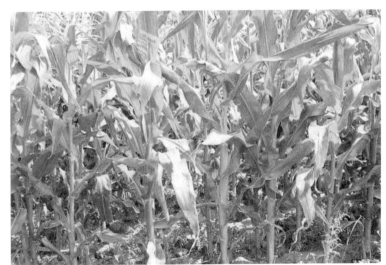

Plant: *Zea mays* L.

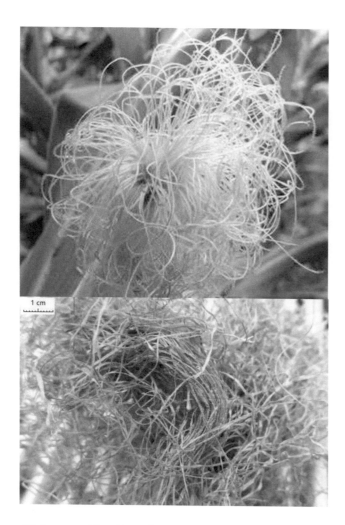

TCM prepared in ready-to-use forms (medicinal parts): it's dried flower stigma. Property and flavor: neutral; sweet, bland. Main and collateral channels: bladder, liver and gallbladder meridians. Administration and dosage: 30-60 g. Indication: edema, jaundice, cholecystitis, gallstones, hypertension, diabetes; lactagogue. (The picture is only for learning and identification the herb; the specific use of the herb please consult the herbalist or health professionals)

Chingma Abutilon Seed (Qingmazi)
Chinese phonetic alphabet/pin yin: qǐng má zǐ
Chinese characters simplified/traditional:苘麻子/苘麻子
Chinese nickname's alphabet (Nickname's Chinese characters): Qingmazi/ Yemianhuazi/ Baimazi (青麻子/野棉花子/白麻子)
Latin: Abutili Semen (Common name: Chingma Abutilon Seed)

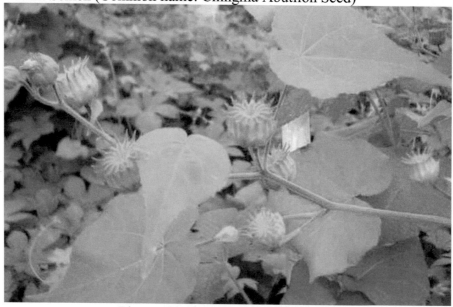

Plant: *Abutilon theophrastii* Medic.

TCM prepared in ready-to-use forms (medicinal parts): it's dried mature seed.

Property and flavor: neutral; bitter.

Main and collateral channels: large intestine, small intestine and bladder meridians.

Administration and dosage: 3-9 g.

Indication: dysentery, stranguriy with difficulty and pain, swell abscess, various skin infection and blurring vision.

(The picture is only for learning and identification the herb; the specific use of the herb please consult the herbalist or health professionals)

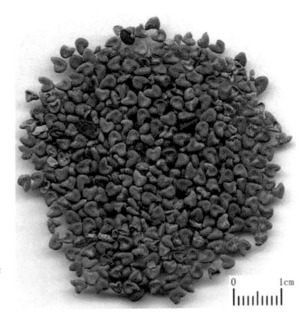

Alpine Yarrow Herb (Shicao)

Chinese phonetic alphabet/pin yin: shī cǎo

Chinese characters simplified/traditional:蓍草/蓍草

Chinese nickname's alphabet (Nickname's Chinese characters): Yizhihao/ Juchicao/ Wugongcao (一支蒿/锯齿草/蜈蚣草)

Latin: Achilleae Herba (Common name: Alpine Yarrow Herb or Milfoil)

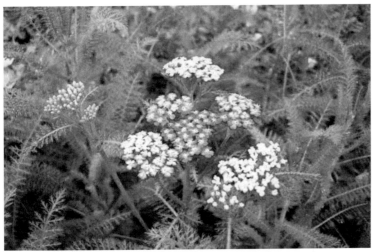

Plant: *Achillea alpina* L.

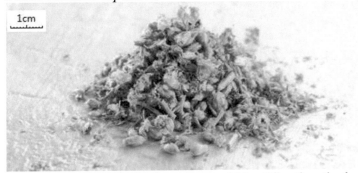

TCM prepared in ready-to-use forms (medicinal parts): it's dried up-ground-part which harvested in autumn.

Property and flavor: neutral; bitter, acidity.

Main and collateral channels: lung, spleen and bladder meridians.

Administration and dosage: 15-45 g.

Indication: tonsillitis, diarrhea, intestinal abscess with abdominal pain, dysuria and pain, insect or snake bites.

(The picture is only for learning and identification the herb; the specific use of the herb please consult the herbalist or health professionals)

Asiatic Pennywort Herb (Jixuecao)
Chinese phonetic alphabet/pin yin: jī xuě cǎo
Chinese characters simplified/traditional:积雪草/積雪草
Chinese nickname's alphabet (Nickname's Chinese characters): Tongqiancao(铜钱草)

Latin: Centellae Herba (Common name: Asiatic Pennywort Herb)

1cm

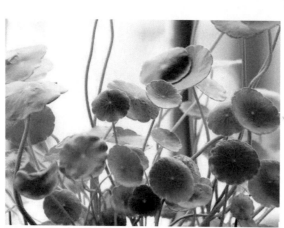

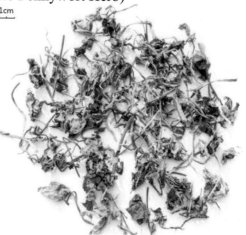

Plant: *Centella asiatica* (L.) Urb.

TCM prepared in ready-to-use forms (medicinal parts): it's dried whole herb which harvested in summer or autumn.

Property and flavor: cold; bitter, pungent.
Main and collateral channels: liver, spleen and kidney meridians.
Administration and dosage: 15-30 g.
Indication: jaundice, diarrhea, urolithiasis, hematuria, swelling abscess, traumatic injuries, sore and toxin.
(The picture is only for learning and identification the herb; the specific use of the herb please consult the herbalist or health professionals)

Snowbellleaf Tickclover Herb (Guangjinqiancao)
Chinese phonetic alphabet/pin yin: guǎng jīn qián cǎo
Chinese characters simplified/traditional:广金钱草/廣金錢草
Chinese nickname's alphabet (Nickname's Chinese characters): Luodijinqian/ Matixiang(落地金钱/马蹄香)
Latin: Desmodii Styracifolii Herba (Common name: Snowbellleaf Tickclover Herb)

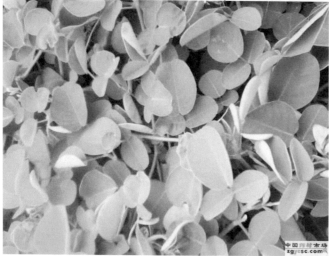

Plant: *Desmodium styracifolium* (Osb.) Merr.
TCM prepared in ready-to-use forms (medicinal parts): it's dried aerial part which harvested in summer or autumn.

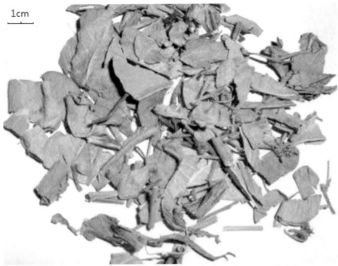

1cm

Property and flavor: cool; sweet, bland.
Main and collateral channels: liver, kidney and bladder meridians.
Administration and dosage: 15-30 g.

Indication: jaundice, pyretic stranguria, urolithiasis, edema, difficult and painful urination.
(The picture is only for learning and identification the herb; the specific use of the herb please consult the herbalist or health professionals)

Fenneflower Seed (Heizhongcaozi)
Chinese phonetic alphabet/pin yin: hēi zhǒng cǎo zǐ
Chinese characters simplified/traditional:黑种草子/黑種草子
Chinese nickname's alphabet (Nickname's Chinese characters): Sailanahebu(赛拉纳赫布)
Latin: Nigellae Semen (Common name: Fenneflower Seed)

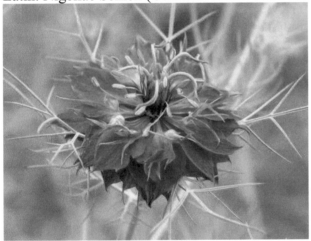

Plant: *Nigella glandulifera* Freyn et Sint.

1 cm

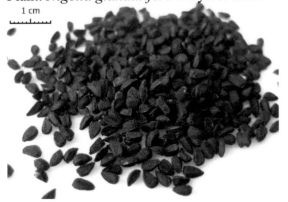

TCM prepared in ready-to-use forms (medicinal parts): it's dried seed.
Property and flavor: warm; sweet, pungent.
Administration and dosage: 2-6 g.
Indication: tinnitus, forgetfulness, amenorrhea, oligogalactia, pyretic stranguria and urolithiasis.
Precaution and warning: contraindicated during pregnancy and patients with febrile disease.
(The picture is only for learning and identification the herb; the specific use of the herb please consult the herbalist or health professionals)

Chinese Lizardtail Herb (Sanbaicao)

Chinese phonetic alphabet/pin yin: sān bái cǎo
Chinese characters simplified/traditional:三白草/三白草
Chinese nickname's alphabet (Nickname's Chinese characters): Tangbian'ou/
Baishegu(塘边藕/白舌骨)
Latin: Saururi Herba (Common name: Chinese Lizardtail Herb)

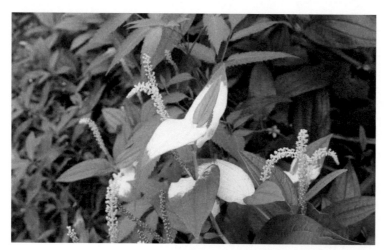

Plant: *Saururus chinensis* (Lour.) Baill.
TCM prepared in ready-to-use forms (medicinal parts): it's dried aerial part which harvested all year round.
Property and flavor: cold; sweet, pungent.

Main and collateral channels: lung and bladder meridians.
Administration and dosage: 15-30 g.
Indication: edema, anuresis and abnormal vaginal discharge; external use for sore, ulcer, eczema, swelling and toxin.

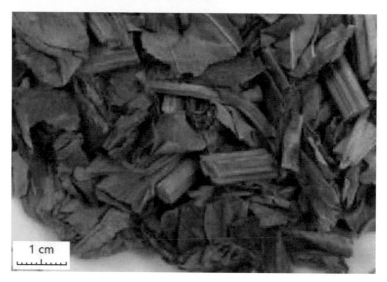

1 cm

(The picture is only for learning and identification the herb; the specific use of the herb please consult the herbalist or health professionals)

Chinaroot Greenbrier Rhizome (Baqia)

Chinese phonetic alphabet/pin yin: bá qià
Chinese characters simplified/traditional:菝葜/菝葜
Chinese nickname's alphabet (Nickname's Chinese characters): Jingangteng/
Tielingjiao/ Majiale(金刚藤/铁菱角/马加勒)
Latin: Smilacis Chinae Rhizoma (Common name: Chinaroot Greenbrier Rhizome)

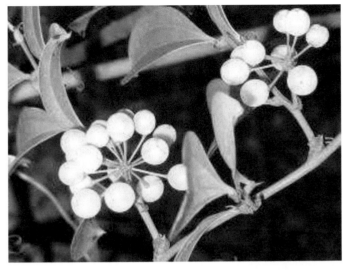

Plant: *Smilax china* L.
TCM prepared in ready-to-use forms (medicinal parts): it's dried rhizome which harvested in autumn to next spring.

Property and flavor: neutral; sweet, mild bitter and astringent.
Main and collateral channels: liver and kidney meridians.
Administration and dosage: 10-15 g.

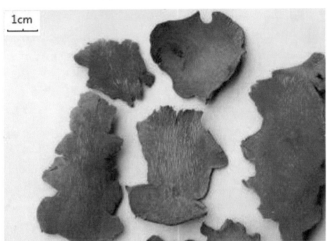

Indication: turbid stranguria, painful *bi* disorder, boil and sore, swelling abscess.
(The picture is only for learning and identification the herb; the specific use of the herb please consult the herbalist or health professionals)

Stachyurus Pith (Xiaotongcao)

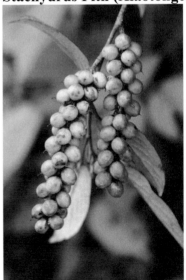

Chinese phonetic alphabet/pin yin: xiǎo tōng cǎo
Chinese characters simplified/ traditional: 小通草/小通草
Chinese nickname's alphabet (Nickname's Chinese characters):
Xiaotonghua/ Yupaoton(小通花/鱼泡通)
Latin: Stachyuri Medulla seu Helwingiae Medulla (Common name: Stachyurus Pith or Japanese Helwingia Pith)
Plant: *Stachyurus himalaicus* Hook. f. et. Thoms. (or *Stachyurus chinensis* Franch., *Helwingia japonica* (Thunb.) Dietr.)

TCM prepared in ready-to-use forms (medicinal parts): it's dried stem pith which harvested in autumn.

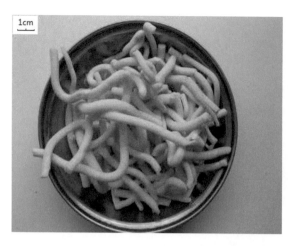

Property and flavor: cold; sweet, bland.
Main and collateral channels: lung and stomach meridians.
Administration and dosage: 3-6 g.
Indication: anuria, stranguria and agalactia.
(The picture is only for learning and identification the herb; the specific use of the herb please consult the herbalist or health professionals)

Chinese Wax Gourd Seed (Dongguaren)
Chinese phonetic alphabet/pin yin: dōng guā rén
Chinese characters simplified/traditional:冬瓜仁/冬瓜仁
Chinese nickname's alphabet (Nickname's Chinese characters): Dongguazi(冬瓜子)
Latin: Benincasae Semen (Common name: Chinese Wax Gourd Seed)

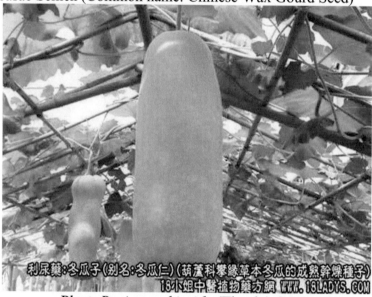

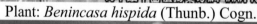

Plant: *Benincasa hispida* (Thunb.) Cogn.

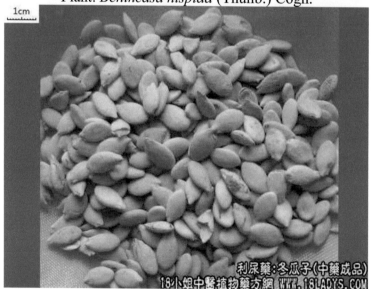

TCM prepared in ready-to-use forms (medicinal parts): it's dried ripe seed.
Property and flavor: cool; sweet.
Administration and dosage: 10-15 g.
Indication: cough, lung and intestinal abscess; diuresis.
(The picture is only for learning and identification the herb; the specific use of the herb please consult the herbalist or health professionals)

Galabash Gourd (Hulu)
Chinese phonetic alphabet/pin yin: hú lù
Chinese characters simplified/traditional:葫芦/葫蘆
Chinese nickname's alphabet (Nickname's Chinese characters): Gabeizhebu(嘎贝哲布)
Latin: Lagenariae Pericarpium (Common name: Galabash Gourd)

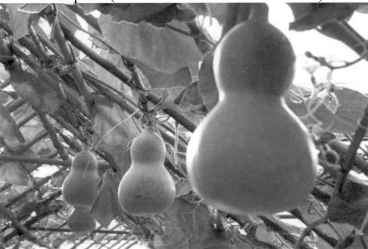

Plant: *Lagenaria siceraria* (Molina.) Standl.

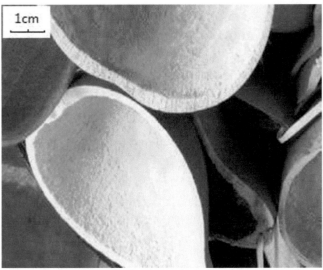

TCM prepared in ready-to-use forms (medicinal parts): it's dried ripe fruit.
Property and flavor: neutral; sweet, acidity and astringent.
Main and collateral channels: lung, stomach and kidney meridians.
Administration and dosage: 6-30 g.
Indication: edema; diuresis.

(The picture is only for learning and identification the herb; the specific use of the herb please consult the herbalist or health professionals)

Wen Li Yao(温里药)-Warm herbs
Wen Li Yao is a kind of herbs which's the major functions are dispelling cold, abdominal pain or stomachache caused by cold/chill (*Hanliang*); some of them can antiemetic, cardiac, treat excessive phlegm.

Prepared Common Monkshood Daughter Root (Fuzi)
Chinese phonetic alphabet/pin yin: fù zǐ
Chinese characters simplified/traditional:附子/附子
Chinese nickname's alphabet (Nickname's Chinese characters): Cezi/ Tianxiong(侧子/天雄)
Latin: Aconiti Lateralis Radix Praeparata (Common name: Prepared Common Monkshood Daughter Root)

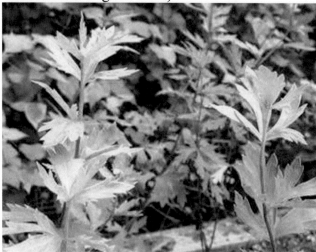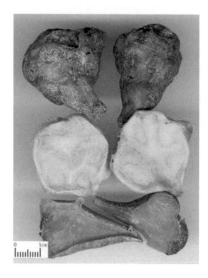

Plant: *Aconitum carmichaeli* Debx.
TCM prepared in ready-to-use forms (medicinal parts): it's processed product of the root which harvested between June and August.
Process: it can be processed by follow variety ways:
(Method 1) Soak the cleaned herb over night in liquor of mineral salt preparation (main components are sodium chloride, potassium chloride, magnesium chloride, calcium chloride, magnesium sulfate and magnesium bromide). Add salt (sodium chloride), soak and take it out to sun-dry and air-dry per day. Gradually prolong the time for dryness until a lot of salt is crystallized on the surface of the herb and its texture become hard. It is known as "yanfuzi".
(Method 2) Cut the cleaned herb into suitable size, and soak in liquor of mineral salt preparation (main components are sodium chloride, potassium chloride, magnesium chloride, calcium chloride, magnesium sulfate and magnesium bromide) for several days. Boil in the infusion thoroughly. Take out, rinse in water, cut into about 0.5 cm thickness slice. Rinse in water again. Stain the slice dark brown (by fried brown sugar and rape-seed oil, or black bean juice) and steam them until the slice turn into be oily and lustrous. Bake the slice to half-dryness, and then sun-dry or bake to complete dryness. It is known as "heifupian"
(Method 3) Soak the cleaned herb in liquor of mineral salt preparation (main components are sodium chloride, potassium chloride, magnesium chloride, calcium chloride, magnesium sulfate and magnesium bromide) for several days. Boil in the infusion thoroughly. Take out, remove the bark and cut into slice about 0.3 cm in thickness. After soaking and rinsing in water, take out, steam thoroughly, sun-dry to dryness. It is known as "baifupian" .
Property and flavor: highly hot; pungent and sweet.
Main and collateral channels: heart, kidney and spleen meridians.
Administration and dosage: 3-15 g. It should be decocted first and for long time.
Indication: the death collapse, icy cold limbs, weak pulse, impotence, edema, body coldness, rheumatic and arthralgia.

It is key herb to treat extreme critically ill caused by cold/chill (*Hanliang*).
Precaution and warning: toxic. Unprocessed one should be used cautiously for oral administration. Used cautiously for pregnant woman. Incompatible with Pinellia Tuber, Snakegourd Fruit, Snakegourd seed, Snakegourd peel, Snakegourd Root, Tendrilleaf Fritilary Bulb, Thunberg Fritillary Bulb, Ussuri Fritillary Bulb, Sinkiang Fritillary Bulb, Hubei Fritillary Bulb, Japanese Ampelopsis Root and Common Bletilla Tuber.
(The picture is only for learning and identification the herb; the specific use of the herb please consult the herbalist or health professionals)

Dried Ginger (Ganjiang)

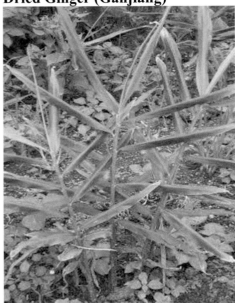

Chinese phonetic alphabet/
pin yin: gān jiāng
Chinese characters simplified/traditional:
干姜/乾薑
Chinese nickname's alphabet
(Nickname's Chinese characters):
Baijiang/ Junjiang/ Ganshengjiang(白姜/
均姜/干生姜)
Latin: Zingiberis Rhizoma (Common name: Dried Ginger or Zingiber)
Plant: *Zingiber officinale* Rosc.
TCM prepared in ready-to-use forms (medicinal parts): it's dried rhizome which harvested in winter.

Property and flavor: hot; pungent.
Main and collateral channels: spleen, stomach, kidney, heart and lung meridians.
Administration and dosage: 3-10 g.
Indication: abdominal pain caused by cold/chill (*Hanliang*), vomiting, diarrhea, weak pulse, icy cold limbs, phlegm and cough.
It is key herb to treat vomiting, abdominal pain, diarrhea and food stagnation.

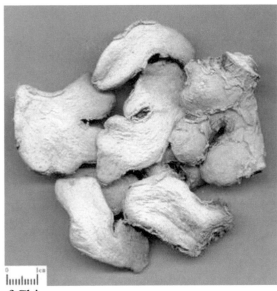

It is taken as seasoning in some part of China.
Attention: to protect the rare wild plant, please don't use the herb from wild plant.
(The picture is only for learning and identification the herb; the specific use of the herb please consult the herbalist or health professionals)

Cassia Bark (Rougui)

Chinese phonetic alphabet/pin yin: ròu guì

Chinese characters simplified/traditional:肉桂/肉桂

Chinese nickname's alphabet (Nickname's Chinese characters): Mugui/ Guipi/ Yugui(牡桂/桂皮/玉桂)

Latin: Cinnamomi Cortex (Common name: Cassia Bark or Cinnamon)

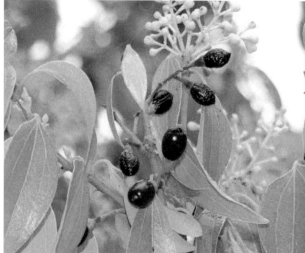

Plant: *Cinnamomum cassia* Presl.

TCM prepared in ready-to-use forms (medicinal parts): it's dried stem bark which harvested in autumn. Property and flavor: highly hot; pungent, sweet.

Main and collateral channels: kidney, spleen, heart and liver meridians. Administration and dosage: 1-5 g.

Indication: impotence, cold in the loins and knee, dizziness, red eyes, sore throat, cold pain in the heart, vomiting, diarrhea, cold hernia, amenorrhea and dysmenorrhea.

It is key herb to treat sexual hypofunction and metabolism hypofunction. It is taken as seasoning in some part of China.

Precaution and warning: use with caution in pregnant woman and patient prone to bleeding. Incompatible with Red Halloysite.

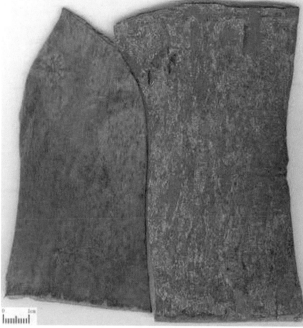

Attention: to protect the rare wild plant, please don't use the herb from wild plant. (The picture is only for learning and identification the herb; the specific use of the herb please consult the herbalist or health professionals)

Medicinal Evodia Fruit (Wuzhuyu)

Chinese phonetic alphabet/pin yin: wú zhū yú

Chinese characters simplified/traditional:吴茱萸/吳茱萸

Chinese nickname's alphabet (Nickname's Chinese characters): Wuyu/ Chala/ Zuoli(吴萸/茶辣/左力)

Latin: Euodiae Fructus (Common name: Medicinal Evodia Fruit)

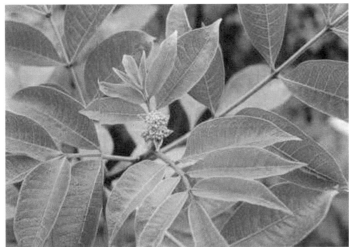

Plant: *Euodia rutaecarpa* (Juss.) Benth. (or *Euodia rutaecarpa* (Juss.) Benth. var. *officinalis* (Dode.) Huang., *Euodia rutaecarpa* (Juss.) Benth. var. *bodinieri* (Dode.) Huang., *Tetradium ruticarpum* (Juss.) Benth.)

TCM prepared in ready-to-use forms (medicinal parts): it's dried nearly ripe fruit.

Property and flavor: hot; bitter, pungent.

Main and collateral channels: liver, spleen, stomach and kidney meridians.

Administration and dosage: 2-5 g. Appropriate amount for topical application.

Indication: headache, abdominal pain caused by cold/chill (*Hanliang*), beriberi, vomiting, acid reflux, diarrhoea and hypertension; external use for ulcer.

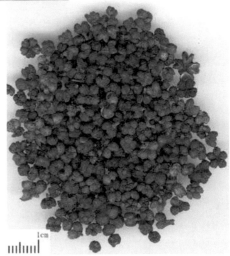

It is key herb to treat sour regurgitation, cold limbs, dysmenorrheal and irregular menstruation.

Precaution and warning: slightly toxin.

(The picture is only for learning and identification the herb; the specific use of the herb please consult the herbalist or health professionals)

Pricklyash Peel (Huajiao)

Chinese phonetic alphabet/ pin yin: huā jiāo

Chinese characters simplified/traditional: 花椒/花椒

Chinese nickname's alphabet (Nickname's Chinese characters): Hui/ Qinjiao/ Shujiao(檓/秦椒/ 蜀椒)

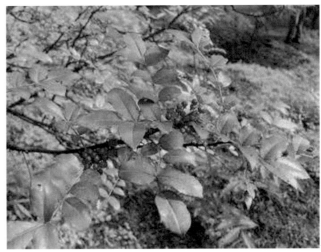

Latin: Zanthoxyli Pericarpium

(Common name: Pricklyash Peel or Sichuan Pepper)

Plant: *Zanthoxylum bungeanum* Maxim. (or *Zanthoxylum schinifolium* Sieb et Zucc.)

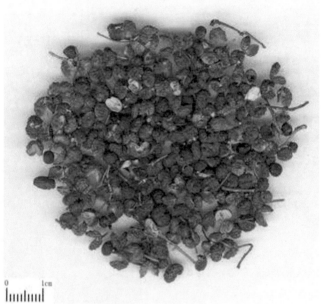

TCM prepared in ready-to-use forms (medicinal parts): it's dried percarp of ripe fruit.
Property and flavor: warm; pungent.
Main and collateral channels: spleen, stomach and kidney meridians.
Administration and dosage: 3-6 g. Appropriate amount for topical application. It can be decocted for fuming-washing therapy.
Indication: abdominal pain caused by cold/chill (*Hanliang*), vomiting, diarrhea, intestinal parasites; external use for eczema.
It is taken as seasoning in some part of China.
Precaution and warning: slightly toxin.
(The picture is only for learning and identification the herb; the specific use of the herb please consult the herbalist or health professionals)

Clove (Dingxiang)

Chinese phonetic alphabet/pin yin: dīng xiāng
Chinese characters simplified/traditional: 丁香/丁香
Chinese nickname's alphabet (Nickname's Chinese characters): Dingzixiang/ Zhijiexiang/ Gongdingxiang(丁子香/支解香/公丁香)
Latin: Caryophylli Flos (Common name: Clove)

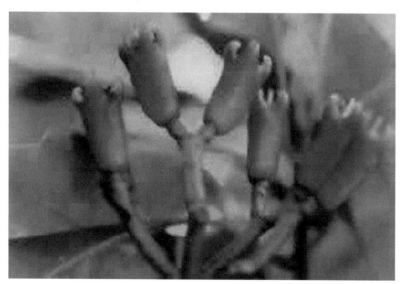

Plant: *Eugenia caryophyllata* Thunb. (or *Syzygium aromaticum* (L.) Merr. et Perry.)

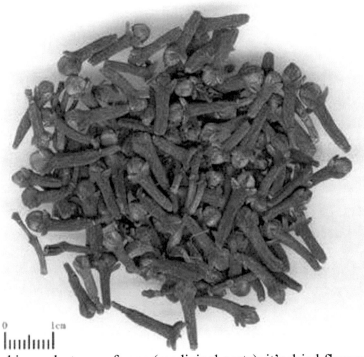

TCM prepared in ready-to-use forms (medicinal parts): it's dried flower bud.

Property and flavor: warm; pungent.

Main and collateral channels: spleen, stomach, lung and kidney meridians.

Administration and dosage: 1-3 g. For oral administration or ground it into powder for topical application.

Indication: vomiting, hiccup, cold pain in heart, diarrhea and impotence; appetizer. It is key herb to treat vomiting, nausea.

It is taken as seasoning in some part of China

Precaution and warning: incompatible with Turmeric Root Tuber.

(The picture is only for learning and identification the herb; the specific use of the herb please consult the herbalist or health professionals)

Clove Fruit (Mudingxiang)

Chinese phonetic alphabet/pin yin: mǔ dīng xiāng

Chinese characters simplified/traditional:母丁香/母丁香

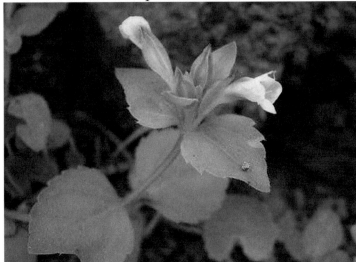

Chinese nickname's alphabet (Nickname's Chinese characters): Jishexiang/ Tingjiongdusheng/ Cidingxiang(鸡舌香 /亭炅独生/雌丁香)
Latin: Caryophylli Fructus (Common name: Clove Fruit)
Plant: *Eugenia caryophyllata* Thunb.

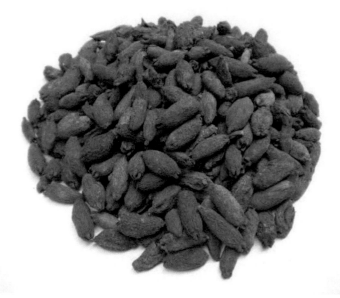

1 cm

TCM prepared in ready-to-use forms (medicinal parts): it's dried fruit.
Property and flavor: warm; pungent.
Main and collateral channels: spleen, stomach, lung and kidney meridians.

.

Administration and dosage: 1-3 g. For oral administration or ground it into powder for topical application.

Indication: hiccup, vomiting, heart and abdomen caused by cold/chill (*Hanliang*), impotence.

Precaution and warning: incompatible with Turmeric Root Tuber.

(The picture is only for learning and identification the herb; the specific use of the herb please consult the herbalist or health professionals)

Fennel (Xiaohuixiang)

Chinese phonetic alphabet/pin yin: xiǎo huí xiāng

Chinese characters simplified/traditional:小茴香/小茴香

Chinese nickname's alphabet (Nickname's Chinese characters): Huixiang/ Guhuixiang/ Xiangzi(茴香/谷茴香/香子)

Latin: Foeniculi Fructus (Common name: Fennel)
Plant: *Foeniculum vuLgare* Mil.

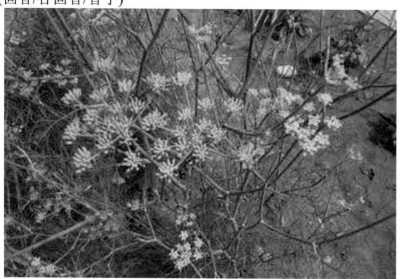

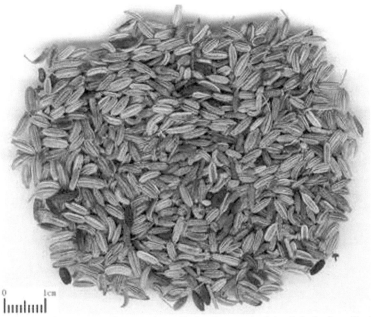

TCM prepared in ready-to-use forms (medicinal parts): it's dried ripe fruit.

Property and flavor: warm; pungent.

Main and collateral channels: liver, kidney, spleen and stomach meridians.

Administration and dosage: 3-6 g.

Indication: abdominal pain and distension caused by cold/chill (*Hanliang*), dysmenorrhea; appetizer.

It is taken as seasoning in some part of China.

(The picture is only for learning and identification the herb; the specific use of the herb please consult the herbalist or health professionals)

Lesser Galangal Rhizome (Gaoliangjiang)

Chinese phonetic alphabet/pin yin: gāo liáng jiāng

Chinese characters simplified/traditional:高良姜/高良薑

Chinese nickname's alphabet (Nickname's Chinese characters): Xiaoliangjiang/ Liangjiang(小良姜/良姜)

Latin: Alpiniae Officinarum Rhizoma (Common name: Lesser Galangal Rhizome)

Plant: *Alpinia officinarum* Hance.

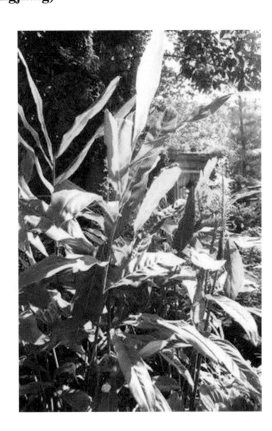

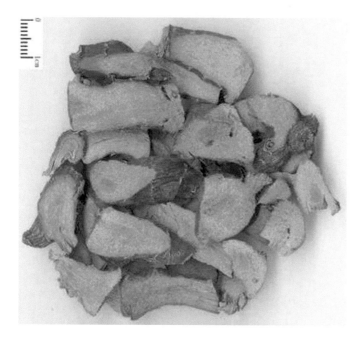

TCM prepared in
ready-to-use forms
(medicinal parts):
it's dried rhizome
which harvested in
summer or autumn.
Property and flavor:
hot; pungent.
Main and collateral
channels: spleen and
stomach meridians.

Administration and dosage: 3-6 g.
Indication: abdominal and epigastrium pain and distension caused by cold/chill
(*Hanliang*), vomiting and acid regurgitation.
It is taken as seasoning in some part of China.
(The picture is only for learning and identification the herb; the specific use of the
herb please consult the herbalist or health professionals)

Long Pepper (Bibo)
Chinese phonetic alphabet/pin yin: bì bō
Chinese characters simplified/traditional:荜茇/蓽菝

Chinese
nickname's
alphabet
(Nickname's
Chinese
characters):
Shensheng/
Shuwei(椹圣/鼠
尾)
Latin: Piperis
Longui Fructus
(Common name:
Long Pepper)
Plant: *Piper
longum* L.

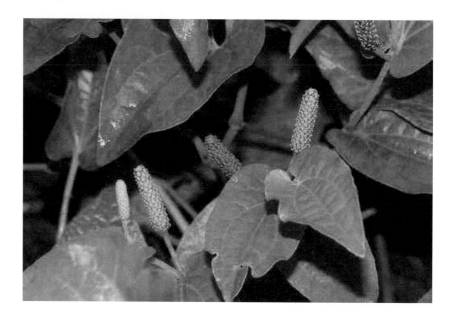

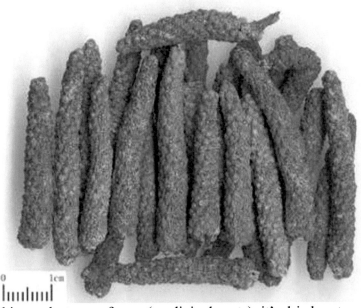

TCM prepared in ready-to-use forms (medicinal parts): it's dried mature ear or fruit-spike.

Property and flavor: hot; pungent.

Main and collateral channels: stomach and large intestine meridians.

Administration and dosage: 1-3 g. Topical application in appropriate amount, ground into powder to stuff dental caries.

Indication: epigastrium and abdominal pain and distension caused by cold/chill (*Hanliang*), vomiting, diarrhea, migraine and heart pain; external used for toothache. It is taken as seasoning in some part of China.

(The picture is only for learning and identification the herb; the specific use of the herb please consult the herbalist or health professionals)

Galanga Resurrectionlily Rhizome (Shannai)

Chinese phonetic alphabet/pin yin: shān nài

Chinese characters simplified/traditional:山柰/山柰

Chinese nickname's alphabet (Nickname's Chinese characters): Shannai/ Sannaizi/ Sanlai/ Shanla/ Shajiang(山奈/三柰子/三赖/山辣/沙姜)

Latin: Kaempferiae Rhizoma (Common name: Galanga Resurrectionlily Rhizome)

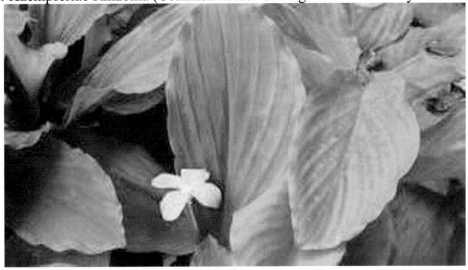

Plant: *Kaempferia galanga* L.

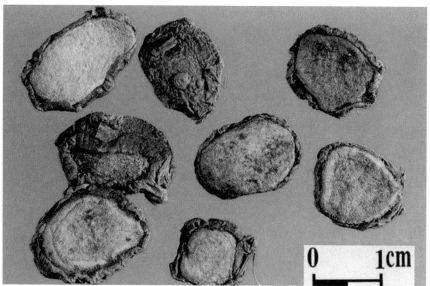

TCM prepared in ready-to-use forms (medicinal parts): it's dried rhizome which harvest in winter.

Property and flavor: warm; pungent.

Main and collateral channels: stomach meridian.

Administration and dosage: 6-9 g.

Indication: chest tightness, cold pain in epigastrium and abdominal, indigestion and dyspepsia.

It is taken as seasoning in some part of China.

(The picture is only for learning and identification the herb; the specific use of the herb please consult the herbalist or health professionals)

Mountain Spicy Fruit (Bichengqie)

Chinese phonetic alphabet/pin yin: bì chéng qié

Chinese characters simplified/traditional:荜澄茄/蓽澄茄

Chinese nickname's alphabet (Nickname's Chinese characters): Pilinqiezi/ Biqie/ Shanjijiao(毗陵茄子/毕茄/山鸡椒)

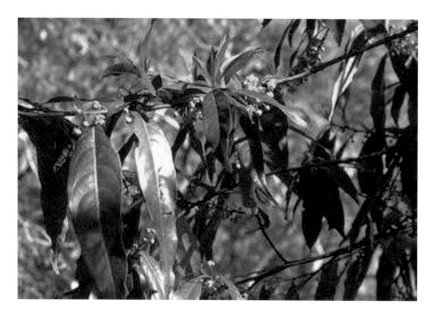

Latin: Litseae Fructus (Common name: Mountain Spicy Fruit) Plant: *Litsea cubeba* (Lour.) Pers.

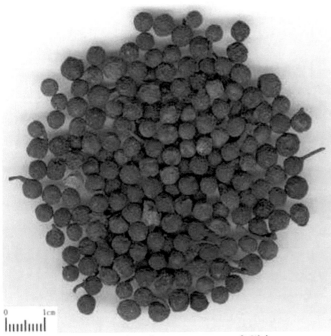

TCM prepared in ready-to-use forms (medicinal parts): it's dried mature fruit.
Property and flavor: warm; pungent.
Main and collateral channels: spleen, stomach, kidney and bladder meridians.
Administration and dosage: 1-3 g.
Indication: stomach and abdominal pain caused by cold/chill (*Hanliang*), vomiting, hiccups, hernia, turbid urine.

It is taken as seasoning in some part of China.
(The picture is only for learning and identification the herb; the specific use of the herb please consult the herbalist or health professionals)

Chinese Star Anise (Bajiaohuixiang)
Chinese phonetic alphabet/pin yin: bā jiǎo huí xiāng
Chinese characters simplified/traditional:八角茴香/八角茴香
Chinese nickname's alphabet (Nickname's Chinese characters): Bohuixiang/ Bajao/ Dahuixiang(舶茴香/八角/大茴香)
Latin: Anisi Stellati Fructus (Common name: Chinese Star Anise)

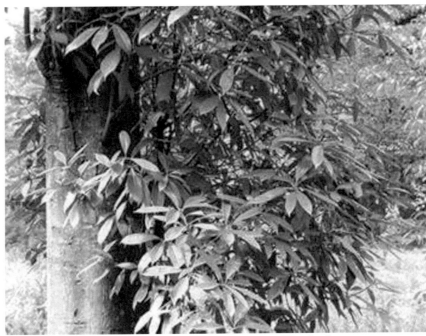

Plant: *Illicium verum* Hook. f.

TCM prepared in ready-to-use forms (medicinal parts): it's dried mature fruit. Property and flavor: warm; pungent. Main and collateral channels: liver, kidney, spleen and stomach meridians.

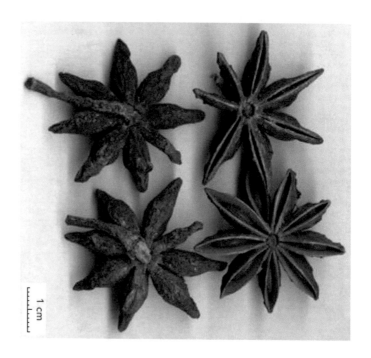

Administration and dosage: 3-6 g, used in alcohol preparation, for oral administration or for topical application.

Indication: hernia, abdominal and stomach pain caused by cold/chill (*Hanliang*), lumbago, vomiting.

It is taken as seasoning in some part of China.

(The picture is only for learning and identification the herb; the specific use of the herb please consult the herbalist or health professionals)

Tibet Sweetflag Rhizome (Zangchangpu)

Chinese phonetic alphabet/pin yin: zàng chāng pú

Chinese characters simplified/traditional:藏菖蒲/藏菖蒲

Chinese nickname's alphabet (Nickname's Chinese characters): Pujian/ Baichang (蒲剑/白菖)

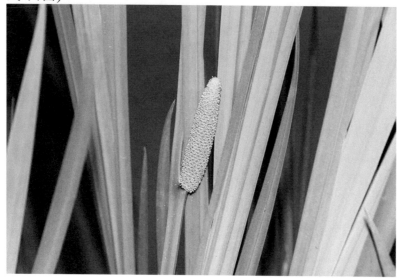

Latin: Acori Calami Rhizoma (Common name: Tibet Sweetflag Rhizome)
Plant: *Acorus calamus* L.

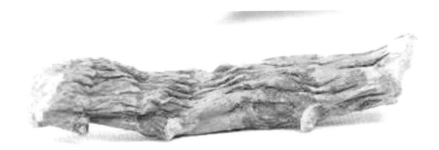

1cm

TCM prepared in ready-to-use forms (medicinal parts): it's dried rhizome which harvested in autumn or winter.

Flavor: pungent, bitter.

Administration and dosage: 3-6 g.

Indication: dyspepsia, diphthera, anhtrax and indigestion.

(The picture is only for learning and identification the herb; the specific use of the herb please consult the herbalist or health professionals)

Jack Bean (Daodou)

Chinese phonetic alphabet/pin yin: dāo dòu

Chinese characters simplified/traditional:刀豆/刀豆

Chinese nickname's alphabet (Nickname's Chinese characters): Xiejiandou/ Daodoujiao(挟剑豆/刀豆角)

Latin: Canavaliae Semen (Common name: Jack Bean)

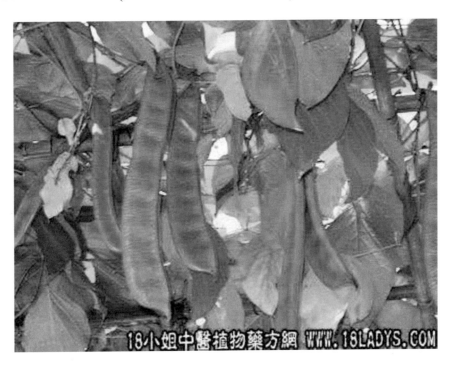

Plant: *Canavalia gladiata* (Jacq.) DC.

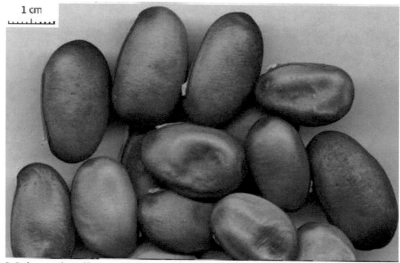

TCM prepared in ready-to-use forms (medicinal parts): it's dried ripe seed. Property and flavor: warm; sweet.

Main and collateral channels: stomach and kidney meridians.
Administration and dosage: 6-9 g.
Indication: hiccup and vomiting.
It is taken as food in some part of China.
(The picture is only for learning and identification the herb; the specific use of the herb please consult the herbalist or health professionals)

Hot Pepper (Lajiao)
Chinese phonetic alphabet/pin yin: là jiāo
Chinese characters simplified/traditional:辣椒/辣椒
Chinese nickname's alphabet (Nickname's Chinese characters): Lazi/ Qinjiao/ Haijiao(辣子/秦椒/海椒)
Latin: Capsici Fructus (Common name: Hot Pepper)

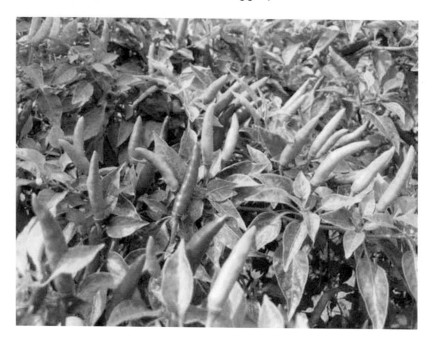

Plant: *Capsicum annuum* L. (or its cultivated varieties)

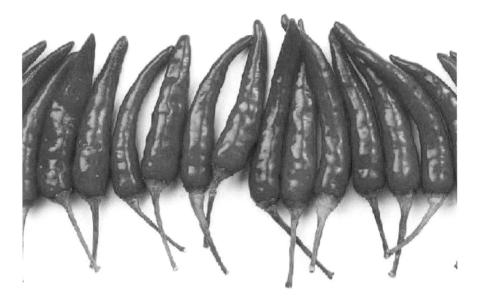

TCM prepared in ready-to-use forms (medicinal parts): it's dried mature fruit.
Property and flavor: hot; pungent.
Main and collateral channels: heart and spleen meridians.
Administration and dosage: 0.9-2.4 g. Appropriate amount for topical application.
Indication: abdominal pain caused by cold/chill (*Hanliang*), vomiting, diarrhea and dysentery, frostbite, loss appetite.
It is taken as seasoning in some part of China.
(The picture is only for learning and identification the herb; the specific use of the herb please consult the herbalist or health professionals)

Galanga Galangal Fruit (Hongdoukou)
Chinese phonetic alphabet/pin yin: hóng dòu kòu
Chinese characters simplified/traditional:红豆蔻/紅豆蔻
Chinese nickname's alphabet (Nickname's Chinese characters): Daliangjiang/
Shanjiang(大良姜/山姜)

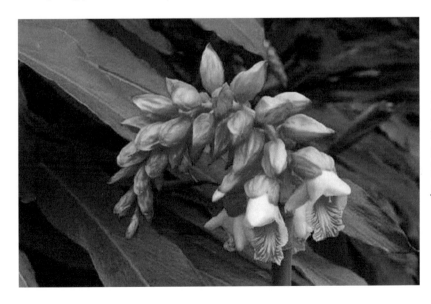

Latin: Galangae Fructus (Common name: Galanga Galangal Fruit)
Plant: *Alpinia galanga* Willd.

222

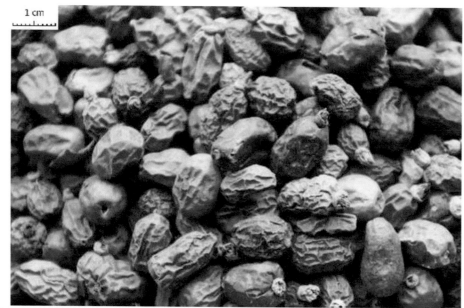

TCM prepared in ready-to-use forms (medicinal parts): it's dried mature fruit.

Property and flavor: warm; pungent.

Main and collateral channels: spleen and lung meridians.

Administration and dosage: 3-6 g.

Indication: epigastrium and abdomen pain caused by cold/chill (*Hanliang*), indigestion, vomiting, diarrhea, alcohol abuse.

Attention: to protect the rare wild plant, please don't use the herb from wild plant. (The picture is only for learning and identification the herb; the specific use of the herb please consult the herbalist or health professionals)

Pepper Fruit (Hujiao)

Chinese phonetic alphabet/pin yin: hú jiāo

Chinese characters simplified/traditional:胡椒/胡椒

Chinese nickname's alphabet (Nickname's Chinese characters): Meilvzhi/ Pilei(昧履支/披垒)

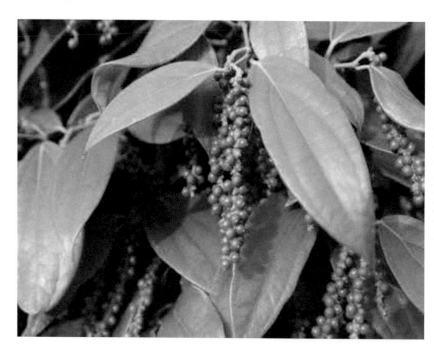

Latin: Piperis Fructus (Common name: Pepper Fruit)
Plant: *Piper nigrum* L.

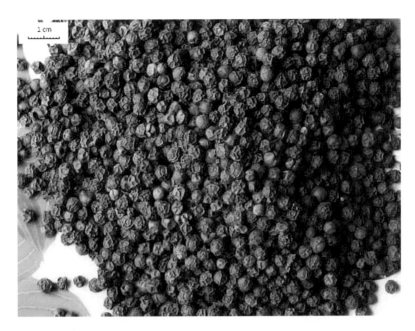

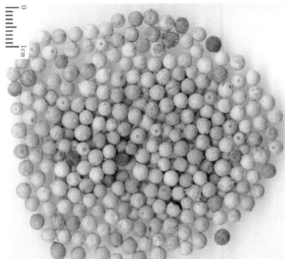

TCM prepared in ready-to-use forms (medicinal parts): it's dried mature fruit.
Property and flavor: hot; pungent.
Main and collateral channels: stomach and large intestine meridians.
Administration and dosage: 0.6-1.5 g, ground into powder for oral administration.
Topical application in appropriate amount.

Indication: vomiting caused by cold/chill (*Hanliang*), diarrhea, loss of appetite, epilepsy, excessive phlegm.
It is taken as seasoning in some part of China.
White pepper is harvested until the fruit is ripe and is removed red skin by mechanical or water washing, then dried the remaining white seeds. Black pepper is dried the whole one, its original red skin become black after dried, so it is black.
(The picture is only for learning and identification the herb; the specific use of the herb please consult the herbalist or health professionals)

Li *Qi* Yao(理气药)-Qi regulating herbs
Li *Qi* Yao is a kind of herbs which's the major functions are to treat distention and fullness, some of them can treat colic or hernia, amenorrhea and dysmenorrhea, vomit, acid regurgitation.

Dried Tangerine Peel (Chenpi)
Chinese phonetic alphabet/pin yin: chén pí
Chinese characters simplified/traditional:陈皮/陳皮
Chinese nickname's alphabet (Nickname's Chinese characters): Jupi/ Guangchenpi

(橘皮/广陈皮)
Latin:Citri Reticulatae Pericarpium (Common name: Dried Tangerine Peel or Dried Orange Peel)

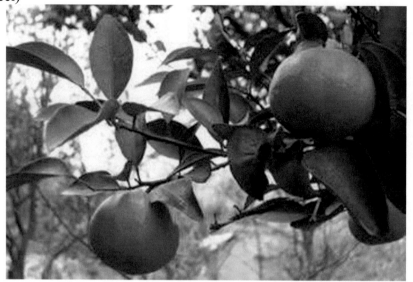

Plant: *Citrus reticulata* Blanco. (or its cultivars)

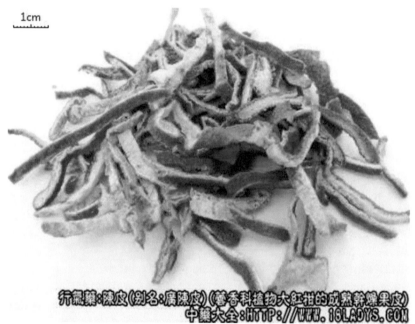

行气药:陈皮(别名:广陈皮)(芸香科植物大红柑的成熟干燥果皮)
中药大全:HTTP://WWW.16LADYS.COM

TCM prepared in ready-to-use forms (medicinal parts): it's dried pericarp of mature fruit.

Property and flavor: warm; pungent, bitter.

Main and collateral channels: lung and spleen meridians.

Administration and dosage: 3-10 g.

Indication: epigastrium and abdominal distension, vomit, diarrhea, cough with asthma and excessive phlegm; appetizer.

It is key herb to promote digestion and reduce phlegm.

(The picture is only for learning and identification the herb, the specific use of the herb please consult the herbalist or health professionals)

Immature Orange Fruit (Zhishi)

Chinese phonetic alphabet/pin yin: zhì shí

Chinese characters simplified/traditional:枳实/枳實

Chinese nickname's alphabet (Nickname's Chinese characters): Dongting/ Nianci(洞庭/黏刺)

Latin: Aurantii Fructus Immaturus (Common name: Immature Orange Fruit)

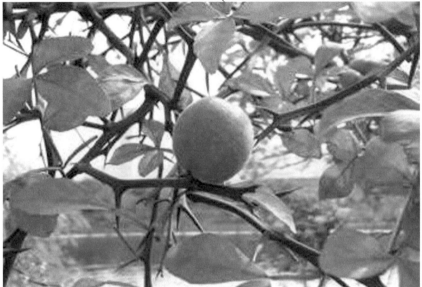

Plant: *Citrus aurantium* L. (or *Citrus sinensis* Osbeck.)

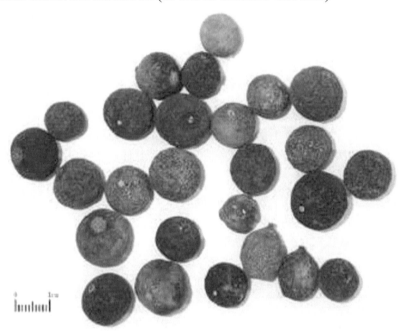

TCM prepared in ready-to-use forms (medicinal parts): it's dried young fruit.

Property and flavor: mild cold; bitter, pungent and acidity.

Main and collateral channels: spleen and stomach meridians.

Administration and dosage: 3-10 g

Indication: abdominal distension, vomit, diarrhea, dysentery, excessive phlegm, constipation; appetizer.

It is key herb to treat gastrointestinal stagnation and phlegm stagnation.

Precaution and warning: use with caution during pregnancy.

(The picture is only for learning and identification the herb; the specific use of the herb please consult the herbalist or health professionals)

Common Aucklandia Root (Muxiang)
Chinese phonetic alphabet/pin yin: mù xiāng
Chinese characters simplified/traditional:木香/木香
Chinese nickname's alphabet (Nickname's Chinese characters): Mixiang/ Wuxiang/
Wumuxiang(蜜香/五香/五木香)
Latin: Aucklandiae Radix (Common name: Common Aucklandia Root)

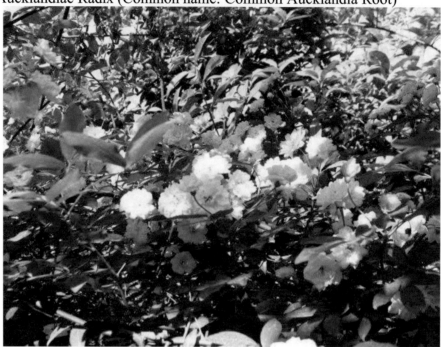

Plant: *Aucklandia lappa* Decne. (or *Saussurea costus* (Falc.) Lipschitz)

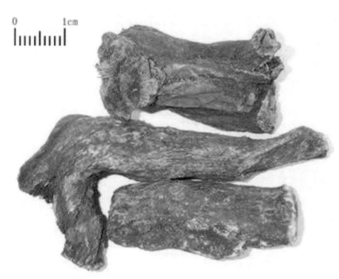

TCM prepared in ready-to-use forms (medicinal parts): it's dried root which harvested in spring or winter.
Property and flavor: warm; pungent, bitter.
Main and collateral channels: spleen, stomach, large intestine, triple energizer and gallbladder meridians.

Administration and dosage: 3-6 g.
Indication: epigastrium and abdominal pain and distension, diarrhea, dysentery and indigestion.
It is key herb to treat epigastria and abdomen pain and distention.
Attention: to protect the rare wild plant, please don't use the herb from wild plant.
(The picture is only for learning and identification the herb; the specific use of the herb please consult the herbalist or health professionals)

Nutgrass Galingale Rhizome (Xiangfu)

Chinese phonetic alphabet/pin yin: xiāng fù

Chinese characters simplified/traditional:香附/香附

Chinese nickname's alphabet (Nickname's Chinese characters): Shacaogen/ Xiangfuzi/ Leigongtou(莎草根/香附子/雷公头)

Latin: Cyperi Rhizoma (Common name: Nutgrass Galingale Rhizome)

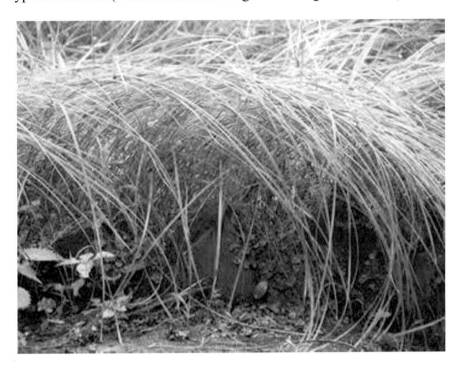

Plant: *Cyperus rotundus* L.

TCM prepared in ready-to-use forms (medicinal parts): it's dried rhizome which harvested in autumn.

Property and flavor: neutral; pungent, mild bitter and mild sweet.

Main and collateral channels: liver, spleen and triple energizers meridians.

Administration and dosage: 6-10 g.

Indication: epigastrium and abdominal pain and distension, indigestion, mastitis, irregular menstruation, amenorrhea and dysmenorrhea.

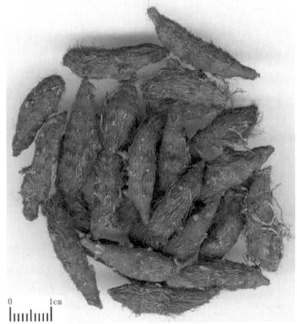

It is key herb to treat hypochondriac distress and pain, chest oppression, dysmenorrheal and amenorrhea.

(The picture is only for learning and identification the herb; the specific use of the herb please consult the herbalist or health professionals)

Chinese Eaglewood Wood (Chenxiang)
Chinese phonetic alphabet/pin yin: chén xiāng
Chinese characters simplified/traditional:沉香/沉香
Chinese nickname's alphabet (Nickname's Chinese characters): Chenshuixiang(沉水香)
Latin: Aquilariae Lignum Resinatum (Common name: Chinese Eaglewood Wood)

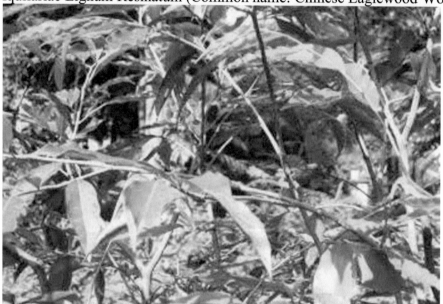

Plant: *Aquilaria sinensis* (Lour.) Gilg.

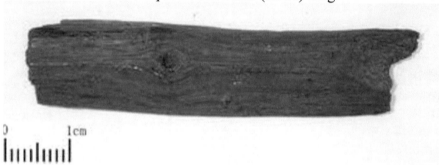

0   1cm

TCM prepared in ready-to-use forms (medicinal parts): it's wood contains resin which harvested all year round.
Property and flavor: mild warm; pungent, bitter.
Main and collateral channels: spleen, stomach and kidney meridians.
Administration and dosage: 1-5 g, added when the decoction nearly done.
Indication: abdominal pain and distension caused by cold, vomit, dyspnea.
Attention: to protect the rare wild plant, please don't use the herb from wild plant.
(The picture is only for learning and identification the herb; the specific use of the herb please consult the herbalist or health professionals)

Szechwan Chinaberry Fruit (Chuanlianzi)
Chinese phonetic alphabet/pin yin: chuān liàn zǐ
Chinese characters simplified/traditional:川楝子/川楝子
Chinese nickname's alphabet (Nickname's Chinese characters): Jinlingzi/ Lianshi(金铃子/楝实)

Latin: Toosendan Fructus (Common name: Szechwan Chinaberry Fruit)

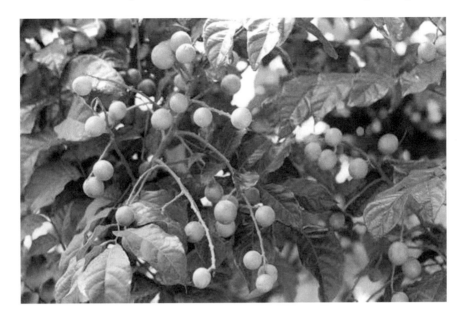

Plant: *Melia toosendan* Sieb. et Zucc.

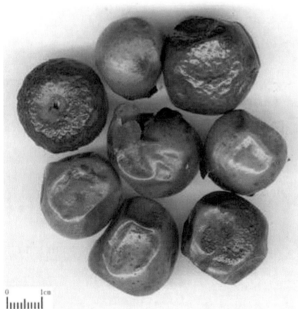

TCM prepared in ready-to-use forms (medicinal parts): it's mature fruit.
Property and flavor: cold; bitter.
Main and collateral channels: liver, small intestine and bladder meridians.
Administration and dosage: 5-10 g. Topical application in appropriate amount, ground into powder as liniment.

Indication: epigastrium and abdominal pain and distension, colic, intestinal parasites.
Precaution and warning: slightly toxic.
(The picture is only for learning and identification the herb; the specific use of the herb please consult the herbalist or health professionals)

Longstamen Onion Bulb (Xiebai)
Chinese phonetic alphabet/pin yin: xiè bái
Chinese characters simplified/traditional:薤白/薤白
Chinese nickname's alphabet (Nickname's Chinese characters): Xiaogencai/ Xiaodusuan/ Yesuan(小根菜/小独蒜/野蒜)
Latin: Allii Macrostemonis Bulbus (Common name: Longstamen Onion Bulb)

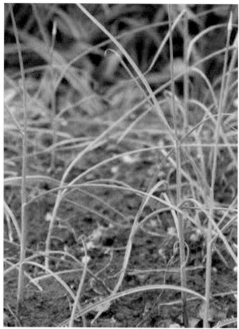

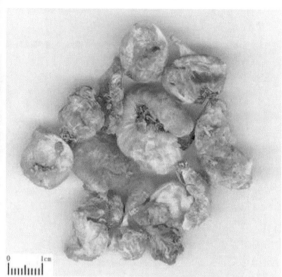

Plant: *Allium macrostemon* Bunge. (or *Allium chinensis* G. Don.)

TCM prepared in ready-to-use forms (medicinal parts): it's subterranean bulb which harvested in summer or autumn.

Property and flavor: warm; pungent, bitter.

Main and collateral channels: heart, lung, stomach and large intestine meridians.

Administration and dosage: 5-10 g.

Indication: chest pain of impediment, diarrhea and dysentery.

It is key herb to treat thoracic obstruction.

It is taken as food in some part of China.

(The picture is only for learning and identification the herb; the specific use of the herb please consult the herbalist or health professionals)

Pummelo Peel (Huajuhong)

Chinese phonetic alphabet/pin yin: huà jú hóng

Chinese characters simplified/traditional:化橘红/化橘紅

Chinese nickname's alphabet (Nickname's Chinese characters): Huazhoujuhong(化州橘红)

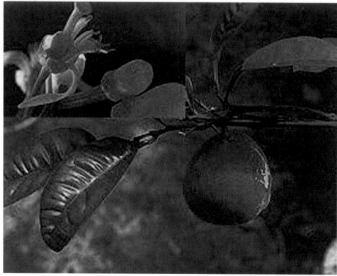

Latin:
Citri Grandis
Exocarpium
(Common name:
Pummelo Peel)
Plant: *Citrus grandis*
Tomentosa. (or *Citrus grandis* (L.) Osbeck.)

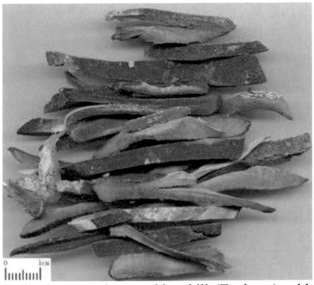

TCM prepared in ready-to-use forms (medicinal parts): it's dried exocarp of almost ripe fruit.
Property and flavor: warm; pungent, bitter.
Main and collateral channels: lung and spleen meridians.
Administration and dosage: 3-6 g.

Indication: cough caused by chill *(Fenhang)* cold, excessive phlegm, indigestion, vomiting, distension; alleviate a hangover .
It is taken as seasoning in some part of China.
(The picture is only for learning and identification the herb; the specific use of the herb please consult the herbalist or health professionals)

Dried Immaturity Tangerines Peel (Qingpi)

Chinese phonetic alphabet/pin yin: qīng pí
Chinese characters simplified/traditional:青皮/青皮
Chinese nickname's alphabet (Nickname's Chinese characters): Qingjupi/ Qingpizi(青橘皮/青皮子)
Latin: Citri Reticulatae Pericarpium Viride (Common name: Dried Immaturity Tangerines Peel or Green Tangerine Peel)

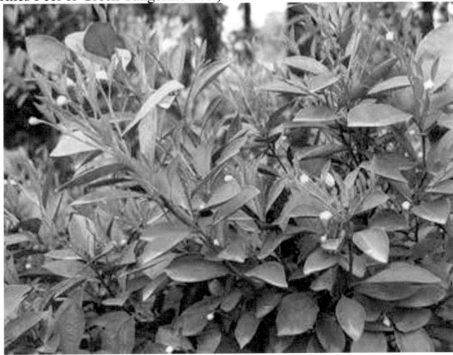

Plant: *Citrus reticulata* Blanco. (or its cultivars)

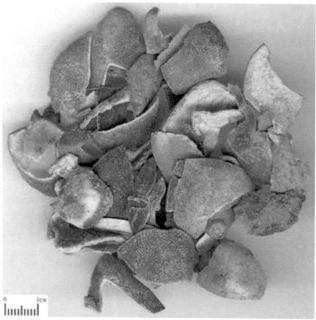

TCM prepared in ready-to-use forms (medicinal parts): it's dried pericarp of unripe fruit.
Property and flavor: warm; pungent, bitter.
Main and collateral channels: liver, gallbladder and stomach meridians.
Administration and dosage: 3-10 g.
Indication: chest and abdominal pain and distension, hernia, mastitis and dyspepsia; lactagogue.

(The picture is only for learning and identification the herb; the specific use of the herb please consult the herbalist or health professionals)

Finger Citron (Foshou)

Chinese phonetic alphabet/pin yin: fó shǒu
Chinese characters simplified/traditional:佛手/佛手
Chinese nickname's alphabet (Nickname's Chinese characters): Foshougan/ Wuzhigan(佛手柑/五指柑)
Latin: Citri Sarcodactylis Fructus (Common name: Finger Citron or Bergamot)

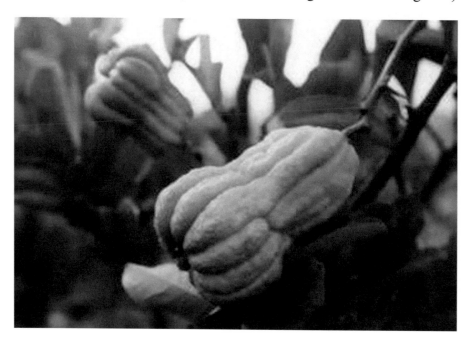

Plant: *Citrus medica* L. var. *sarcodactylis* Swingle.

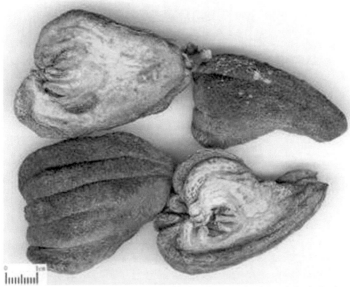

TCM prepared in ready-to-use forms (medicinal parts): it's dried fruit.

Property and flavor: warm; pungent, bitter and acidity.

Main and collateral channels: liver, stomach, lung and spleen meridians.

Administration and dosage: 3-10 g.

Indication: chest and abdominal pain and distension, vomiting and cough and profuse sputum; appetizer.

It is taken as food in some part of China.

(The picture is only for learning and identification the herb; the specific use of the herb please consult the herbalist or health professionals)

Combined Spicebush Root (Wuyao)

Chinese phonetic alphabet/pin yin: wū yào

Chinese characters simplified/traditional:乌药/烏藥

Chinese nickname's alphabet (Nickname's Chinese characters): Pangqi/ Aizhang(旁其/矮樟)

Latin: Linderae Radix (Common name: Combined Spicebush Root)

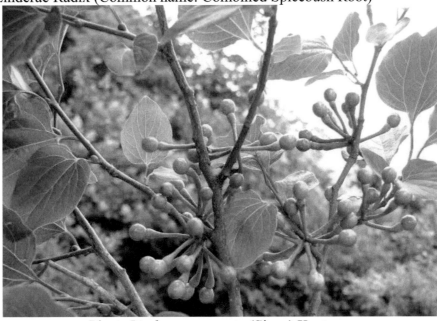

Plant: *Lindera aggregata* (Sims.) Kosterm.

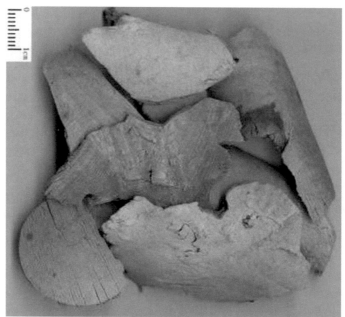

TCM prepared in ready-to-use forms (medicinal parts): it's dried root tuber which harvested all year round.

Property and flavor: warm; pungent.

Main and collateral channels: lung, spleen, kidney and bladder meridians.

Administration and dosage: 6-10 g.

Indication: chest and abdominal pain and distension, wheezing, dyspnea, frequent micturition and hernia.

(The picture is only for learning and identification the herb; the specific use of the herb please consult the herbalist or health professionals)

Lychee Seed (Lizhihe)

Chinese phonetic alphabet/pin yin: lì zhī hé
Chinese characters simplified/traditional: 荔枝核/荔枝核
Chinese nickname's alphabet (Nickname's Chinese characters):
Liren/ Zhihe/ Dalihe(荔仁/枝核/大荔核)
Latin: Litchi Semen
(Common name: Lychee Seed)
Plant: *Litchi chinensis* Sonn.

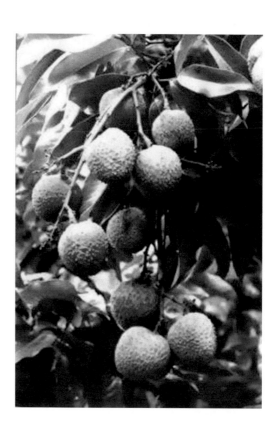

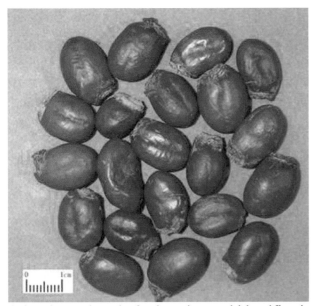

TCM prepared in ready-to-use forms (medicinal parts): it's dried mature seed.
Property and flavor: warm; sweet, mild bitter.
Main and collateral channels: liver and kidney meridians.
Administration and dosage: 5-10 g.
Indication: cold hernia, abdominal pain, testicular swelling and pain.

(The picture is only for learning and identification the herb; the specific use of the herb please consult the herbalist or health professionals)

Nardostachys Root (Gansong)
Chinese phonetic alphabet/pin yin: gān sōng
Chinese characters simplified/traditional:甘松/甘松
Chinese nickname's alphabet (Nickname's Chinese characters): Xiangsong(香松)
Latin: Nardostachyos Radix et Rhizoma (Common name: Nardostachys Root)

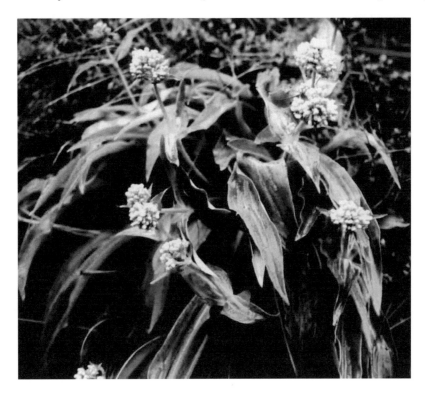

Plant: *Nardostachys jatamansi* DC.

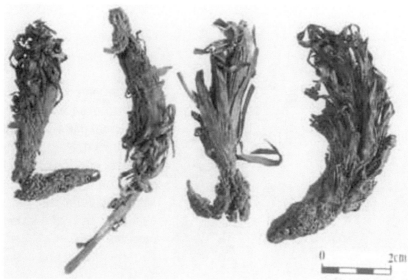

TCM prepared in ready-to-use forms (medicinal parts): it's dried root and rhizome which harvested in spring and autumn.

Property and flavor: warm; pungent, sweet.

Main and collateral channels: spleen and stomach meridians.

Administration and dosage: 3-6 g. Topical application in appropriate amount, brewed for gargle or decocted for rinsing, or ground into powder for applying to the *pars affecta*.

Indication: epigastrium and abdominal distension, loss of appetite and vomiting; external use for toothache, disperse swollen.

Attention: to protect the rare wild plant, please don't use the herb from wild plant. (The picture is only for learning and identification the herb; the specific use of the herb please consult the herbalist or health professionals)

Red Tangerine Peel (Juhong)

Chinese phonetic alphabet/pin yin: jú hóng

Chinese characters simplified/traditional:橘红/橘紅

Chinese nickname's alphabet (Nickname's Chinese characters): Yunpi/ Yunhong(芸皮/芸红)

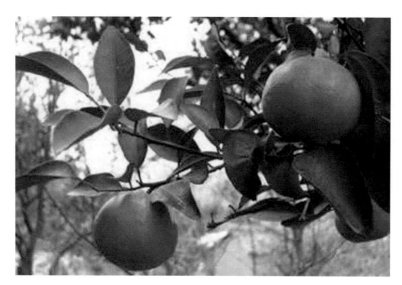

Latin: Citri Exocarpium Rubrum (Common name: Red Tangerine Reel)
Plant: *Citrus reticulata* Blanco. (or its cultivars)

TCM prepared in ready-to-use forms (medicinal parts): it's dried ripe epicarp (exocarp).

Property and flavor: warm; pungent, bitter.

Main and collateral channels: lung and spleen meridians.

Administration and dosage: 3-10 g.

Indication: cough caused by chill (*Fenghan*) cold, itchy throat, excessive phlegm, drink over, vomiting, distension.

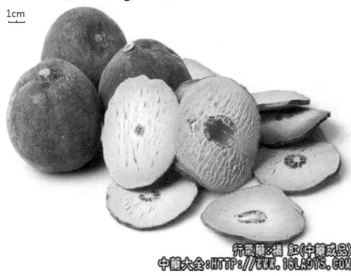

It is taken as seasoning in some part of China. (The picture is only for learning and identification the herb; the specific use of the herb please consult the herbalist or health professionals)

Orange Fruit (Zhiqiao)

Chinese phonetic alphabet/pin yin: zhǐ qiào

Chinese characters simplified/traditional:枳壳/枳殼

Chinese nickname's alphabet (Nickname's Chinese characters): Suanchengke/ Daidaihuaguoke (酸橙壳/代代花果壳)

Latin: Aurantii Fructus (Common name: Orange Fruit, Fruit of Citron or Trifoliate Orange)

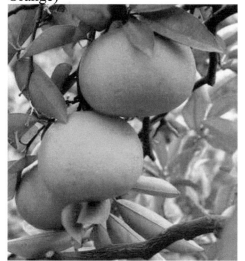

Plant: *Citrus aurantium* L. (or its cultivated varieties)

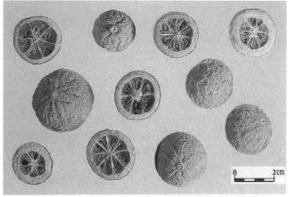

TCM prepared in ready-to-use forms (medicinal parts): it's dried immature fruit.

Property and flavor: mild cold; bitter, pungent and acidity.

Main and collateral channels: spleen and stomach meridians.

Administration and dosage: 3-10 g.

Indication: chest pain and fullness, dyspepsia, sputum retention and splanchnoptosis.

Precaution and warning: use with caution during pregnancy.

(The picture is only for learning and identification the herb; the specific use of the herb please consult the herbalist or health professionals)

Persimmon Calyx (Shidi)

Chinese phonetic alphabet/pin yin: shì dì

Chinese characters simplified/traditional: 柿蒂/柿蒂

Chinese nickname's alphabet (Nickname's Chinese characters): Shiding/ Shiziba(柿丁/柿子把)

Latin: Kaki Calyx (Common name: Persimmon Calyx)

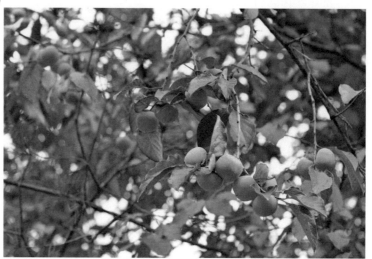

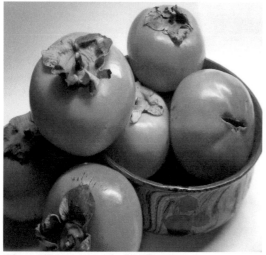
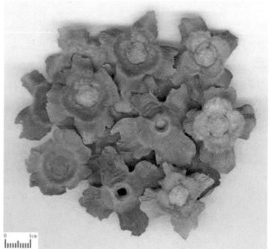

Plant: *Diospyros kaki* Thunb.

TCM prepared in ready-to-use forms (medicinal parts): it's dried ripe fruit pedicel/ persistent calyx.

Property and flavor: neutral; bitter, astringent.

Main and collateral channels: stomach meridian.

Administration and dosage: 5-10 g.

Indication: hiccups.

It is key herb to relieve hiccup.

(The picture is only for learning and identification the herb; the specific use of the herb please consult the herbalist or health professionals)

Dutchmanspipe Root (Qingmuxiang)

Chinese phonetic alphabet/pin yin: qīng mù xiāng

Chinese characters simplified/traditional:青木香/青木香

Chinese nickname's alphabet (Nickname's Chinese characters): Tuqingmuxiang/ Qingtengxiang/ Limuxiang/ Tianxiangen(土青木香/青藤香/理木香/天仙根)

Latin: Aristolochiae Radix (Common name: Dutchmanspipe Root)

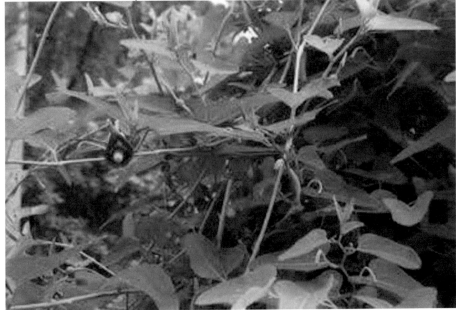

Plant: *Aristolochia debilis* Sieb. et Zucc. (or *Aristolochia contorta* Bge.)

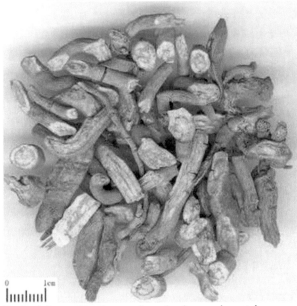

TCM prepared in ready-to-use forms (medicinal parts): it's dried root which harvested in spring or autumn.
Property and flavor: cold; bitter, pungent.
Main and collateral channels: liver and stomach meridians.
Administration and dosage: 3-10 g. Topical application in appropriate amount, ground into powder and apply to the *pars affecta*.

Indication: dizziness, headache, epigastrium and abdominal pain, carbuncle, insect and snake bites.
Precaution and warning: slightly toxic.
(The picture is only for learning and identification the herb; the specific use of the herb please consult the herbalist or health professionals)

Citron Fruit (Xiangyuan)
Chinese phonetic alphabet/pin yin: xiāng yuán
Chinese characters simplified/traditional:香橼/香櫞
Chinese nickname's alphabet (Nickname's Chinese characters): Juyuan/ Juyuanzi(枸橼/枸櫞子)
Latin: Citri Fructus (Common name: Citron Fruit)

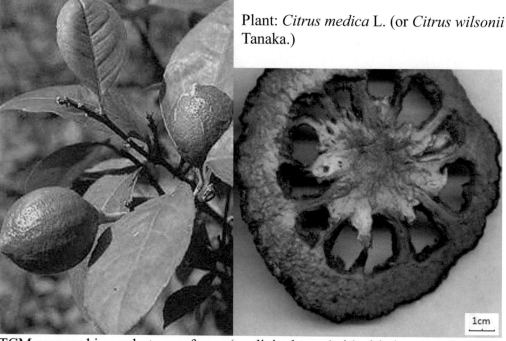

Plant: *Citrus medica* L. (or *Citrus wilsonii* Tanaka.)

TCM prepared in ready-to-use forms (medicinal parts): it's dried mature fruit.
Property and flavor: warm; pungent, bitter and acidity.
Main and collateral channels: liver, spleen and lung meridians.
Administration and dosage: 3-10 g.
Indication: chest and abdominal pain and distension, ructation, vomiting, cough, belching and excessive phlegm.
It is taken as food in some part of China.
(The picture is only for learning and identification the herb; the specific use of the herb please consult the herbalist or health professionals)

Rose Flower (Meiguihua)
Chinese phonetic alphabet/pin yin: méi guì huā
Chinese characters simplified/traditional:玫瑰花/玫瑰花
Chinese nickname's alphabet (Nickname's Chinese characters):Paihuaihua/ Cimeihua(徘徊花/刺玫花)
Latin: Rosae Rugosae Flos (Common name: Rose Flower)
Plant: *Rosa rugosa* Thunb.

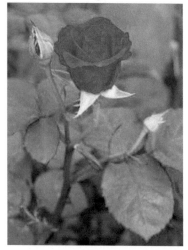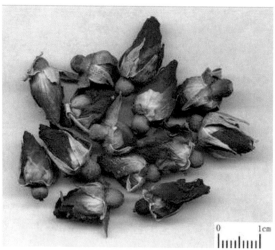

TCM prepared in ready-to-use forms (medicinalparts): it's dried flower bud.
Property and flavor: warm; sweet, mild bitter.
Main and collateral channels: liver and spleen meridians.
Administration and dosage: 3-6 g.
Indication: stomachache, vomiting, irregular menstruation, traumatic injury; dispel melancholy; appetizer.
It is taken as food in some part of China.
(The picture is only for learning and identification the herb; the specific use of the herb please consult the herbalist or health professionals)

Plum Flower (Meihua)

Chinese phonetic alphabet/pin yin: méi huā
Chinese characters simplified/traditional:梅花/梅花
Chinese nickname's alphabet (Nickname's Chinese characters): Baimeihua/ Lv'emei(白梅花/绿萼梅)
Latin: Mume Flos seu Pruni Mume Flos (Common name: Plum Flower or Plum Blossom)

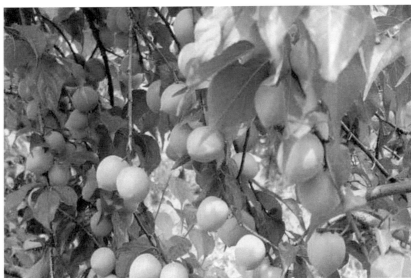

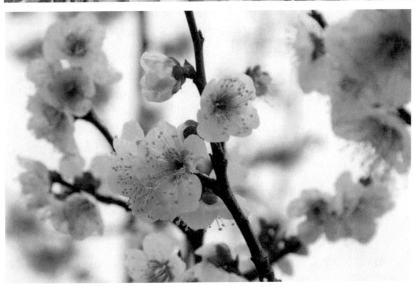

Plant: *Prunus mume* (Sieb.) Sieb et Zucc. (or *Armeniaca mume* Sieb.)

TCM prepared in ready-to-use forms (medicinal parts): it's dried flower bud.

Property and flavor: neutral; mild acidity.

Main and collateral channels: liver, stomach and lung meridians.

Administration and dosage: 3-5 g.

Indication: globus hystericus, liver and stomach pain, loss of appetite, dizziness scrofula, sore and skin infection.

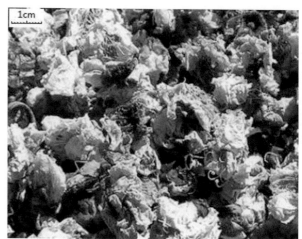

(The picture is only for learning and identification the herb; the specific use of the herb please consult the herbalist or health professionals)

Chinese Asafetida (Awei)

Chinese phonetic alphabet/ pin yin: a wèi

Chinese characters simplified/traditional: 阿魏/阿魏

Chinese nickname's alphabet (Nickname's Chinese characters): Xunqu/ Haxini(熏渠/ 哈昔泥)

Latin: Ferulae Resina (Common name: Chinese Asafetida)

Plant: *Ferula sinkiangensis* K. Shen. (or *Ferula fukanensis* K. M. Shen.)

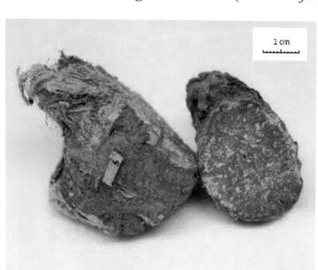

TCM prepared in ready-to-use forms (medicinal parts): it's dried resin.

Property and flavor: warm; bitter, pungent.

Main and collateral channels: lung and stomach meridians.

Administration and dosage: 1-1.5 g, usually used in pill or powder, or paste for topical application.

Indication: mass and lump, intestinal parasites, dyspepsia, cold pain and static blood.

Precaution and warning: contraindicated during pregnancy.

(The picture is only for learning and identification the herb; the specific use of the

herb please consult the herbalist or health professionals)

Secretion of Sperm Whale (Longxianxiang)
Chinese phonetic alphabet/pin yin: lóng xián xiāng
Chinese characters simplified/traditional:龙涎香/龍涎香
Chinese nickname's alphabet (Nickname's Chinese characters): Longfuxiang(龙腹香)
Latin: Ambergris (Common name: Secretion of Sperm Whale)

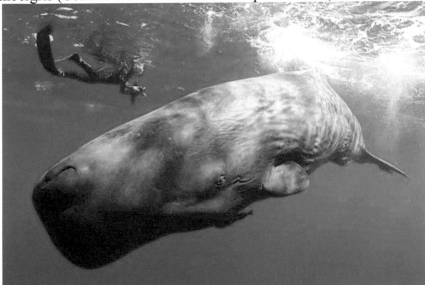

Animal: *Physeter macrocephalus* L.

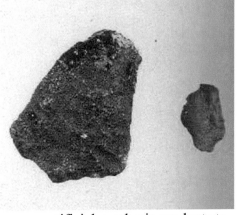

TCM prepared in ready-to-use forms (medicinal parts): it's sperm whale's intestinal secretions.
Property and flavor: warm; sweet, acidity.
Main and collateral channels: liver meridian.
Administration and dosage: 0.3-0.6 g (artificial synthesis products), usually used in pill or powder, or paste for topical application.
Indication: cough, chest and abdominal pain, coma and dizziness.

Attention: to protect the rare wild animals, please use artificial synthesis products to substitute.
(The picture is only for learning and identification the herb; the specific use of the herb please consult the herbalist or health professionals)

Hedgehog Skin (Ciweipi)
Chinese phonetic alphabet/pin yin: cì wěi pí
Chinese characters simplified/traditional:刺猬皮/刺猬皮
Chinese nickname's alphabet (Nickname's Chinese characters): Weipi/ Xianrenyi(猥皮/仙人衣)
Latin: Erinaceus Corium (Common name: Hedgehog Skin)

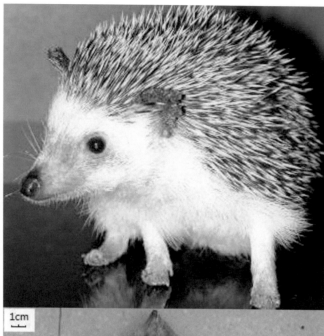

Animal: *Erinaceus amurensis* Schrenk. (or *Erinaceus europaeus* L., *Hemichianus dauricus* Sundevall., *Hemichianus auritus* Gmelin.)

TCM prepared in ready-to-use forms (medicinal parts): it's dried skin and hair.

Property and flavor: neutral; bitter, sweet.

Main and collateral channels: stomach, large intestine and kidney meridians.

Administration and dosage: 6-9 g.

Indication: vomiting, epigastrium and abdominal pain, anal fistula, spermatorrhea and hemorrhoids.

Precaution and warning: slight toxin.

Attention: to protect the rare wild animals, please don't use it from wild animals. (The picture is only for learning and identification the herb; the specific use of the herb please consult the herbalist or health professionals)

Buckeye Seed (Suoluozi)

Chinese phonetic alphabet/pin yin: suō luó zǐ
Chinese characters simplified/traditional:娑罗子/娑羅子
Chinese nickname's alphabet (Nickname's Chinese characters): Suopozi/Wuji(娑婆子/武吉)
Latin: Aesculi Semen (Common name: Buckeye Seed)

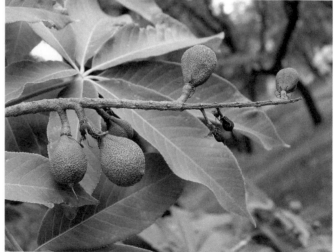

Plant: *Aesculus chinensis* Bge. (or *Aesculus chinensis* Bge. var. *chekiangensis* (Hu. et Fang) Fang., *Aesculus wilsonii* Rehd.)

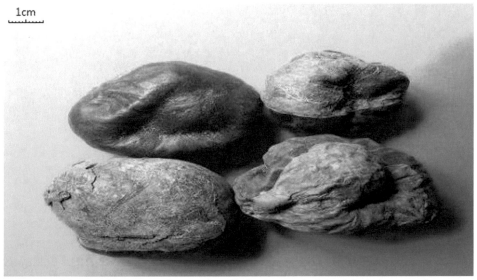

TCM prepared in ready-to-use forms (medicinal parts): it's dried ripe seed.

Property and flavor: warm; sweet.

Main and collateral channels: liver and stomach meridians.

Administration and dosage: 3-9 g.

Indication: it can harmonize the stomach and relieve pain.

(The picture is only for learning and identification the herb; the specific use of the herb please consult the herbalist or health professionals)

Akebia Fruit (Yuzhizi)

Chinese phonetic alphabet/pin yin: yù zhī zǐ

Chinese characters simplified/traditional:预知子/預知子

Chinese nickname's alphabet (Nickname's Chinese characters): Bayuegua/ Bayuezha/ Yajingzi(八月瓜/八月炸/压惊子)

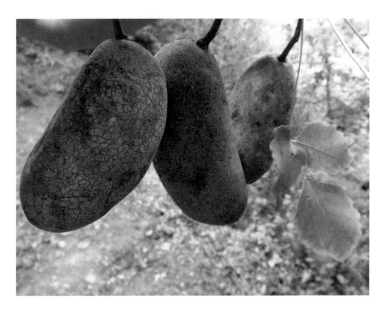

Latin: Akebiae Fructus (Common name: Akebia Fruit)
Plant: *Akebia quinata* (Thunb.) Decne. (or *Akebia trifoliata* (Thunb.) Koidz., *Akebia trifoliata* (Thunb.) Koidz. var. *australis* (Diels.) Rehd.)

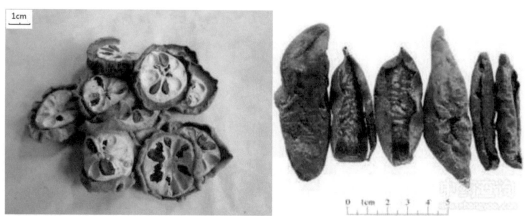

TCM prepared in ready-to-use forms (medicinal parts): it's dried mature fruit.
Property and flavor: cold; bitter.
Main and collateral channels: liver, gallbladder, stomach and bladder meridians.
Administration and dosage: 3-9 g.
Indication: epigastric and abdominal distending pain, dysmenorrhea and amenorrhea, phlegm nodule and stuffy masses, inhibited urination.
(The picture is only for learning and identification the herb; the specific use of the herb please consult the herbalist or health professionals)

Dutchmanspipe Vine (Tianxianteng)

Chinese phonetic alphabet/pin yin:
tiān xiān téng
Chinese characters
simplified/traditional:天仙藤/天仙藤
Chinese nickname's alphabet
(Nickname's Chinese characters):
Dulinteng/ Sanbailiangyin/
Doulinmiao(都淋藤/三百两银/兜铃苗)
Latin: Aristolochiae Herb (Common
name: Dutchmanspipe Vine)

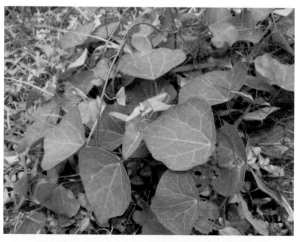

Plant: *Aristolochia debilis* Sieb et Zucc. (or *Aristolochia contora* Bge.)

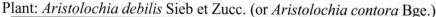

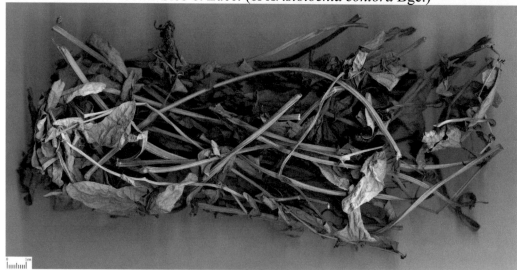

TCM prepared in ready-to-use forms (medicinal parts): it's dried up-ground-part which harvested in autumn.
Property and flavor: warm; bitter.
Main and collateral channels: liver, kidney and spleen meridians.
Administration and dosage: 3-6 g.
Indication: painful *bi* disorder, acute pain in epigastrium and abdomen.
Precaution and warning: the herb contain aristolochic acid which may induce kidney damage. It should be used cautiously for child and aged. Contraindicated for pregnant woman, infant and the patients suffering from renal insufficiency.
(The picture is only for learning and identification the herb; the specific use of the herb please consult the herbalist or health professionals)

Stink-bug (Jiuxiangchong)

Chinese phonetic alphabet/pin yin: jiǔ xiāng chóng
Chinese characters simplified/traditional: 九香虫/九香蟲
Chinese nickname's alphabet (Nickname's Chinese characters): Heidouchong/ Guaheichun(黑兜虫/ 瓜黑蝽)
Latin: Aspongopus (Common name: Stink-bug)

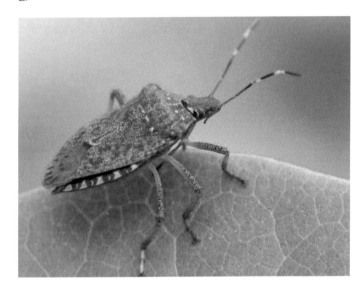

Animal: *Aspongopus chinensis* Dallas.

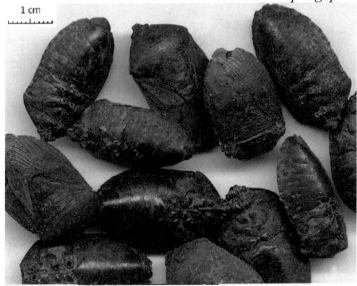

TCM prepared in ready-to-use forms (medicinal parts): it's dried body which harvested in autumn.
Property and flavor: warm; salty.
Main and collateral channels: liver, spleen and kidney meridians.
Administration and dosage: 3-9 g.

Indication: stomach distending and pain caused by cold/chill (*Hanliang*), impotence, sore pain in the waist and knees.
(The picture is only for learning and identification the herb; the specific use of the herb please consult the herbalist or health professionals)

Inula Herb (Jinfeicao)

Chinese phonetic alphabet/pin yin: jīn fēi cǎo
Chinese characters simplified/traditional:金沸草/金沸草
Chinese nickname's alphabet (Nickname's Chinese characters): Jinfocao/ Baizhihu/ Xuanfucao(金佛草/白芷胡/旋复草)
Latin: Inulae Herba (Common name: Inula Herb)

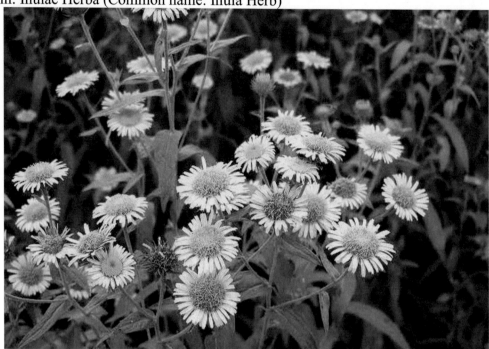

Plant: *Inula linariifolia* Turcz. (or *Inula japonica* Thunb.)

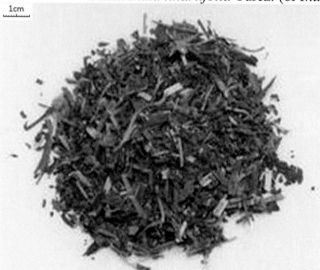

TCM prepared in ready-to-use forms (medicinal parts): it's dried aerial part which harvested in summer or autumn.
Property and flavor: warm; bitter, pungent and salty.
Main and collateral channels: lung and large intestine meridians.
Administration and dosage: 5-10 g.

Indication: chill (*Fenghan*) cold, wheezing and cough, profuse sputum, stuffiness and fullness in the chest and the diaphragm.
(The picture is only for learning and identification the herb; the specific use of the herb please consult the herbalist or health professionals)

Inula Root (Tumuxiang)

Chinese phonetic alphabet/pin yin: tǔ mù xiāng
Chinese characters simplified/traditional:土木香/土木香
Chinese nickname's alphabet (Nickname's Chinese characters): Qimuxiang(祁木香)

Latin: Inulae Radix (Common name: Inula Root)

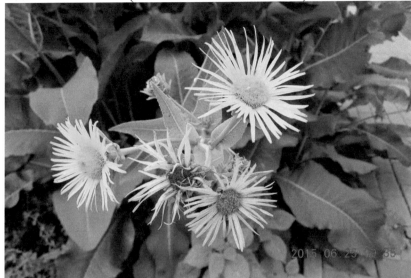

Plant: *Inula helenium* L. TCM prepared in ready-to-use forms (medicinal parts): it's dried root which harvested in autumn.

Property and flavor: warm; bitter, pungent.
Main and collateral channels: liver and spleen meridians.
Administration and dosage: 3-9 g, usually used in pills and powder.
Indication: distending pain in chest, hypochondrium, vomitting, diarrhea, dysentery and fetal irritability.
(The picture is only for learning and identification the herb; the specific use of the herb please consult the herbalist or health professionals)

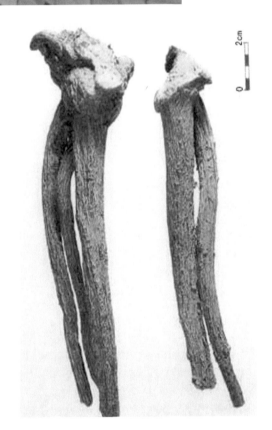

Murraya Jasminorage (Jiulixiang)
Chinese phonetic alphabet/pin yin: jiǔ lǐ xiāng
Chinese characters simplified/traditional:九里香/九裡香
Chinese nickname's alphabet (Nickname's Chinese characters): Shilajiao/ Jiuyuexiang/ Yueju(石辣椒/九秋香/月橘)
Latin: Murrayae Folium et Cacumen (Common name: Murraya Jasminorage)

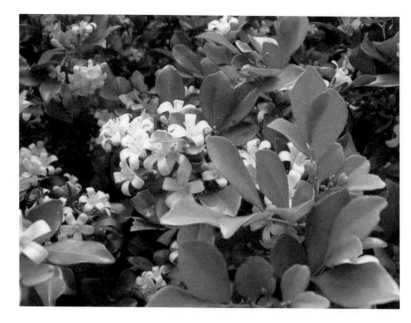

Plant: *Murraya exotica* L. (or *Murraya paniculata* (L.) Jack.) TCM prepared in ready-to-use forms (medicinal parts): it's dried leaf and young foliferous branch which harvested all year round.

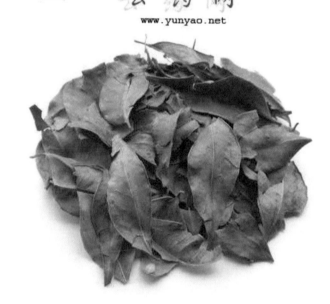

Property and flavor: warm; mild bitter, pungent.
Main and collateral channels: liver and kidney meridians.
Administration and dosage: 6-12 g.

Indication: stomachache, arthralgia; external use for toothache, swelling, traumatic injuries, insect or snake bites.
Precaution and warning: slightly toxic.
(The picture is only for learning and identification the herb; the specific use of the herb please consult the herbalist or health professionals)

Jatamans Valeriana Rhizome (Zhizhuxiang)
Chinese phonetic alphabet/pin yin: zhī zhū xiāng
Chinese characters simplified/traditional:蜘蛛香/蜘蛛香
Chinese nickname's alphabet (Nickname's Chinese characters): Matixiang/ Tuxixin(马蹄香/土细辛)
Latin: Valerianae Jatamansi Rhizoma et Radix (Common name: Jatamans Valeriana Rhizome)

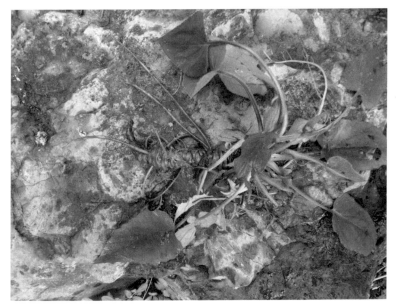

Plant: *Valeriana jatamansi* Jones. TCM prepared in ready-to-use forms (medicinal parts): it's dried rhizome and root which harvested in autumn.

1cm

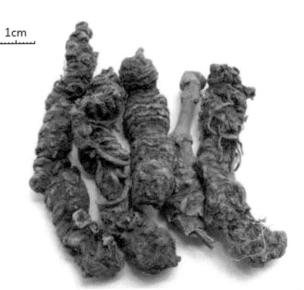

Property and flavor: warm; mild bitter, pungent.
Main and collateral channels: heart, spleen and stomach meridians.
Administration and dosage: 3-6 g.

Indication: epigastrium and abdomen pain, indigest, diarrhea, dysentery, painful *bi* disorder, insomnia, soreness and weakness in the lower back and knees.
(The picture is only for learning and identification the herb; the specific use of the herb please consult the herbalist or health professionals)

Common Vladimiria Root (Chuanmuxiang)
Chinese phonetic alphabet/pin yin: chuān mù xiāng
Chinese characters simplified/traditional:川木香/川木香
Chinese nickname's alphabet (Nickname's Chinese characters): Tieganmuxiang/
Caozimuxiang(铁杆木香/槽子木香)
Latin: Vladimiriae Radix (Common name: Common Vladimiria Root)

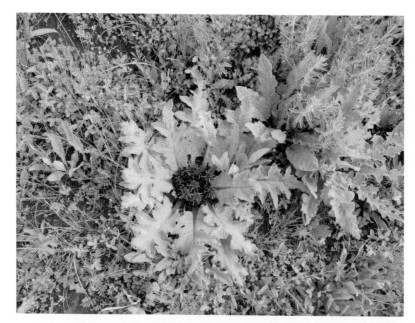

Plant: *Vladimiria souliei* (Franch.) Ling. (or *Vladimiria souliei* (Franch.) Ling. var. *cinerea* Ling.)

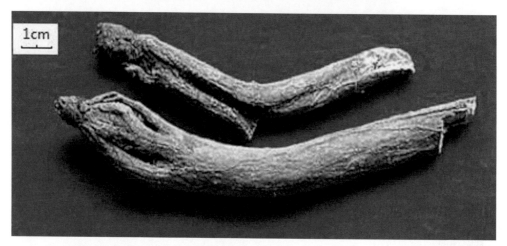

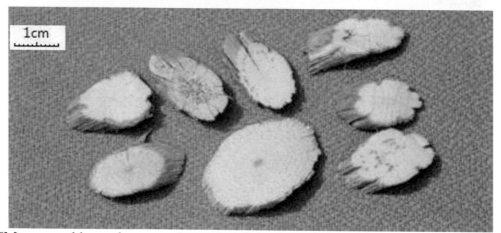

TCM prepared in ready-to-use forms (medicinal parts): it's dried root which harvested in autumn.

Property and flavor: warm; bitter, pungent.

Main and collateral channels: spleen, stomach, large intestine and gallbladder meridians.

Administration and dosage: 3-9 g.

Indication: diarrhea, epigastrium and abdomen pain.

(The picture is only for learning and identification the herb; the specific use of the herb please consult the herbalist or health professionals)

Xiao Shi Yao(消食药)-digestant herbs
Xiao Shi Yao is a kind of herbs which's the major function is promote digestion.

Hawthorn Fruit (Shanzha)
Chinese phonetic alphabet/pin yin: shān zhā
Chinese characters simplified/traditional:山楂/山楂
Chinese nickname's alphabet (Nickname's Chinese characters): Shanlihong/
Shanlihongguo(山里红/山里红果)
Latin: Crataegi Fructus (Common name: Hawthorn Fruit)

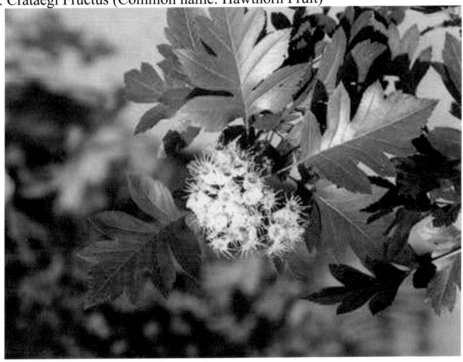

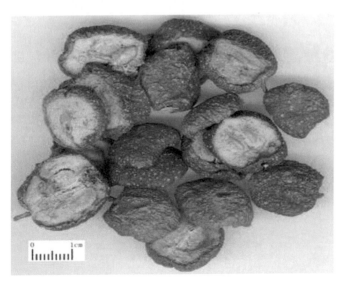

Plant: *Crataegus pinnatifida* Bunge. (or *Crataegus pinnatifida* Bunge. var. *major* N. E. Br.)
TCM prepared in ready-to-use forms (medicinal parts): it's dried mature fruit.

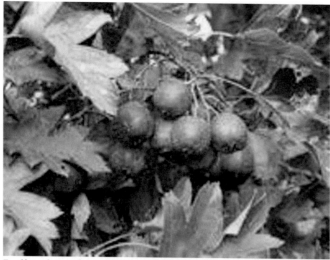

Property and flavor: mild warm; acidity, sweet.
Main and collateral channels: spleen, stomach and liver meridians.
Administration and dosage: 9-12 g.
Fried one is better at promoting digestion.

Indication: dyspepsia, epigastrium and abdominal distension and pain, diarrhea, amenorrhea, heart pain, hernia pain and hyperlipidemia.
It is key herb to treat indigestion caused by intake too much meat or fat.
It is taken as food in some part of China.
(The picture is only for learning and identification the herb; the specific use of the herb please consult the herbalist or health professionals)

Germinated Barly (Maiya)

Chinese phonetic alphabet/pin yin: mài yá

Chinese characters simplified/traditional:麦芽/麥芽

Chinese nickname's alphabet (Nickname's Chinese characters): Damaiya/ Mainie(大麦芽/麦蘖)

Latin: Hordei Fructus Germinatus (Common name: Germinated Barly or Malt)

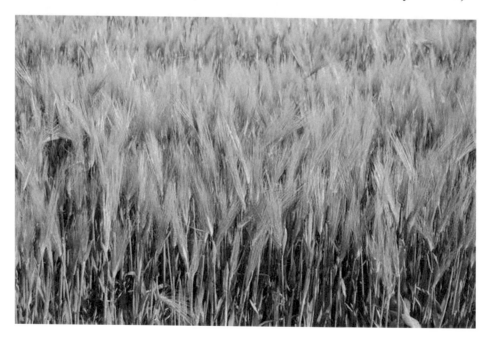

Plant: *Hordeum vulgare* L.

TCM prepared in ready-to-use forms (medicinal parts): it's (processed or unprocessed) dried germination ripe fruit.
Property and flavor: neutral; sweet.
Main and collateral channels: spleen and stomach meridians.

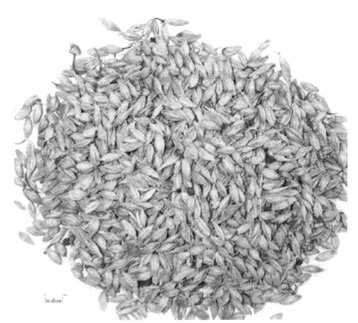

Administration and dosage: 10-15 g; 60 g fried one for lactifuge.
Indication: indigestion, abdominal distention and breast pain; women weaning.
It is taken as food in some part of China.
(The picture is only for learning and identification the herb; the specific use of the herb please consult the herbalist or health professionals)

Radish Seed (Laifuzi)
Chinese phonetic alphabet/pin yin: lái fú zǐ
Chinese characters simplified/traditional:莱菔子/萊菔子
Chinese nickname's alphabet (Nickname's Chinese characters): Luobozi(萝卜子)
Latin: Raphani Semen (Common name: Radish Seed)

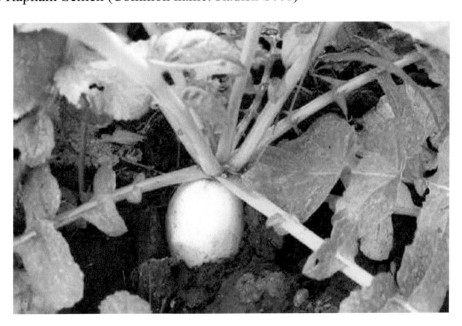

Plant: *Raphanus sativus* L.

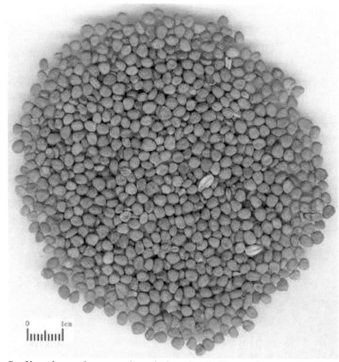

TCM prepared in ready-to-use forms (medicinal parts): it's dried mature seed. Property and flavor: neutral; pungent, sweet. Main and collateral channels: lung, spleen and stomach meridians. Administration and dosage: 5-12 g.

Indication: dyspepsia, abdominal distention, constipation, indigestion, diarrhea, excessive phlegm and cough.
It is taken as food in some part of China.
(The picture is only for learning and identification the herb; the specific use of the herb please consult the herbalist or health professionals)

Chicken's Gizzard-skin (Jineijin)
Chinese phonetic alphabet/pin yin: jī nèi jīn
Chinese characters simplified/traditional:鸡内金/雞內金
Chinese nickname's alphabet (Nickname's Chinese characters): Jishipi/ Jisuzi(鸡食皮/鸡嗉子)
Latin: Galli Gigerii Endothelium Corneum (Common name: Chicken's Gizzard-sink)

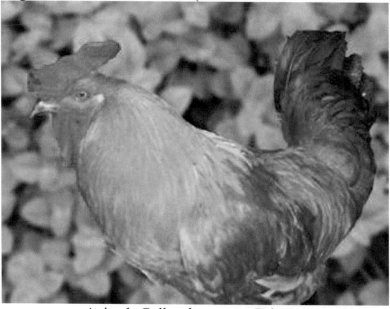

Animal: *Gallus domesticus* Brisson.

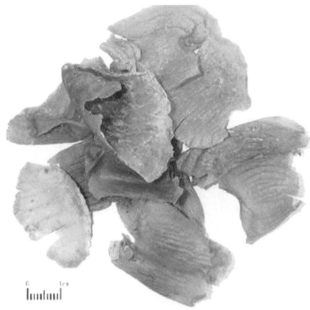

TCM prepared in ready-to-use forms (medicinal parts): it's dried chicken gizzard inner wall.
Property and flavor: neutral; sweet.
Main and collateral channels: spleen, stomach, small intestine and bladder meridians.
Administration and dosage: 3-10 g.
Indication: indigestion, vomiting, diarrhea, infantile malnutrition, spermatorrhea and enuresis.

It is key herb to improve digestion.
It is taken as food in some part of China.
(The picture is only for learning and identification the herb; the specific use of the herb please consult the herbalist or health professionals)

Medicated Leaven (Shenqu)

Chinese phonetic alphabet/pin yin: shén qū

Chinese characters simplified/traditional:神曲/神曲

Chinese nickname's alphabet (Nickname's Chinese characters): Liushenqu(六神曲)

Latin: Massa Medieata Fermentata seu Massa Fermentata Medicinalis (Common name: Medicated Leaven)

TCM prepared in ready-to-use forms (medicinal parts): it is dried fermented mixture product made by wheat flour, bran and the fresh aerial part of Armened Annua, Polygonum Hydropiper and other herbs.
Property and flavor: warm; sweet, pungent.
Main and collateral channels: spleen and stomach meridians.
Administration and dosage: 6-15 g.

Indication: food stagnation syndrome.
(The picture is only for learning and identification the herb; the specific use of the

herb please consult the herbalist or health professionals)

Rice Grain Sprout (Daoya)

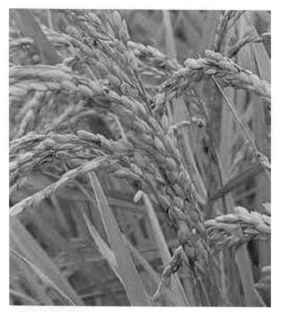

Chinese phonetic alphabet/
pin yin: dào yá
Chinese characters simplified/
traditional:稻芽/稻芽
Chinese nickname's alphabet
(Nickname's Chinese characters):
Niemi/ Gunie/ Daonie(蘖米/谷蘖/
稻蘖)
Latin: Oryzae Fructus Germinatus
(Common name: Rice Grain Sprout)
Plant: *Oryza sativa* L.

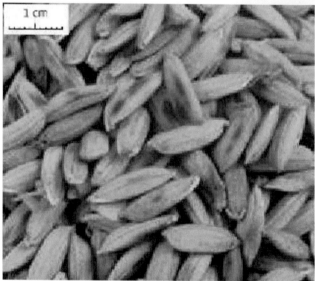

TCM prepared in
ready-to-use forms
(medicinal parts): it's
dried germinated ripe
fruit.
Property and flavor:
warm; sweet.
Main and collateral
channels: spleen and
stomach meridians.

Administration and dosage: 9-15 g. Fired one is better at promoting digestion.
Indication: indigestion, abdominal distension and halitosis; appetizer.
(The picture is only for learning and identification the herb; the specific use of the
herb please consult the herbalist or health professionals)

Seabuckthron Fruit (Shaji)
Chinese phonetic alphabet/pin yin: shā jí
Chinese characters simplified/traditional:沙棘/沙棘
Chinese nickname's alphabet (Nickname's Chinese characters): Heici/ Suanci/
Daribu(黑刺/酸刺/达日布)
Latin: Hippophae Fructus (Common name: Seabuckthron Fruit)

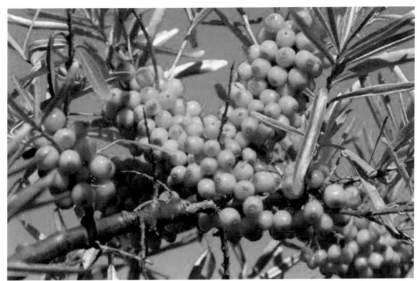

Plant: *Hippophae rhamnoides* L.

1cm

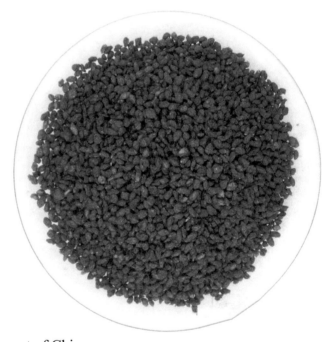

TCM prepared in ready-to-use forms (medicinal parts): it's dried ripe fruit.
Property and flavor: warm; acidity, astringent.
Main and collateral channels: spleen, stomach, lung and heart meridians.
Administration and dosage: 3-10 g.
Indication: cough, profuse sputum, heart pain, blood-stasis, amenorrhea and swelling; appetizer.

It is taken as food in some part of China.
(The picture is only for learning and identification the herb; the specific use of the herb please consult the herbalist or health professionals)

Paniculate Microcos Leaf (Buzhaye)
Chinese phonetic alphabet/pin yin: bù zhā yè
Chinese characters simplified/traditional:布渣叶/布渣葉
Chinese nickname's alphabet (Nickname's Chinese characters): Mabuye (麻布叶)
Latin: Microctis Folium (Common name: Paniculate Microcos Leaf)

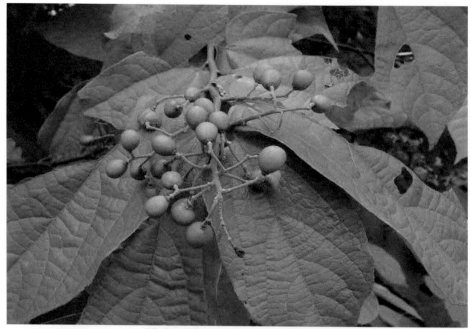

Plant: *Microcos paniculata* L.

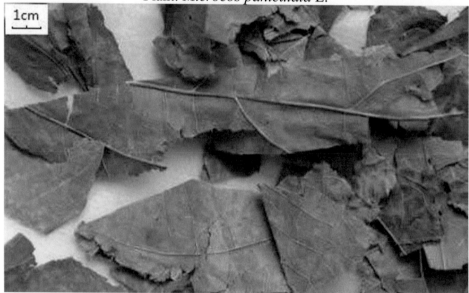

TCM prepared in ready-to-use forms (medicinal parts): it's dried leaf which harvested in summer or autumn.

Property and flavor: cool; mild acidity.

Main and collateral channels: spleen and stomach meridians.

Administration and dosage: 15-30 g.

Indication: indigestion, cold with fever and jaundice.

It is taken as food in some part of China.

(The picture is only for learning and identification the herb; the specific use of the herb please consult the herbalist or health professionals)

Qu Chong Yao(驱虫药)-expelling parasite herbs

Qu Chong Yao is a kind of herbs which's the major function is to expel intestinal parasites.

Rangooncreeper Fruit (Shijunzi)

Chinese phonetic alphabet/pin yin: shǐ jūn zǐ

Chinese characters simplified/traditional:使君子/使君子

Chinese nickname's alphabet (Nickname's Chinese characters): Liuqiuzi/ Wulengzi/ Dongjunzi(留求子/五棱子/冬均子)

Latin: Quisqualis Fructus (Common name: Rangooncreeper Fruit)

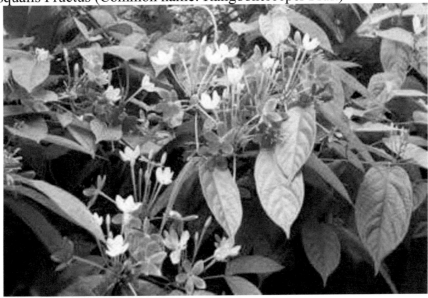

Plant: *Quisqualis indica* Linn.

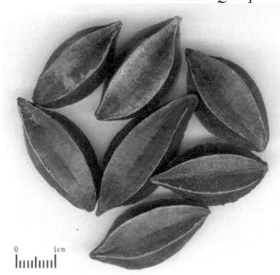

TCM prepared in ready-to-use forms (medicinal parts): it's dried mature fruit.

Property and flavor: warm; sweet.

Main and collateral channels: spleen and stomach meridians. Administration and dosage: 9-12 g, crush to piece for making decoction; 6-9 g of its seeds are usually used in pills and powder, or taken alone, one to two times. Indication: infantile malnutrition, intestinal parasites.

It is key herb to treat infantile malnutrition.

Precaution and warning: incompatible with tea.

(The picture is only for learning and identification the herb; the specific use of the herb please consult the herbalist or health professionals)

Szechwan Chinaberry Bark (Kulianpi)

Chinese phonetic alphabet/pin yin: kǔ liàn pí

Chinese characters simplified/traditional:苦楝皮/苦楝皮

Chinese nickname's alphabet (Nickname's Chinese characters): Kulian/ Lianpi/ Shuangbaipi(苦楝/楝皮/双白皮)

Latin: Meliae Cortex (Common name: Szechwan Chinaberry Bark)

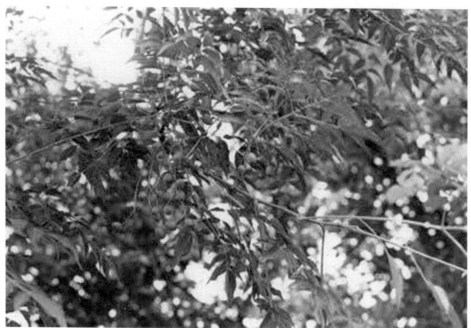

Plant: *Melia toosendan* Sieb.et Zucc. (or *Melia azedarach* L.)

TCM prepared in ready-to-use forms (medicinal parts): it's dried stem bark which harvested in spring or autumn.
Property and flavor: cold; bitter.
Main and collateral channels: liver, spleen and stomach meridians.
Administration and dosage: 3-6 g. Topical application in appropriate amount, ground into powder, mixed it with pig fat for apply to *pars affecta.*
Indication: intestinal parasites; external use for scabies and tinea itching.

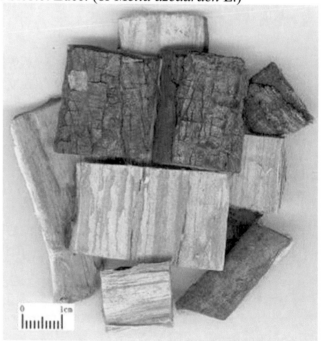

Precaution and warning: toxic. Use with caution during pregnancy and hepatic insufficiency or renal insufficiency.
(The picture is only for learning and identification the herb; the specific use of the herb please consult the herbalist or health professionals)

Areca Seed (Binglang)
Chinese phonetic alphabet/pin yin: bīng láng
Chinese characters simplified/traditional:槟榔/檳榔
Chinese nickname's alphabet (Nickname's Chinese characters): Ganlanzi/ Dafuzi(橄榄子/大腹子)
Latin: Arecae Semen (Common name: Areca Seed or Betel Nut)

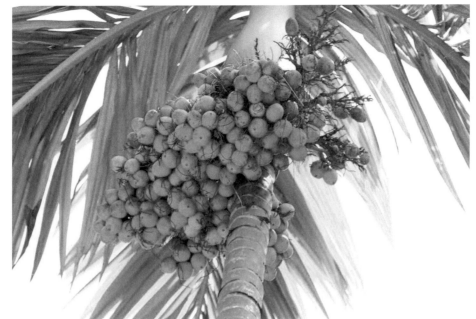

Plant: *Areca catechu* L.

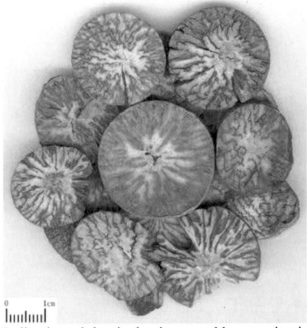

TCM prepared in ready-to-use forms (medicinal parts): it's dried mature fruit.
Property and flavor: warm; pungent, bitter.
Main and collateral channels: stomach and large intestine meridians.
Administration and dosage: 3-10 g. To dispel tape worm and fasciolopsis: 30-60 g.

Indication: abdominal pain caused by parasite, indigestion, diarrhea, tenesmus, edema, tinea pedis and malaria; expel intestinal parasites.
(The picture is only for learning and identification the herb; the specific use of the herb please consult the herbalist or health professionals)

Male Fern Rhizome (Guanzhong)
Chinese phonetic alphabet/pin yin: guàn zhòng
Chinese characters simplified/traditional:贯众/貫眾
Chinese nickname's alphabet (Nickname's Chinese characters): Mianmalinmaojue/ Mianmaguanzhong/ Guanjie/ Guanqu(绵马鳞毛蕨/绵马贯众/贯节/贯渠)
Latin: Dryopteridis Crassirhizomatis Rhizoma (Common name: Male Fern Rhizome)

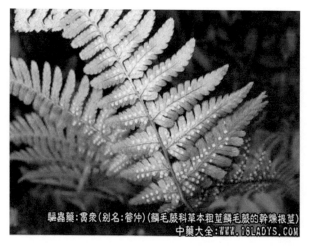

Plant:*Dryopteris crass irhizoma* Nakai. TCM prepared in ready-to-use forms (medicinal parts): it's dried rhizome and frond base which harvested in autumn.

Property and flavor: mild cold; bitter.
Main and collateral channels: liver and stomach meridians.
Administration and dosage: 4.5-9 g.
Indication: sore and ulcer; expel parasite and worm.

Precaution and warning:

slightly toxic.

(The picture is only for learning and identification the herb; the specific use of the herb please consult the herbalist or health professionals)

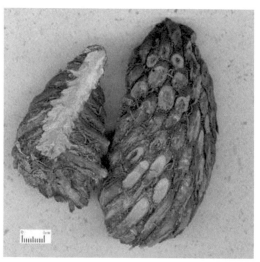

Japanese Osmunda Rhizome (Ziqiguanzhong)

Chinese phonetic alphabet/pin yin: zǐ qí guàn zhòng
Chinese characters simplified/traditional:紫萁贯众/紫萁貫眾
Chinese nickname's alphabet (Nickname's Chinese characters): Weiguanzhong(薇贯众)
Latin: Osmundae Rhizoma (Common name: Japanese Osmunda Rhizome)

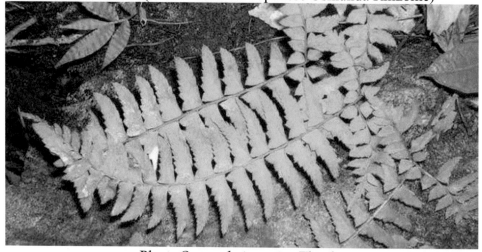

Plant: *Osmunda japonica* Thunb.

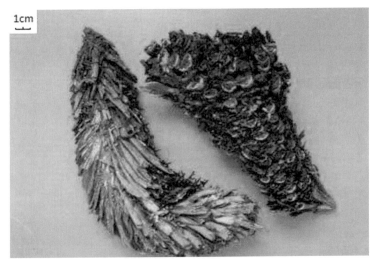

TCM prepared in ready-to-use forms (medicinal parts): it's dried rhizome which harvested in spring or autumn. Property and flavor: mild cold; bitter.

Main and collateral channels: lung, stomach and liver meridians.
Administration and dosage: 5-9 g.
Indication: flu, diarrhea, dysentery, abscess, sore, swelling, toxin, hematemesis, epistaxis, hematochezia, menstrual flooding and spotting, and abdominal pain caused by intestinal parasites.
Precaution and warning: slightly toxic.
(The picture is only for learning and identification the herb; the specific use of the herb please consult the herbalist or health professionals)

Thunder Ball (Leiwan)

Chinese phonetic alphabet/pin yin: léi wán

Chinese characters simplified/traditional:雷丸/雷丸

Chinese nickname's alphabet (Nickname's Chinese characters): Leishi/ Zhulinzi(雷实/竹林子)

Latin: Omphalia (Common name: Thunder Ball)

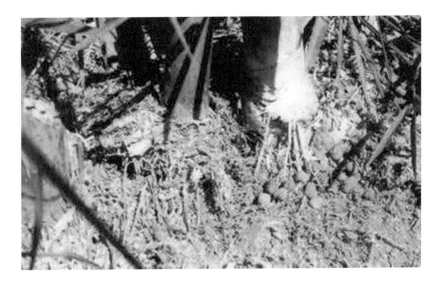

Fungus: *Omphalia lapidescens* Schroet.

TCM prepared in ready-to-use forms (medicinal parts): it's dried sclerotium which harvested in November or December.
Property and flavor: cold; mild bitter.
Main and collateral channels: stomach and large intestine meridians.
Administration and dosage: 15-21 g, it is inadvisable to be added into decoction; usually ground into powder for oral administration, 5-7 g per time, taken with warm water after meal, three times a day, continue for 3 days.

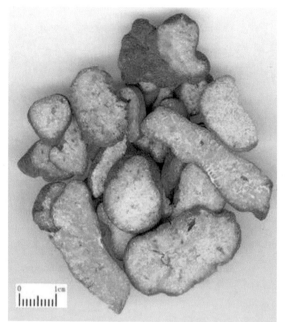

Indication: tapeworm, hookworm, roundworm, abdominal pain caused by parasites and infantile malnutrition.
Precaution and warning: slightly toxic.
(The picture is only for learning and identification the herb; the specific use of the herb please consult the herbalist or health professionals)

Pumpkin Seed (Nanguazi)
Chinese phonetic alphabet/pin yin: nán guā zǐ
Chinese characters simplified/traditional:南瓜子/南瓜子
Chinese nickname's alphabet (Nickname's Chinese characters): Nanguaren/ Baiguazi(南瓜仁/白瓜子)
Latin: Moschatae Semen (Common name: Pumpkin Seed or Cushaw Seed)

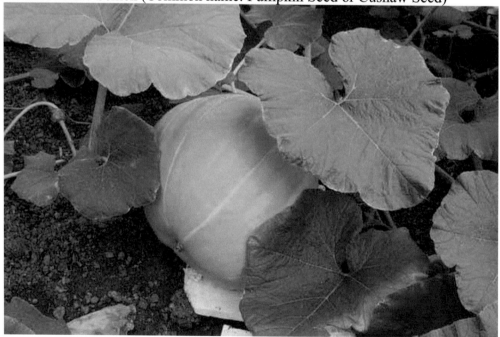

Plant: *Cucurbita moschata* (Duch. ex Lam.) Duch. ex Poiret.

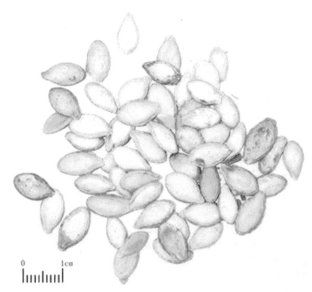

TCM prepared in ready-to-use forms (medicinal parts): it's dried mature seed.
Property and flavor: neutral; sweet.
Main and collateral channels: stomach and large intestine meridians.
Administration and dosage: 60-120 g. It can be decocted for fuming-washing therapy. To dispel schistosome, long-term heavy usage is needed.

Indication: tapeworm, roundworm, schistosomiasis, hookworm, pertussis, abdominal distension, foot edema and hemorrhoids; lactagogue.

It is taken as food in some part of China.

(The picture is only for learning and identification the herb; the specific use of the herb please consult the herbalist or health professionals)

Hairyvein Agrimonia Sprout (Hecaoya)

Chinese phonetic alphabet/pin yin: hè cǎo yá

Chinese characters simplified/traditional:鹤草芽/鶴草芽

Chinese nickname's alphabet (Nickname's Chinese characters): Longyacaoya/(龙芽草芽)

Latin: Agrimoniae Germinatus (Common name: Hairyvein Agrimonia Sprout)

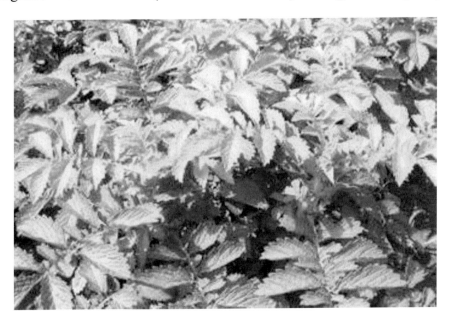

Plant: *Agrimonia pilosa* Ldb.

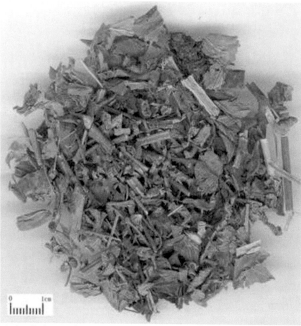

TCM prepared in ready-to-use forms (medicinal parts): it's dried winter sprout. Property and flavor: cool; bitter, astringent. Main and collateral channels: heart meridian.

Administration and dosage: 30-50 g for adult; 0.7-0.8 g/kg for child. Ground into powder for oral administration, one time a day taken before the breakfast.
Indication: tapeworm.
(The picture is only for learning and identification the herb; the specific use of the herb please consult the herbalist or health professionals)

Grand Torreya Seed (Feizi)
Chinese phonetic alphabet/pin yin: fěi zī
Chinese characters simplified/traditional:榧子/榧子
Chinese nickname's alphabet (Nickname's Chinese characters): Feishi/ Yufei(榧实/玉榧)
Latin: Torreyae Semen (Common name: Grand Torreya Seed)

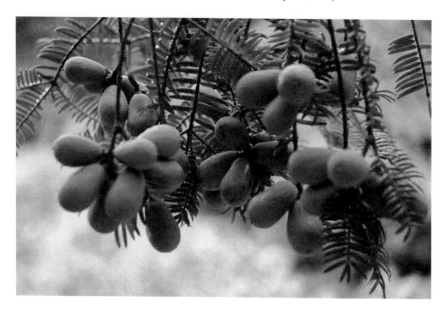

Plant: *Torreya grandis* Fort.

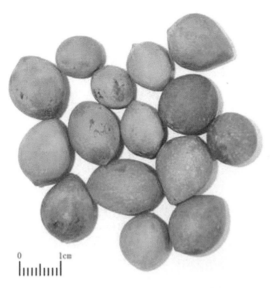

TCM prepared in ready-to-use forms (medicinal parts): it's dried mature seed.
Property and flavor: neutral; sweet.
Main and collateral channels: lung, stomach and large intestine meridians.
Administration and dosage: 9-15 g.
Indication: hookworm, roundworm, tapeworm, abdominal pain caused by inner parasites, infantile malnutrition, constipation and dry cough.

It is taken as food in some part of China.
Attention: to protect the rare wild plant, please don't use the herb from wild plant. (The picture is only for learning and identification the herb; the specific use of the herb please consult the herbalist or health professionals)

Prepared Ulmi Fruit (Wuyi)
Chinese phonetic alphabet/pin yin: wú yí
Chinese characters simplified/traditional:芜荑/蕪荑
Chinese nickname's alphabet (Nickname's Chinese characters): Shanyuzi/ Chouwuyi (山榆子/臭芜荑)
Latin: Ulmus Fructus Preparatum (Common name: Prepared Ulmi Fruit)

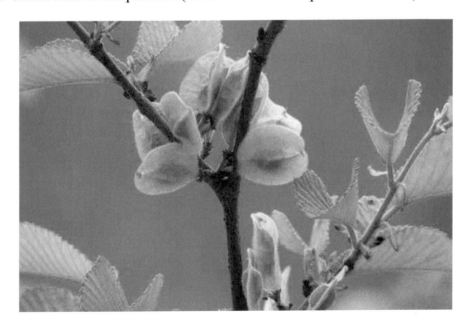

Plant: *Ulmus macrocarpa* Hance.s

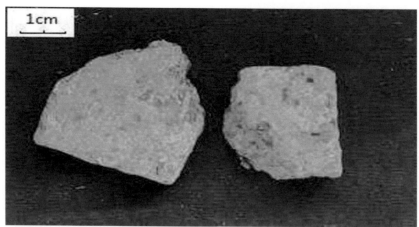

TCM prepared in ready-to-use forms (medicinal parts): it's the processed mature fruit.

Property and flavor: warm; bitter, pungent.

Main and collateral channels: spleen and stomach meridians.

Process: Sun-dried the mature fruit, take out the seed, soak in warm water until the fermented, add the elm bark powder (10 kg), red clay (30 kg) and Chrysanthemum powder (5kg per 55 kg herb), then add some warm water mixed into paste, spread and sun-dry the paste cut into cubes.

Administration and dosage: 3-10g.

Indication: intestinal parasites, infantile malnutrition.

(The picture is only for learning and identification the herb; the specific use of the herb please consult the herbalist or health professionals)

Wild Carrot Fruit (Nanheshi)

Chinese phonetic alphabet/pin yin: nán hè shī
Chinese characters simplified/traditional:南鹤虱/南鶴虱
Chinese nickname's alphabet (Nickname's Chinese characters): Shizicao/ Yehuluobozi(虱子草/野胡萝卜子)
Latin: Carotae Fructus (Common name: Wild Carrot Fruit)

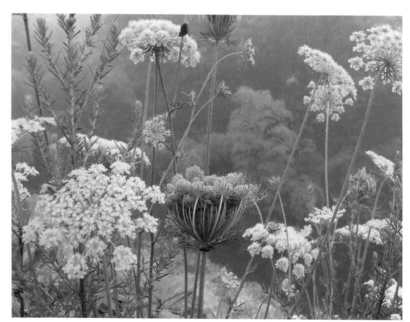

Plant: *Dausus carota* L.

TCM prepared in ready-to-use forms (medicinal parts): it's dried ripe fruit which harvested in autumn.
Property and flavor: neutral; bitter, pungent.
Main and collateral channels: spleen and stomach meridians.
Administration and dosage: 3-9 g.

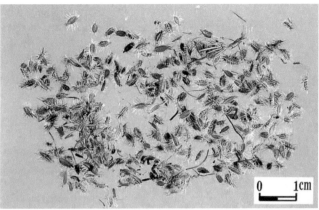

Indication: intestinal parasites, infantile malnutrition with food retention.
Precaution and warning: slightly toxic.
(The picture is only for learning and identification the herb; the specific use of the herb please consult the herbalist or health professionals)

Common Carpesium Fruit (Heshi)

Chinese phonetic alphabet/ pin yin: hè shī
Chinese characters simplified/ traditional:鹤虱/鶴蝨
Chinese nickname's alphabet (Nickname's Chinese characters): Hushi/ Guighi/ Beiheshi(鹄虱/ 鬼虱/北鹤虱)
Latin: Carpesii Fructus (Common name: Common Carpesium Fruit)
Plant: *Carpesium abrotanoides* L.
TCM prepared in ready-to-use forms (medicinal parts): it's dried ripe fruit.
Property and flavor: neutral; bitter, pungent.
Main and collateral channels: spleen and stomach meridians.
Administration and dosage: 3-9 g.
Indication: ascariasis, enterobiasis, taeniasis, abdominal pain caused by intestinal parasites accumulation, infantile malnutrition with indigestion.
Precaution and warning: slightly toxic.
(The picture is only for learning and identification the herb; the specific use of the herb please consult the herbalist or health professionals)

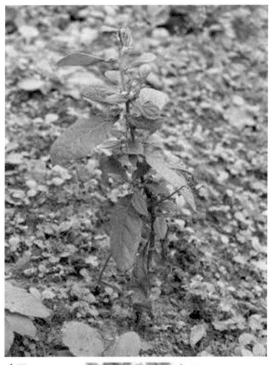

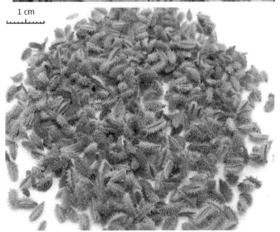

Chinese Honeylocust Spine (Zaojiaoci)

Chinese phonetic alphabet/pin yin: zào jiǎo cì
Chinese characters simplified/traditional:皂角刺/皂角刺
Chinese nickname's alphabet (Nickname's Chinese characters): Zaojiaci/ Zaoci/ Tiading(皂荚刺/皂刺/天丁)
Latin: Gleditsiae Spina (Common name: Chinese Honeylocust Spine)

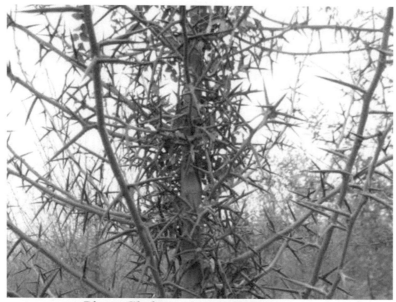

Plant: *Gleditsia sinensis* Lam.

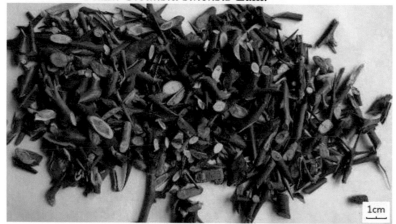

TCM prepared in ready-to-use forms (medicinal parts): it's dried spine which harvested all year round.
Property and flavor: warm; pungent.
Main and collateral channels: liver and stomach meridians.
Administration and dosage: 3-10 g. Topical application in appropriate amount, steamed with vinegar, and the juice is applied to the *pars affecta*.
Indication: abscess, cellulitis, diabrosis; external use for scabies, tinea, leprosy.

(The picture is only for learning and identification the herb; the specific use of the herb please consult the herbalist or health professionals)

Zhi Xue Yao(止血药)-hemostatic herbs

Zhi Xue Yao is a kind of herbs which's the major functions are to treat trauma hemorrhage and nontraumatic bleeding.

Japanese Thistle Herb (Daji)

Chinese phonetic alphabet/pin yin: dà jì
Chinese characters simplified/traditional:大蓟/大薊
Chinese nickname's alphabet (Nickname's Chinese characters): Dacicai/ Laohuci (大刺菜/老虎刺)

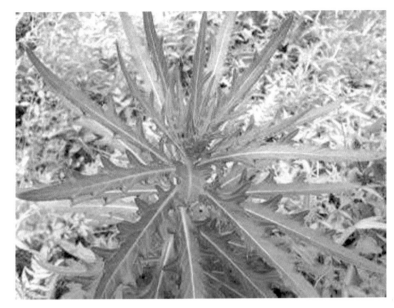

Latin: Cirsii Japonici Herba (Common name: Japanese Thistle Herb)
Plant: *Cirsium japonicum* Fisch. ex DC.

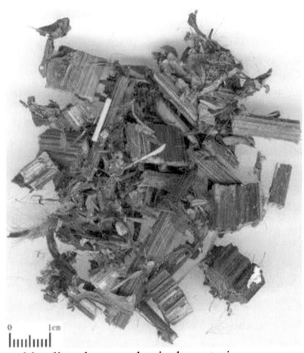

TCM prepared in ready-to-use forms (medicinal parts): it's dried up ground part which harvested in summer or autumn.
Property and flavor: cool; sweet, bitter.
Main and collateral channels: heart and liver meridians.
Administration and dosage: 9-15 g.
Indication: hematemesis, epistaxis, hematuria, hematochezia, external bleeding, carbuncle, sore and skin infection.

It is key herb to treat epistaxis, gum bleeding, hematochezia, hematuria.
(The picture is only for learning and identification the herb; the specific use of the herb please consult the herbalist or health professionals)

Field Thistle Herb (Xiaoji)
Chinese phonetic alphabet/pin yin: xiǎo jì
Chinese characters simplified/traditional:小蓟/小薊
Chinese nickname's alphabet (Nickname's Chinese characters): Ci'ercai(刺儿菜)
Latin: Cirsii Herba (Common name: Field Thistle Herb)

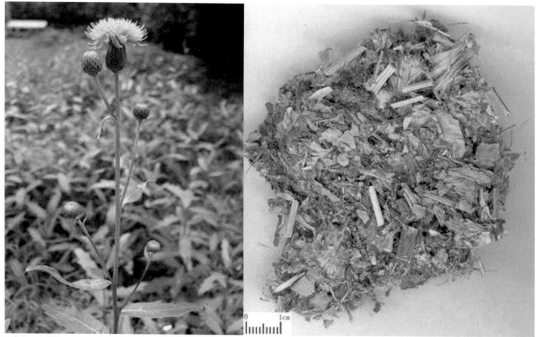

Plant: *Cirsium setosum* (Willd.) MB.

TCM prepared in ready-to-use forms (medicinal parts): it's dried up-ground-part which harvested when it is bloom.

Property and flavor: cool; sweet, bitter.

Main and collateral channels: heart and liver meridians.

Administration and dosage: 5-12 g.

Indication: hematemesis, epistaxis, hematuria, hematochezia, external bleeding, carbuncle, sore and skin infection.

It is taken as food in some part of China.

(The picture is only for learning and identification the herb; the specific use of the herb please consult the herbalist or health professionals)

Garden Burnet Root (Diyu)

Chinese phonetic alphabet/pin yin:
dì yú
Chinese characters simplified/traditional:
地榆/地榆
Chinese nickname's alphabet (Nickname's Chinese characters):
Shandigua/ Zhurenshen/ Shanzaoshen(山地瓜/ 猪人参/山枣参)
Latin: Sanguisorbae Radix (Common name: Garden Burnet Root)

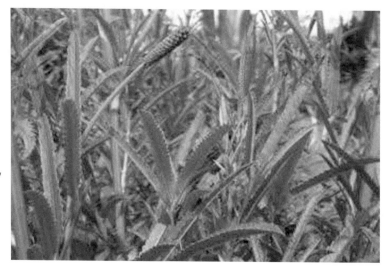

Plant: *Sanguisorba officinalis* L. (or *Sanguisorba officinalis* L. var. *longifolia* (Bert.) Yu. et Li.)

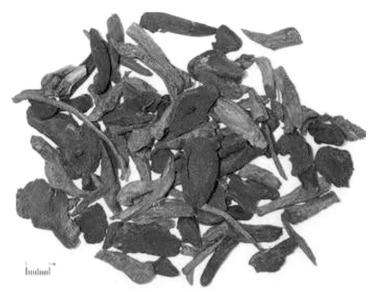

TCM prepared in ready-to-use forms (medicinal parts): it's dried root which harvested in spring or autumn.
Property and flavor: mild cold; bitter, acidity and astringent.
Main and collateral channels: liver and large intestine meridians.

Administration and dosage: 9-15 g. Appropriate amount for topical application, ground into powder for applyment.
Indication: hematochezia, hemorrhoid bleeding, metrorrhagia and spotting, burn, scald, carbuncle, sore and skin infections.
It is key herb to treat burn and scald.
(The picture is only for learning and identification the herb; the specific use of the herb please consult the herbalist or health professionals)

Lalang Grass Rhizome (Baimaogen)

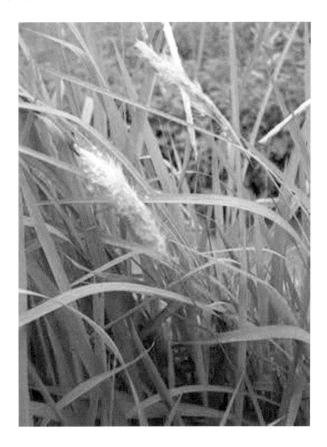

Chinese phonetic alphabet/ pin yin: bái máo gēn
Chinese characters simplified/ traditional:白茅根/白茅根
Chinese nickname's alphabet (Nickname's Chinese characters):
Maocaogen/ Baimaocao(茅草根/白茅草)
Latin: Imperatae Rhizoma (Common name: Lalang Grass Rhizome)
Plant: *Imperata cylindrica* Beauv. var. *major* (Nees.) C. E. Hubb.

TCM prepared in ready-to-use forms (medicinal parts): it's dried rhizome which harvested in spring or autumn.
Property and flavor: cold; sweet.
Main and collateral channels: lung, stomach and bladder meridians.
Administration and dosage: 9-30 g.
Indication: hematemesis, epistaxis, hematuria, fever, jaundice, edema, dysuria, pain and pyretic strangury. It is taken as food in some part of China.

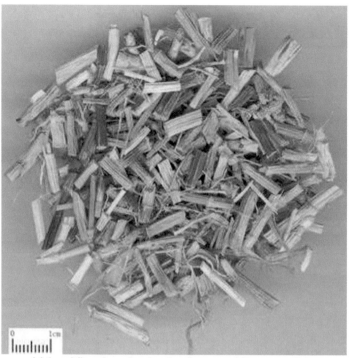

(The picture is only for learning and identification the herb; the specific use of the herb please consult the herbalist or health professionals)

Common Bletilla Tuber (Baiji)

Chinese phonetic alphabet/pin yin: bái jí
Chinese characters simplified/traditional:白芨/白芨
Chinese nickname's alphabet (Nickname's Chinese characters): Baiji/ Baigen/ Gangen/ Ruolan/ Zhulan(白及/白根/甘根/箬兰/朱兰)
Latin: Bletillae Rhizoma (Common name: Common Bletilla Tuber)

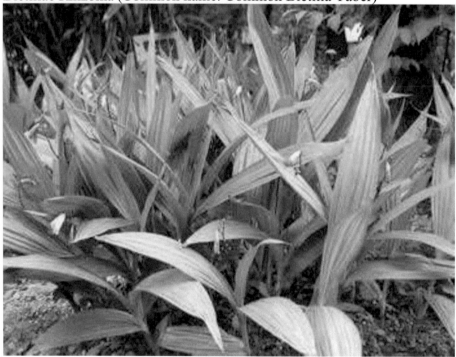

Plant: *Bletilla striata* (Thunb.) Reichb. f.

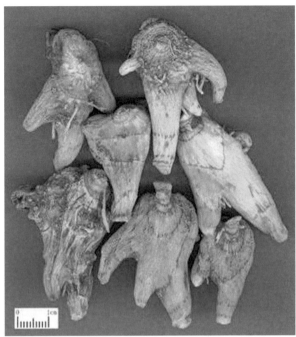

TCM prepared in ready-to-use forms (medicinal parts): it's dried tuber root which harvested in summer or autumn.
Property and flavor: mild cold; bitter, sweet and astringent.
Main and collateral channels: lung, liver and stomach meridians.
Administration and dosage: 6-15 g. Ground into powder for oral administration: 3-6 g. Topical application in appropriate amount.
Indication: hemoptysis, hematemesis, traumatic bleeding, sores, chapped skin, skin infection, sore and ulcer.
It is key herb to stops bleeding.

Precaution and warning: incompatible with Common Monkshood Mother Root, Kusnezoff Monkshood Root, Prepared Common Monkshood Daughter Root, Short-pedicel Aconite Root and their prepared one.
Attention: to protect the rare wild plant, please don't use the herb from wild plant. (The picture is only for learning and identification the herb; the specific use of the herb please consult the herbalist or health professionals)

Sanchi (Sanqi)
Chinese phonetic alphabet/pin yin: sān qī
Chinese characters simplified/traditional:三七/三七
Chinese nickname's alphabet (Nickname's Chinese characters): Tianqi/ Jinbuhuan(田七/金不换)
Latin: Notoginseng Radix et Rhizoma (Common name: Sanchi or Pseudo-Ginseng)

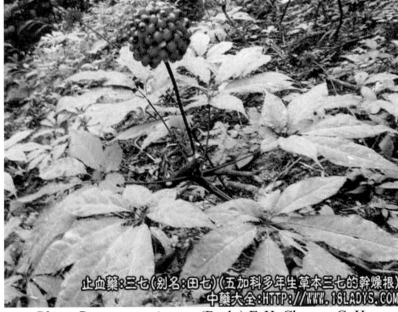

止血藥:三七(別名:田七)(五加科多年生草本三七的幹燥根)
中藥大全:HTTP://WWW.16LADYS.COM

Plant: *Panax notoginseng* (Burk.) F. H. Chen ex C. H.

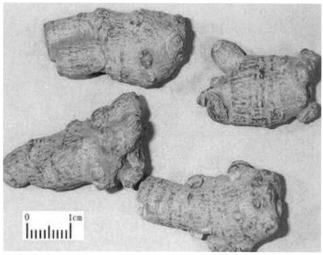

TCM prepared in ready-to-use forms (medicinal parts): it's dried root and rhizome which harvested in spring or winter.
Property and flavor: warm; mild bitter, sweet.
Main and collateral channels: liver and kidney meridians.

Administration and dosage: 3-9 g. Ground into powder for oral administration:1-3 g per time. Appropriate amount for topical application.
Indication: hematemesis, hemoptysis, epistaxis, hematuria, hematochezia, metrorrhagia, external bleeding, chest and abdominal pain, traumatic injury.
It is key herb to treat traumatic injury and bleeding.
Precaution and warning: used with caution during pregnancy.
(The picture is only for learning and identification the herb; the specific use of the herb please consult the herbalist or health professionals)

Indian Madder Root (Qiancao)
Chinese phonetic alphabet/pin yin: qiàn cǎo
Chinese characters simplified/traditional:茜草/茜草
Chinese nickname's alphabet (Nickname's Chinese characters): Xuejianchou/ Hongneixiao(血见愁/红内消)
Latin: Rubiae Radix et Rhizoma (Common name: Indian Madder Root)

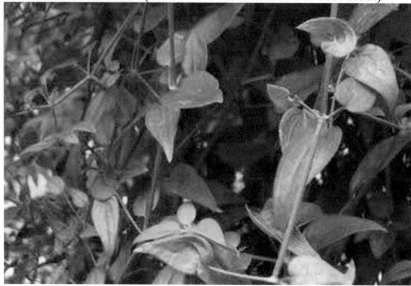

Plant: *Rubia cordifolia* L.
TCM prepared in ready-to-use forms (medicinal parts): it's dried root and rhizome which harvested in spring or summer.
Property and flavor: cold; bittert.
Main and collateral channels: liver meridian.
Administration and dosage: 6-10 g.

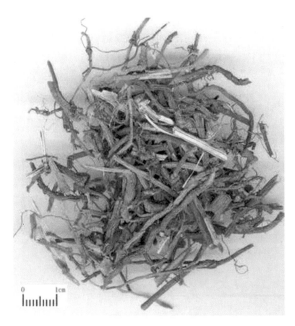

Indication: hematemesis, epistexis, metrorrhagia and spotting, external bleeding, amenorrhea and blood stasis, joint pain, traumatic injury. It is key herb to treat amenorrhea, dysmenorrheal and irregular menstruation. (The picture is only for learning and identification the herb; the specific use of the herb please consult the herbalist or health professionals)

Cattail Pollen (Puhuang)

Chinese phonetic alphabet/pin yin: pú huáng

Chinese characters simplified/traditional:蒲黄/蒲黃

Chinese nickname's alphabet (Nickname's Chinese characters): Pubanghuafen/ Xiangpu (蒲棒花粉/香蒲)

Latin: Typhae Pollen (Common name: Cattail Pollen)

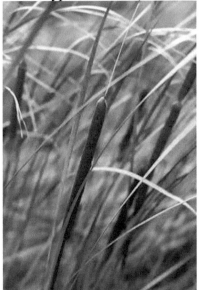

Plant: *Typha angustifolia* L. (or *Typha orientalis* Presl.)

TCM prepared in ready-to-use forms (medicinal parts): it's dried pollen.

Property and flavor: neutral; sweet.

Main and collateral channels: liver and pericardium meridians.

Administration and dosage: 5-10 g, wrap-boiling. Appropriate amount for topical application.

Indication: hematemesis, epistaxis, hemoptysis, hematuria, hematochezia, menstrual flooding and spotting, external bleeding, amenorrhea and dysmenorrhea, abdominal pain, swelling or flutter.

Precaution and warning: use with caution during pregnancy.

(The picture is only for learning and identification the herb; the specific use of the

herb please consult the herbalist or health professionals)

Argy Wormwood Leaf (Aiye)
Chinese phonetic alphabet/pin yin: ài yè
Chinese characters simplified/traditional:艾叶/艾葉
Chinese nickname's alphabet (Nickname's Chinese characters): Aihao(艾蒿)
Latin: Artemisiae Argyi Folium (Common name: Argy Wormwood Leaf or Mugwort Leaf)

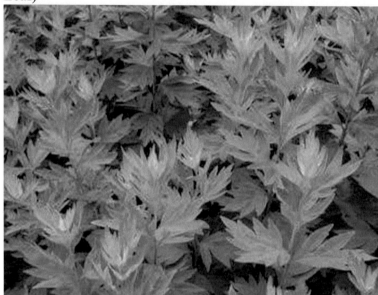

Plant: *Artemisia argyi* Lévl. et Vant.
TCM prepared in ready-to-use forms (medicinal parts): it's dried leaf which harvested in summer.

Property and flavor: warm; pungent, bitter.
Main and collateral channels: liver, spleen and kidney meridians.
Administration and dosage: 3-9 g. Topical application in appropriate amount. It can be used for moxibustion or decocted for fuming-washing therapy.

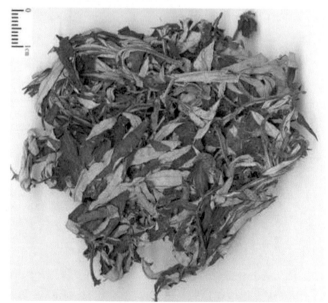

Indication: abdominal pain caused by cold/chill (*Hanliang*), infertility caused by uterine cold, hematemesis, epistaxis, hematuria, metrorrhagia, menstrual irregularities, vaginal bleeding during pregnancy; external use for skin itching.
Precaution and warning: slightly toxic. Use with caution during pregnancy.
(The picture is only for learning and identification the herb; the specific use of the herb please consult the herbalist or health professionals)

Pagoda Tree Flower (Huaihua)

Chinese phonetic alphabet/pin yin: huái huā

Chinese characters simplified/traditional:槐花/槐花

Chinese nickname's alphabet (Nickname's Chinese characters): Jinyaoshuhua/ Huairui/Huaimi(金药树花/槐蕊/槐米)

Latin: Sophorae Flos (Common name: Pagoda Tree Flower)

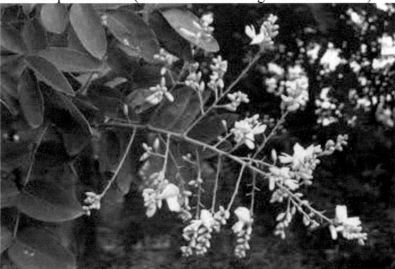

Plant: *Sophora japonica* L.

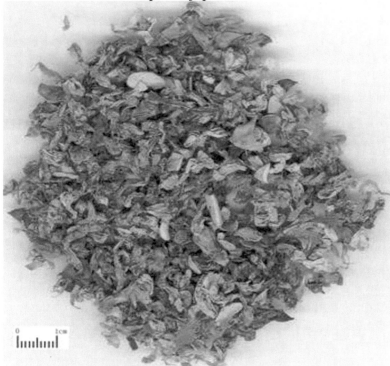

TCM prepared in ready-to-use forms (medicinal parts): it's dried flower and bud. Property and flavor: cold; mild bitter. Main and collateral channels: liver and large intestine meridians. Administration and dosage: 5-10 g. Indication: hematemesis, epistaxis, hematuria, hematochezia, metrorrhagia and spotting, hemorrhoid, red eyes, headache and dizziness. It is taken as food in some part of China.

(The picture is only for learning and identification the herb; the specific use of the herb please consult the herbalist or health professionals)

Chinese Arborvitae Twig and Leaf (Cebaiye)

Chinese phonetic alphabet/pin yin: cè bǎi yè

Chinese characters simplified/traditional:侧柏叶/側柏葉

Chinese nickname's alphabet (Nickname's Chinese characters): Bianbaiye/

Congbaiye(扁柏叶/丛柏叶)
Latin: Platycladi Cacumen (Common name: Chinese Arborvitae Twig and Leaf)

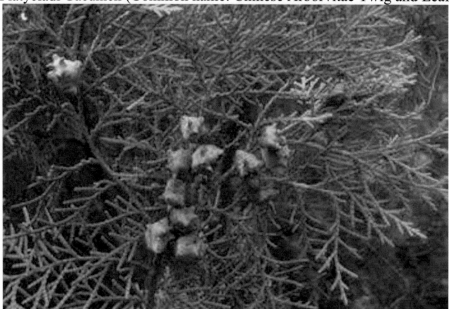

Plant: *Platycladus orientalis* (L.) Franco.

TCM prepared in ready-to-use forms (medicinal parts): it's dried twig and leaf which harvested in summer or autumn.
Property and flavor: cold; bitter, astringent.
Main and collateral channels: lung, liver and spleen meridians.
Administration and dosage: 6-12 g. Topical application in appropriate amount.
Indication: hematemesis, epistaxis, hematuria, hematochezia, metrorrhagia, alopecia, premature graying hairs.

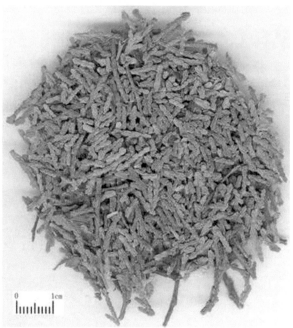

(The picture is only for learning and identification the herb; the specific use of the herb please consult the herbalist or health professionals)

Spikemoss (Juanbai)
Chinese phonetic alphabet/pin yin: juǎn bǎi
Chinese characters simplified/traditional:卷柏/卷柏
Chinese nickname's alphabet (Nickname's Chinese characters): Yibazhua/ Laohuzhua(一把抓/老虎爪)
Latin: Selaginellae Herba (Common name: Spikemoss)

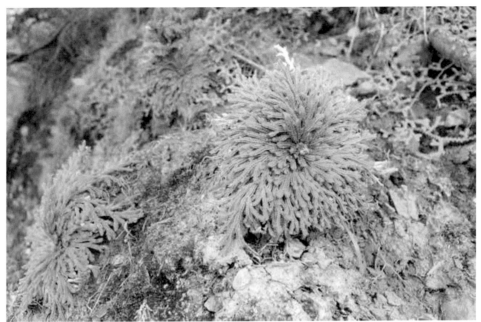

Plant: *Selaginella tamariscina* (Beauv.) Spring. (or *Selaginella pulvinata* (Hook. Et Grev.) Maxim.)

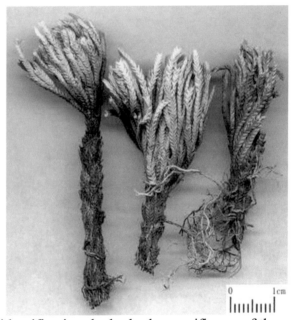

TCM prepared in ready-to-use forms (medicinal parts): it's dried whole herb which harvested all year round.

Property and flavor: neutral; pungent.

Main and collateral channels: liver and heart meridians.

Administration and dosage: 5-10 g.

Indication: amenorrhea, dysmenorrheal, hematochezia, metrorrhagia, aggregation accumulation masses, glomus and traumatic injuries.

Precaution and warnings: use with caution during pregnancy.

(The picture is only for learning and identification the herb; the specific use of the herb please consult the herbalist or health professionals)

Ramie Root (Zhumagen)
Chinese phonetic alphabet/pin yin: zhù má gēn
Chinese characters simplified/traditional:苎麻根/苧麻根
Chinese nickname's alphabet (Nickname's Chinese characters): Yuanma(园麻)
Latin: Boehmeriae Radix (Common name: Ramie Root)

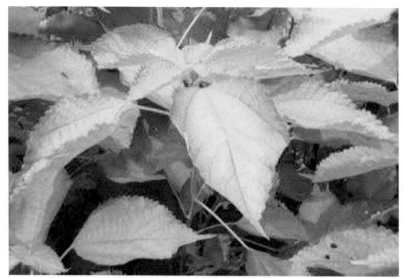

Plant: *Boehmeria nivea* (L.) Gaud.

TCM prepared in ready-to-use forms (medicinal parts): it's dried root which harvested in winter.
Property and flavor: cold; sweet.
Main and collateral channels: heart and liver meridians.
Administration and dosage: 10-30 g. Topical application in appropriate amount, decocted for bathing.
Indication: treat fever, urinary tract infection, nephritis, edema, abdominal pain, fetal irritability; external use for traumatic injuries and fractures.

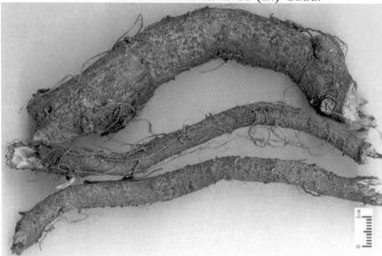

It is key herb to tocolysis.
(The picture is only for learning and identification the herb; the specific use of the herb please consult the herbalist or health professionals)

Hairyvein Agrimonia Herb (Xianhecao)

Chinese phonetic alphabet/pin yin: xiān hè cǎo
Chinese characters simplified/traditional:仙鹤草/仙鶴草
Chinese nickname's alphabet (Nickname's Chinese characters): Longyacao(龙芽草)
Latin: Agrimoniae Herba (Common name: Hairyvein Agrimonia Herb)

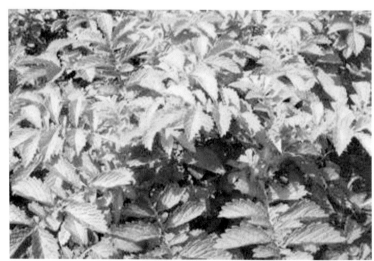

Plant: *Agrimonia pilosa* Ldb.

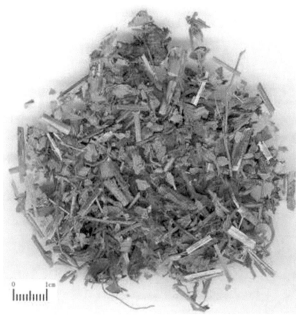

TCM prepared in ready-to-use forms (medicinal parts): it's dried aerial part which harvested in summer or autumn.

Property and flavor: neutral; bitter and astringent.

Main and collateral channels: heart and liver meridians.

Administration and dosage: 6-12 g. Topical application in appropriate amount.

Indication: hemoptysis, hematemesis, metrorrhagia, malaria, dysentery with blood, weakness, carbuncle sore, pruritus vulvae leucorrhea.

(The picture is only for learning and identification the herb; the specific use of the herb please consult the herbalist or health professionals)

Prepared Dried Ginger (Paojiang)
Chinese phonetic alphabet/pin yin: páo jiāng

Chinese characters simplified/traditional:炮姜/炮薑

Chinese nickname's alphabet (Nickname's Chinese characters): Heijiang(黑姜)

Latin: Zingiberis Rhizoma Praeparatum (Common name: Prepared Dried Ginger)

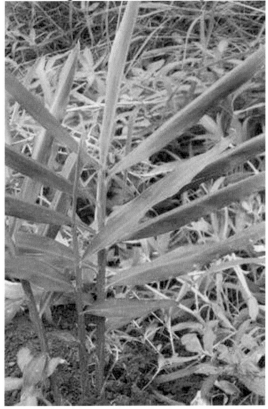

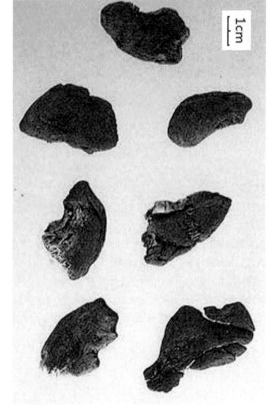

Plant: *Zingiber officinale* Rosc.

TCM prepared in ready-to-use forms (medicinal parts): it's treated root which harvested in winter.

Property and flavor: hot; pungent.

Main and collateral channels: spleen, stomach and kidney meridians.

Procedure: scald the dried Ginger with sand until it become inflated and brown externally.

Administration and dosage: 3-9 g.

Indication: abdominal pain, vomiting, diarrhea, hematemesis, metrorrhagia and spotting.

It is taken as seasoning in some part of China.

Attention: to protect the rare wild plant, please don't use the herb from wild plant.

(The picture is only for learning and identification the herb; the specific use of the herb please consult the herbalist or health professionals)

Carbonized Fortune Windmillpalm Petiole (Zonglyutan)

Chinese phonetic alphabet/pin yin: zōng lǚ tàn

Chinese characters simplified/traditional:棕榈碳/棕櫚碳

Chinese nickname's alphabet (Nickname's Chinese characters): Zonglvtan/Zongpi(棕榈炭/棕皮)

Latin: Trachycarpi Petiolus Carbonisatus (Common name: Carbonized Fortune Windmillpalm Petiole or Carbonized Palm)

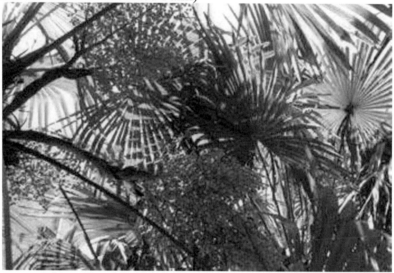

Plant: *Trachycarpus fortunei* (Hook. f.) H. Wendl.

TCM prepared in ready-to-use forms (medicinal parts): it's carbonization petiole.

Property and flavor: neutral; bitter, astringent.

Main and collateral channels: liver, lung and large intestine meridians.

Administration and dosage: 5-15 g.

Indication: hematemesis, existaxis, hematuria, hematochezia and menstrual flooding and spotting.

It is key herb to treat metrorrhagia.

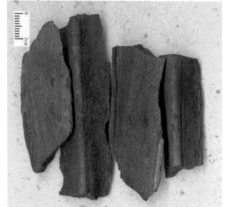

(The picture is only for learning and identification the herb; the specific use of the herb please consult the herbalist or health professionals)

Callicarpa Formosana Leaf (Zizhuye)

Chinese phonetic alphabet/
pin yin: zǐ zhū yè
Chinese characters
simplified/traditional:
紫珠叶/紫珠葉
Chinese nickname's
alphabet (Nickname's
Chinese characters):
Dafengye/ Baigouchang
(大风叶/白狗肠)
Latin: Callicarpae
Formosanae Folium
(Common name:
Callicarpa Formosana
Leaf or Beautyberry Leaf)
Plant: *Callicarpa formosana*
Rolfe.

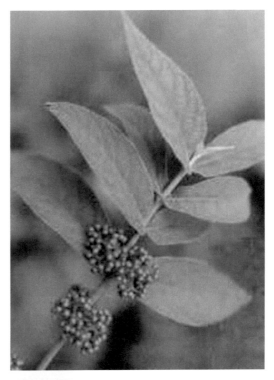

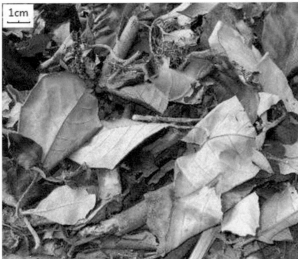

TCM prepared in
ready-to-use forms
(medicinal parts): it's
dried leaf which
harvested in summer or
winter.
Property and flavor:
cool; bitter, astringent.
Main and collateral
channels: liver, lung
and stomach meridians.

Administration and dosage: 3-15 g. Ground into powder for oral administration: 1.5-3 g. Topical application in appropriate amount.
Indication: peptic ulcer bleeding, traumatic hemorrhage, hemoptysis, hematemesis, epistaxis, gingival bleeding, sprain swelling, sore and ulcers, scald and burn.
(The picture is only for learning and identification the herb; the specific use of the herb please consult the herbalist or health professionals)

Kwangtung Beautyberry Stem and Leaf (Guangdongzizhu)
Chinese phonetic alphabet/pin yin: guǎng dōng zǐ zhū
Chinese characters simplified/traditional:广东紫珠/廣東紫珠
Chinese nickname's alphabet (Nickname's Chinese characters): Wannianqing/ Zhixuechai(万年青/止血柴)
Latin: Callicarpae Caulis et Folium (Common name: Kwangtung Beautyberry Stem and Leaf)

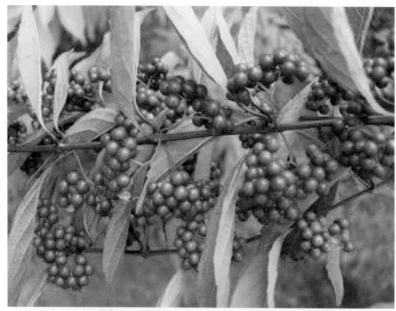

Plant: *Callicarpa kwangtungenis* Chun.

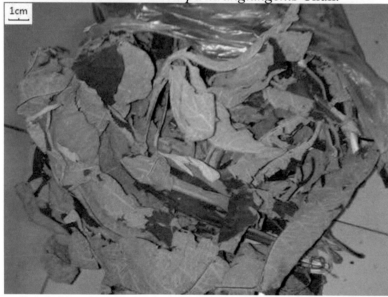

TCM prepared in ready-to-use forms (medicinal parts): it's dried stem, branch and leaf which harvested in summer or autumn.
Property and flavor: cool; bitter, astringent.
Main and collateral channels: liver, lung and stomach meridians.
Administration and dosage: 9-15 g. Appropriate amount for topical application after grinding it into powder.

Indication: epistaxis, hemoptysis, hematemesis, hematochezia, metrorrhagia, cough, swelling and sore throat, sore and ulcer caused by toxin, scald and burn.
(The picture is only for learning and identification the herb; the specific use of the herb please consult the herbalist or health professionals)

Callicarpae Macrophyllae (Dayezizhu)
Chinese phonetic alphabet/pin yin: dà yè zǐ zhū
Chinese characters simplified/traditional:大叶紫珠/大葉紫珠
Latin: Callicarpae Macrophyllae Folium (Common name: Callicarpae Macrophyllae)

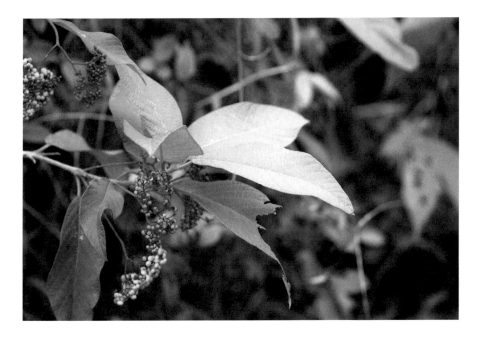

Plant: *Callicarpa macrophylla* Vahl.

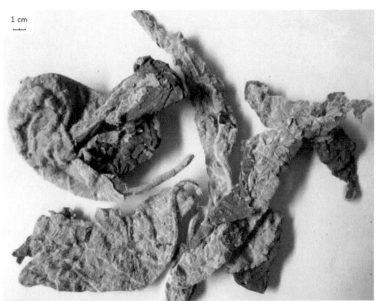

TCM prepared in ready-to-use forms (medicinal parts): it's dried leaf or young foliferous branch which harvested in summer or autumn.
Property and flavor: neutral; pungent, bitter.
Main and collateral channels: liver, lung and stomach meridians.

Administration and dosage: 15-30 g. Appropriate amount for topical application after grinding it into powder.
Indication: bleeding, hemoptysis, hematimesis and traumatic injuries.
(The picture is only for learning and identification the herb; the specific use of the herb please consult the herbalist or health professionals)

Lotus Rhizome Node (Oujie)
Chinese phonetic alphabet/pin yin: ǒu jié
Chinese characters simplified/traditional:藕节/藕節
Chinese nickname's alphabet (Nickname's Chinese characters): Oujieba(藕节巴)
Latin: Nelumbinis Rhizomatis Nodus (Common name: Lotus Rhizome Node or Lotus Joint)

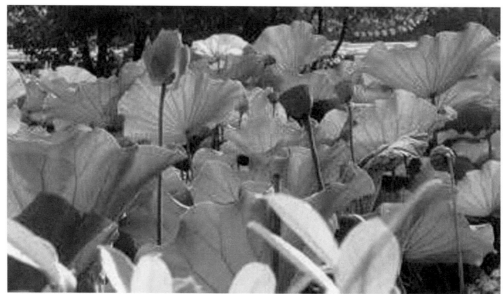

Plant: *Nelumbo nucifera* Gaertn.

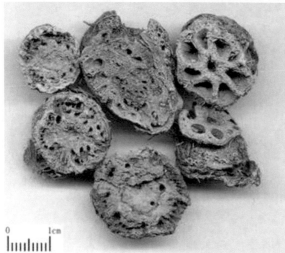

TCM prepared in ready-to-use forms (medicinal parts): it's dried rhizome node which harvested in autumn or winter.

Property and flavor: neutral; sweet, astringent.

Main and collateral channels: liver, lung and stomach meridians.

Administration and dosage: 9-15 g.

Indication: hemoptysis, hematemesis, epistaxis, hematuria, uterine bleeding and menstrual flooding and spotting.

(The picture is only for learning and identification the herb; the specific use of the herb please consult the herbalist or health professionals)

Stonecrop Notoginseng Herb (Jingtiansanqi)

Chinese phonetic alphabet/pin yin: jǐng tiān sān qī

Chinese characters simplified/traditional:景天三七/景天三七

Chinese nickname's alphabet (Nickname's Chinese characters): Feicai/Tusanqi(费菜/土三七)

Latin: Sedum Herba (Common name: Stonecrop Notoginseng Herb)

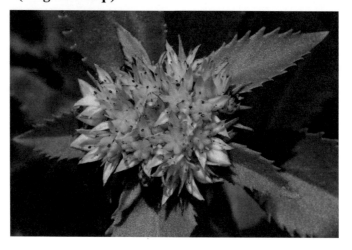

Plant: *Sedum aizoon* L.

TCM prepared in ready-to-use forms (medicinal parts): it's dried whole herb which harvested in summer or autumn.
Property and flavor: neutral; sweet, mild acidity.
Main and collateral channels: heart and liver meridians.
Administration and dosage: 10-15 g. Appropriate amount for topical application.

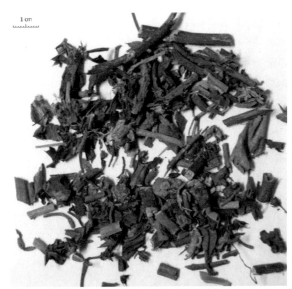

Indication: hemoptysis, hematemesis, epistaxis, hematuria, uterine bleeding, traumatic injuries and insomnia.
(The picture is only for learning and identification the herb; the specific use of the herb please consult the herbalist or health professionals)

Carbonized Hair (Xueyutan)

Chinese phonetic alphabet/pin yin: xuě yú tàn
Chinese characters simplified/traditional:血余炭/血餘炭
Chinese nickname's alphabet(Nickname's Chinese characters): Toufatan(头发碳)
Latin: Crinis Carbonisatus
(Common name: Carbonized Hair)

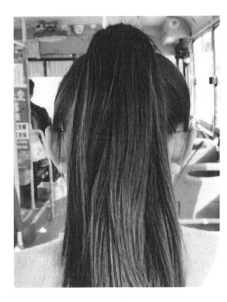

hair

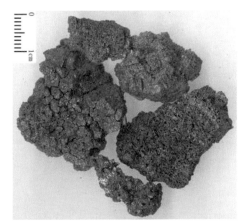

TCM prepared in ready-to-use forms (medicinal parts): it's carbonized human hair.
Property and flavor: neutral; bitter.
Main and collateral channels: liver and stomach meridians.
Administration and dosage: 5-10 g.
Indication: hemoptysis, hematemesis, epistaxis, hematuria, uterine bleeding, external bleeding.

(The picture is only for learning and identification the herb; the specific use of the herb please consult the herbalist or health professionals)

Cockcomb Flower (Jiguanhua)

Chinese phonetic alphabet/pin yin: jī guān huā

Chinese characters simplified/traditional:鸡冠花/雞冠花

Chinese nickname's alphabet (Nickname's Chinese characters): Jijihua(鸡髻花)

Latin: Celosiae Cristatae Flos (Common name: Cockcomb Flower or Coxcomb)

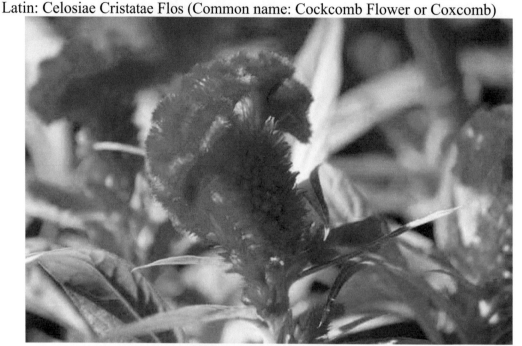

Plant: *Celosia cristata* L.

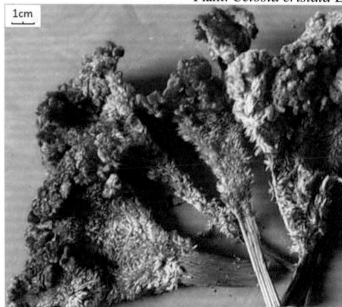

TCM prepared in ready-to-use forms (medicinal parts): it's dried flower or capitulum.

Property and flavor: cool; sweet, astringent.

Main and collateral channels: liver and large intestine meridians.

Administration and dosage: 6-12 g.

Indication: hematemesis, bloody stool, metrorrhagia, leucorrhea and chronic dysentery.

(The picture is only for learning and identification the herb; the specific use of the herb please consult the herbalist or health professionals)

Stove Subsoil (Fulonggan)

Chinese phonetic alphabet/pin yin: fú lóng gān

Chinese characters simplified/traditional:伏龙肝/伏龍肝

Chinese nickname's alphabet (Nickname's Chinese characters): Zaoxintu(灶心土)

Latin: Terra Flava Usta (Common name: Stoves Subsoil)

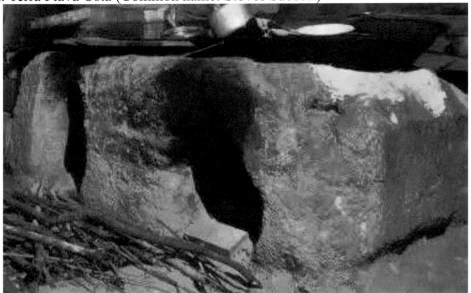

Traditional Chinese Stove

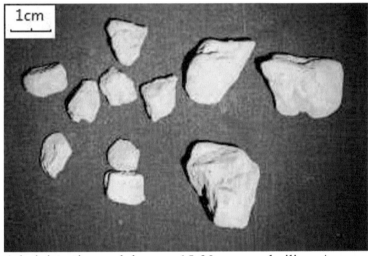

TCM prepared in ready-to-use forms (medicinal parts): it's the yellow or brown scorched earth in the center of the bottom of traditional Chinese stoves.
Property and flavor: warm; pungent.
Main and collateral channels: spleen and stomach meridians.

Administration and dosage: 15-30 g, wrap boiling. Appropriate amount for topical application, ground into powder and apply to the *pars affecta*.
Indication: hematochezia, uterine bleeding, vomiting, nausea.
(The picture is only for learning and identification the herb; the specific use of the herb please consult the herbalist or health professionals)

Rosewood (Jiangxiang)
Chinese phonetic alphabet/pin yin: jiàng xiāng
Chinese characters simplified/traditional:降香/降香
Chinese nickname's alphabet (Nickname's Chinese characters): Jiangzhenxiang/ Zijiangxiang(降真香/紫降香)
Latin: Dalbergiae Odoriferae Lignum (Common name: Rosewood or Dalbergia Wood)

Plant: *Dalbergia odorifera* T. Chen. TCM prepared in ready-to-use forms (medicinal parts): it's heartwood of the trunk and root.
Property and flavor: warm; pungent.
Main and collateral channels: liver and spleen meridians.

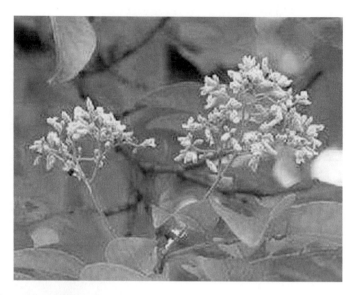

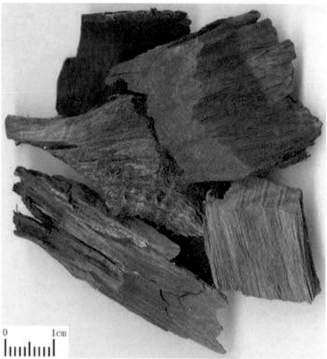

Administration and dosage: 9-15 g, add when the decoction is nearly done. Appropriate amount for topical application after grounding it into extreme fine powder.
Indication: hematemesis, epistaxis, traumatic bleeding, abdominal pain, liver and chest pain, traumatic injury and vomiting.

Attention: to protect the rare wild plant, please don't use the herb from wild plant. (The picture is only for learning and identification the herb; the specific use of the herb please consult the herbalist or health professionals)

Japanese Pagodatree Pod (Huaijiao)
Chinese phonetic alphabet/pin yin: huái jiǎo
Chinese characters simplified/traditional:槐角/槐角
Chinese nickname's alphabet (Nickname's Chinese characters): Huaishi/ Huaizi/ Huaidou/ Tiandou(槐实/槐子/槐豆/天豆)
Latin: Sophorae Fructus (Common name: Japanese Pagodatree Pod or Pod of Pagoda Tree)

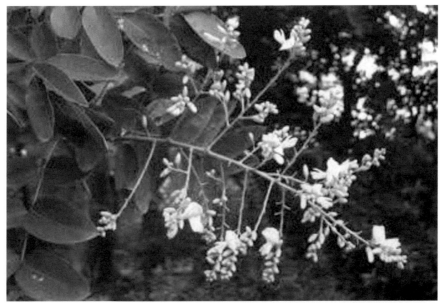

Plant: *Sophora japonica* L.

TCM prepared in ready-to-use forms (medicinal parts): it's dried ripe fruit.
Property and flavor: cold; bitter.
Main and collateral channels: liver and large intestine meridians.
Administration and dosage: 6-9 g.
Indication: hemorrhoids, hematochezia, headache, dizziness, red eyes.
(The picture is only for learning and identification the herb; the specific use of the herb please consult the herbalist or health professionals)

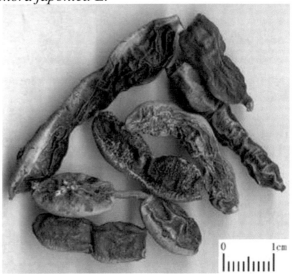

Sunset Abelmoschus Flower (Huangshukuihua)

Chinese phonetic alphabet/pin yin: huáng shǔ kuí huā
Chinese characters simplified/traditional:黄蜀葵花/黄蜀葵花
Chinese nickname's alphabet (Nickname's Chinese characters): Huangkui/ Cejinzhan (黄葵/侧金盏)
Latin: Abelmoschi Corolla (Common name: Sunset Abelmoschus Flower)

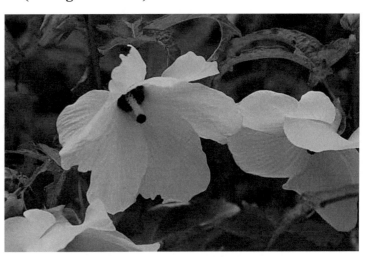

Plant: *Abelmoschus manihot* (L.) Medic.

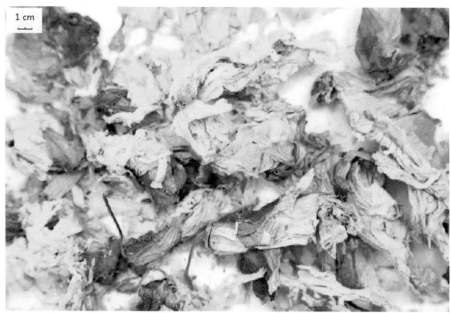

TCM prepared in ready-to-use forms (medicinal parts): it's dried corolla.

Property and flavor: cold; sweet.

Main and collateral channels: kidney and bladder meridians.

Administration and dosage: ground into powder for oral administration: 10-30 g. Appropriate amount for topical application after grinding in into powder.

Indication: turbid strangruy, edema, hematemesis, epistaxis, uterine bleeding, external used for skin infection, burn and scald.

Precaution and warning: use with caution during pregnancy.

(The picture is only for learning and identification the herb; the specific use of the herb please consult the herbalist or health professionals)

Bergenia Rhizome (Yanbaicai)

Chinese phonetic alphabet/pin yin: yán bái cài

Chinese characters simplified/traditional:岩白菜/巖白菜

Chinese nickname's alphabet (Nickname's Chinese characters): Yanbicai/ Yanqi(岩壁菜/岩七)

Latin: Bergniae Rhizoma (Common name: Bergenia Rhizome)

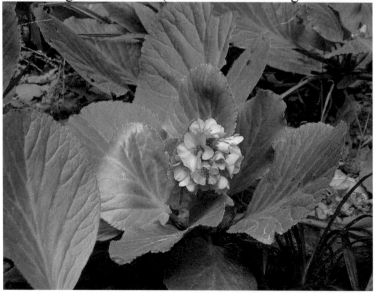

Plant: *Bergenia purpurascens* (Hook. f. et Thoms.) Engl. TCM prepared in ready-to-use forms (medicinal parts): it's dried rhizome which harvested in autumn or winter.

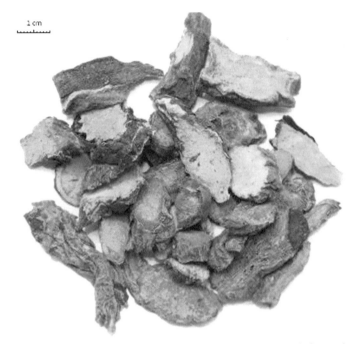

Property and flavor: neutral; bitter and astringent.
Main and collateral channels: lung, liver and spleen meridians.
Administration and dosage: 6-12 g.
Appropriate amount for topical application.

Indication: diarrhea, dysentery, bleeding, cough in pulmonary tuberculosis or tracheitis, rheumatic and traumatic injuries.
(The picture is only for learning and identification the herb; the specific use of the herb please consult the herbalist or health professionals)

Common Cissampelos Herb (Yahunu)

Chinese phonetic alphabet/pin yin: yà hū nú
Chinese characters simplified/traditional: 亚乎奴/亞乎努
Chinese nickname's alphabet (Nickname's Chinese characters): Xishengteng(锡生藤)
Latin: Cissampelotis Herba (Common name: Common Cissampelos Herb)

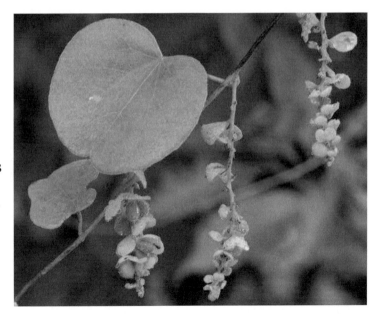

Plant: *Cissampelos pareira* L.var. *hirsuta* (Buch. ex DC.) Forman.

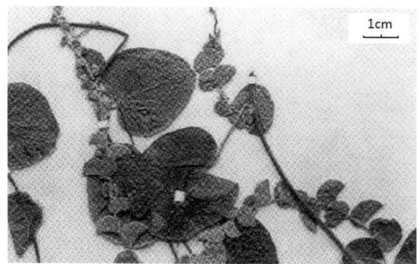

TCM prepared in ready-to-use forms (medicinal parts): it's dried whole plant which harvested in spring or summer.

Property and flavor: warm; sweet, bitter.

Administration and dosage: for swelling and pain caused by trauma, dry powder mixed with appropriate amount of liquor or egg white for being applied to the *pars affecta*; for external bleeding, appropriate amount of dry powder for applyment, once a day.

Indication: swelling, pain, traumatic bleeding.

(The picture is only for learning and identification the herb; the specific use of the herb please consult the herbalist or health professionals)

Clinopodium Herb (Duanxueliu)

Chinese phonetic alphabet/pin yin: duàn xuě liú

Chinese characters simplified/traditional:断血流/斷血流

Chinese nickname's alphabet (Nickname's Chinese characters): Denglongcao/ Fengluncai(灯笼草/风轮菜)

Latin: Clinopodii Herba (Common name: Clinopodium Herb)

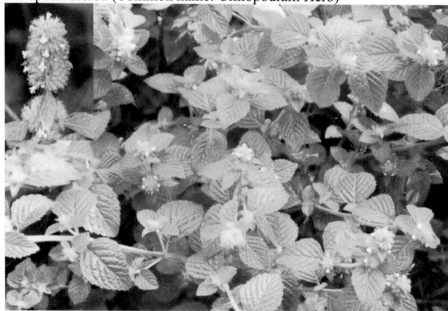

Plant: *Clinopodium polycephalum* (Vaniot) C. Y. Wu et Hsuan. (*Clinopodiurn chinensis* (Benth.) O. Kuntze.)

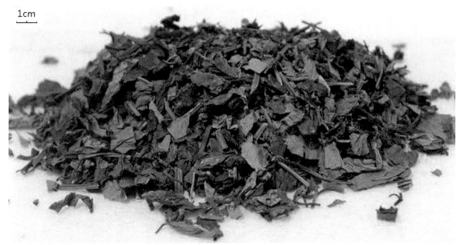

TCM prepared in ready-to-use forms (medicinal parts): it's dried aerial part which harvested in summer.

Property and flavor: cool; mild bitter, astringent.

Main and collateral channels: liver meridian.

Administration and dosage: 9-15 g. Appropriate amount for topical application after grinding it into powder.

Indication: menstrual flooding, spotting, hematuria, epistaxis, gingival bleeding, external bleeding.

(The picture is only for learning and identification the herb; the specific use of the herb please consult the herbalist or health professionals)

Ophicalcite (Huaruishi)

Chinese phonetic alphabet/pin yin: huā ruǐ shí

Chinese characters simplified/traditional:花蕊石/花蕊石

Chinese nickname's alphabet (Nickname's Chinese characters): Huangrushi/ Baiyunshi(花乳石/白云石)

Latin: Ophicalcitum (Common name: Ophicalcite)

Mineral: main component $CaCO_3$

TCM prepared in ready-to-use forms (medicinal parts): it's cleaned mineral.

Property and flavor: neutral; acidity, astringent.

Main and collateral channels: liver meridian.

Administration and dosage: 4.5-9 g, usually ground into powder for oral administration.

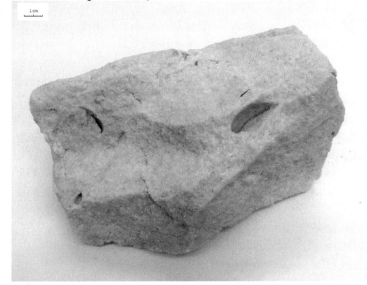

Topical application in appropriate amount.

Indication: hemoptysis, hematemesis and traumatic injuries.

(The picture is only for learning and identification the herb; the specific use of the herb please consult the herbalist or health professionals)

Fimbriate Orostachys Herb (Wasong)

Chinese phonetic alphabet/pin yin: wǎ sōng
Chinese characters simplified/traditional:瓦松/瓦松
Chinese nickname's alphabet (Nickname's Chinese characters): Wahua/Xiangtiancao(瓦花/向天草)
Latin: Orostachyis Fimbriatae Herba (Common name: Fimbriate Orostachys Herb)
Plant: *Orostachys fimbriatus* (Turcz.) Berg.

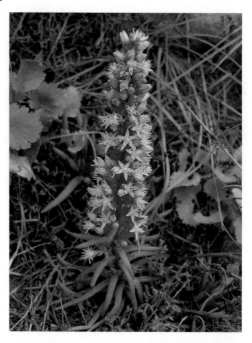

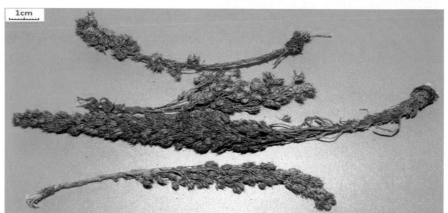

TCM prepared in ready-to-use forms (medicinal parts): it's dried up-ground-part which harvested in summer or autumn.
Property and flavor: cool; acidity, bitter.
Main and collateral channels: liver, lung and spleen meridians.
Administration and dosage: 3-9 g. Topical application in appropriate amount, usually ground into powder for application.
Indication: epistaxis, blood dysentery, stool with blood, hemorrhoid bleeding and unhealing sore.
(The picture is only for learning and identification the herb; the specific use of the herb please consult the herbalist or health professionals)

Japanese Milkwort Herb (Guazijin)
Chinese phonetic alphabet/pin yin: guā zǐ jīn
Chinese characters simplified/traditional:瓜子金/瓜子金
Chinese nickname's alphabet (Nickname's Chinese characters): Chenshacao/Jinsuoshi(辰砂草/金锁匙)
Latin: Polygalae Japonicae Herba (Common name: Japanese Milkwort Herb)

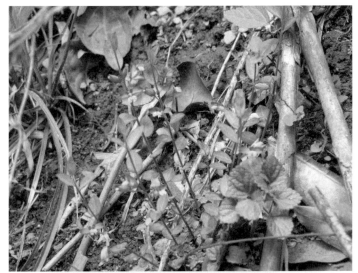

Plant: *Polygala japonica* Houtt.

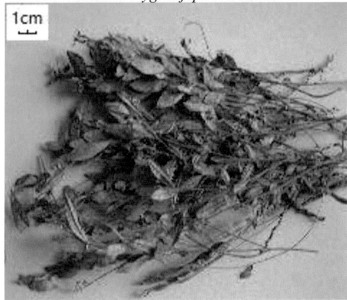

TCM prepared in ready-to-use forms (medicinal parts): it's dried whole herb which harvested in spring.
Property and flavor: neutral; bitter, pungent.
Main and collateral channels: lung meridian.
Administration and dosage: 15-30 g.
Indication: cough, excessive phlegm, swelling and sore throat; external use for traumatic injuries, swelling, boils and sore, insect or snake bites.
(The picture is only for learning and identification the herb; the specific use of the herb please consult the herbalist or health professionals)

Decumbent Bugle Herb (Jingucao)

Chinese phonetic alphabet/pin yin: jīn gǔ cǎo
Chinese characters simplified/traditional:筋骨草/筋骨草
Chinese nickname's alphabet (Nickname's Chinese characters): Baimaoxiakucao/ Toujincao(白毛夏枯草/透筋草)

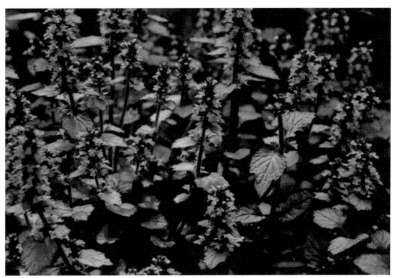

Plant: *Ajuga decumbens* Thunb.

Latin: Ajugae Herba (Common name: Decumbent Bugle Herb or Carpet Bugle)

TCM prepared in ready-to-use forms (medicinal parts): it's dried whole herb which harvested in spring.
Property and flavor: cold; bitter.
Main and collateral channels: lung meridian.
Administration and dosage: 15-30 g. Topical application in appropriate amount, mashed for application.

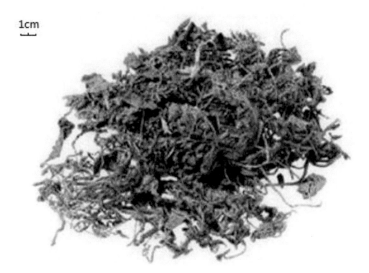

1cm

Indication: sore throat, hemoptysis, traumatic injuries and pain.
(The picture is only for learning and identification the herb; the specific use of the herb please consult the herbalist or health professionals)

INDEX

Special thanks

Thank the follow websites generous support the pictures for this book:

http://www.tcm166.com (国医在线)

http://www.18ladys.com (中药大全)

https://www.cndzys.com (大众养生网)

http://www.tmyy.net (天马(安徽)国药科技股份有限公司)

http://www.yunyao.net (云药网)

http://www.zgycsc.com (中国药材市场)

http://www.qnong.com.cn (黔农网)

http://zhongyao.aipinkd.com (问药堂)

http://www.zhongyoo.com (中药查询)

http://zhongyibaike.com (中医百科)

https://aglbyc.1688.com (安国冷背药材有限公司)

http://www.xyzyw.cn (信誉藏药网)

Some pictures were bought from http://www.plantphoto.cn(中国植物图像库)

The pictures of this book are proofreaded by Huang Hongying (Chief pharmacist of Qinghai Hospital of Traditional Chinese Medicine, China) and Lu Xue-feng (professor of Northwest Institute of Planteau Biology, China).

Thanks for Ma Mingfang's (Qinghai Province Institute for Food Control, China) help to edit this book.

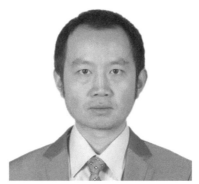

Chen Rui is a senior engineer of food and herb test, pharmacist, and master of botany.